Library and Resource Centre
Calderstones NHS Trust
Mitton Road
Whalley
Clitheron BB7 9PE

APPLETON & LANGE

REVIEW OF

PSYCHIATRY

SEVENTH EDITION

D0313828

CALDERSTONES LIBRARY
TC00545

Notice

Medicine is an ever-changing science. As new research and clinical experience broaden our knowledge, changes in treatment and drug therapy are required. The authors and the publisher of this work have checked with sources believed to be reliable in their efforts to provide information that is complete and generally in accord with the standards accepted at the time of publication. However, in view of the possibility of human error or changes in medical sciences, neither the authors nor the publisher nor any other party who has been involved in the preparation or publication of this work warrants that the information contained herein is in every respect accurate or complete, and they disclaim all responsibility for any errors or omissions or for the results obtained from use of the information contained in this work. Readers are encouraged to confirm the information contained herein with other sources. For example and in particular, readers are advised to check the product information sheet included in the package of each drug they plan to administer to be certain that the information contained in this work is accurate and that changes have not been made in the recommended dose or in the contraindications for administration. This recommendation is of particular importance in connection with new or infrequently used drugs.

APPLETON & LANGE

REVIEW OF

PSYCHIATRY

SEVENTH EDITION

Ivan Oransky, MD

Joseph R. Check, MD
Vladimir Coric, MD
Louis Sanfilippo, MD

Appleton & Lange/McGraw-Hill
Medical Publishing Division

New York   Chicago   San Francisco   Lisbon   London   Madrid   Mexico City   Milan
New Delhi   San Juan   Seoul   Singapore   Sydney   Toronto

McGraw-Hill

A Division of The McGraw·Hill Companies

Appleton & Lange Review of Psychiatry, Seventh Edition

Copyright © 2003 by The **McGraw-Hill Companies,** Inc. All rights reserved. Printed in the United States of America. Except as permitted under the United States Copyright Act of 1976, no part of this publication may be reproduced or distributed in any form or by any means, or stored in a data base or retrieval system, without the prior written permission of the publisher.

Previous editions copyright © 1999, 1996 by Appleton & Lange

1 2 3 4 5 6 7 8 9 0   VHVH   0 9 8 7 6 5 4 3

ISBN: 0-07-140253-5

TC00545

This book was set in Palatino at Rainbow Graphics.
The editors were Catherine A. Johnson and John M. Morriss.
Project supervision was done by Rainbow Graphics.
The production supervisor was Lisa Mendez.
The cover design was Aimee Nordin.
Von Hoffmann was the printer and binder.

Library of Congress Cataloging-in-Publication Data

Appleton & Lange review of psychiatry.–7th ed. / [edited by] Ivan Oransky . . . [et al.].
    p. ; cm.
    Rev. ed. of: Appleton & Lange's review of psychiatry / [edited by] Ivan Oransky. 6th ed. c2001.
    Includes bibliographical references.
    ISBN 0-07-140253-5 (alk. paper)
    1. Psychiatry–Examinations, questions, etc. I. Title: Appleton and Lange review of psychiatry. II. Title: Review of psychiatry. III. Oransky, Ivan. IV. Appleton & Lange's review of psychiatry.
    [DNLM: 1. Mental Disorders–therapy–Examination Questions. 2. Psychiatry–Examination Questions. WM 18.2 A649 2003]
RC457.E18 2003
616.89'0076–dc21   2002032560

Contents

Contributors

Joseph R. Check, MD
Assistant Clinical Professor of Psychiatry
Yale University
New Haven, Connecticut

Vladimir Coric, MD
Chief of Inpatient Services, Clinical Neuroscience
Research Unit
Assistant Clinical Professor of Psychiatry
Yale University
New Haven, Connecticut

Louis Sanfilippo, MD
Assistant Clinical Professor of Psychiatry
Yale University
New Haven, Connecticut

Raziya Sunderji, MD
Resident, Department of Psychiatry
Yale University
New Haven, Connecticut

Chung-Che Charles Wang, MD
Resident, Department of Psychiatry
Yale University
New Haven, Connecticut

Contributors to the Sixth Edition

R. Andrew Chambers, MD
Resident, Department of Psychiatry
Yale University School of Medicine
New Haven, Connecticut

Joseph R. Check, MD
Resident, Department of Psychiatry
Yale University School of Medicine
New Haven, Connecticut

Vladimir Coric, MD
Resident, Department of Psychiatry
Yale University School of Medicine
New Haven, Connecticut

Frank G. Fortunati, MD, JD
Resident, Department of Psychiatry
Yale University School of Medicine
New Haven, Connecticut

Brian Greenlee, MD
Resident, Department of Psychiatry
University of Kentucky
Lexington, Kentucky

Julie E. Peters, MD
Resident, Department of Psychiatry
Yale University School of Medicine
New Haven, Connecticut

Greer Richardson, MD
Resident, Department of Psychiatry
Yale University School of Medicine
New Haven, Connecticut

William Roman, MD
Resident, Department of Psychiatry
Yale University School of Medicine
New Haven, Connecticut

Louis Sanfilippo, MD
Resident, Department of Psychiatry
Yale University School of Medicine
New Haven, Connecticut

Blake Taggart, MD
Resident, Department of Psychiatry
Yale University School of Medicine
New Haven, Connecticut

Elizabeth Walter, MD
Resident, Department of Psychiatry
Yale University School of Medicine
New Haven, Connecticut

Preface

In revising the sixth edition of *Appleton & Lange's Review of Psychiatry*, we had two important tasks: updating the material to reflect changes in psychiatry since the last edition was written and updating our format to better reflect the ever-changing USMLE Step 2 exam. Despite these changes, however, we wanted to be sure that this book remained useful not only to those 100,000 fourth-year medical students and medical school graduates who sit for Step 2, but also to any medical students taking psychiatry clerkships.

Our basic approach in preparing the seventh edition remained the same. The book consists of more than 950 questions similar to those appearing on recent administrations of the exam. The 10 chapters include those on topics such as adult psychopathology, biologic therapies, and differential diagnoses, and two final chapters are practice tests of 120 questions each that simulate the real exam.

Because so many students rely heavily or solely on books of questions such as this, answers include, in addition to a discussion of the correct answer, a discussion of why the incorrect answers were wrong. That way, learning is not restricted to one term or discussion per question. All diagnostic criteria refer to the American Psychiatric Association's *Diagnostic and Statistical Manual of Mental Disorders*, 4th ed., Text Revision (DSM-IV-TR), the most recent edition. A list of references is included for those students who wish to pursue further reading, but is not indexed directly to questions because many students will be using this book—as we did—at the last minute before their exams.

As much as possible, we have done our best to replicate the format of the exam. That means that the vast majority of questions are clinical vignettes, and that there are nearly no negatively phrased questions (e.g., "EXCEPT," "LEAST LIKELY"). Still, because there is some fundamental or important material that is difficult to present otherwise, a few non-vignette and negatively phrased questions remain. For example, there are definitions that any student of psychiatry should learn.

A few words on how best to use this book. If you are first picking it up within a few weeks of Step 2 and don't have time to review the entire book, I'd recommend hitting Chapters 9 and 10, the practice exams. These best reflect what you'll see on the exam and will point out gaps in your knowledge.

If you have more time—say, a few months—pick some questions from each chapter other than 9 and 10 to test your knowledge of each subject, then concentrate on those chapters in which you're weakest.

Finally, if you're using this book during your clerkship, it's probably best to work through all the chapters and save Chapters 9 and 10 for the end of your clerkship review. You'll find basic questions that will help you master the material but that may not appear on Step 2.

Best of luck.

Ivan Oransky, MD
New York, New York
December 2002

Acknowledgments

This book reflects the hard work and dedication of a large group of contributors—5 for this edition, and 11 for the last edition. Thanks to medical student Deborah Lam, who made helpful suggestions on how to improve from the sixth edition. Thanks also to Trish Casey, who began the process of revising this edition, and the ever-patient Catherine Johnson, our editor at McGraw-Hill. Finally, Sean I. Savitz, MD, neurology resident extraordinaire, once again provided last-minute help with the neurology material.

CHAPTER 1

Definitions

Questions

Brian Greenlee, MD, and William Roman, MD

DIRECTIONS (Questions 1 through 72): Each of the numbered items or incomplete statements in this section is followed by answers or by completions of the statement. Select the ONE lettered answer or completion that is BEST in each case.

Questions 1 and 2

A compulsive gambler tells her psychiatrist that once she begins to play the slot machines, she cannot stop, particularly if she wins a few times.

1. The slot machine provides what type of reinforcement schedule?

   (A) fixed interval
   (B) fixed ratio
   (C) variable interval
   (D) variable ratio
   (E) continuous reinforcement

2. One explanation for why the patient has difficulty stopping is

   (A) her behavior is difficult to extinguish
   (B) her behavior is easily extinguished
   (C) habituation
   (D) classical conditioning
   (E) pavlovian conditioning

Questions 3 and 4

A 34-year-old electrical engineer complains to his doctor that he has been feeling suicidal. He feels guilty over the breakup of his marriage; he cannot concentrate; and he feels hopeless and helpless and has a subjective feeling of sadness and depression. He has lost 25 pounds in the last 3 months because his "appetite isn't the same."

3. Which of these symptoms constitute a neurovegetative sign of depression?

   (A) guilt
   (B) hopelessness and helplessness
   (C) decreased concentration
   (D) suicidality
   (E) decreased appetite

4. A diagnosis of depression is made, and he is started on an antidepressant. Which symptom can be expected to improve most quickly?

   (A) guilt
   (B) hopelessness and helplessness
   (C) decreased concentration
   (D) suicidality
   (E) decreased appetite

Questions 5 and 6

A patient in the emergency department tells the physician that over the past 3 weeks, his television has been talking directly to him.

5. This demonstrates

   (A) disorder of thought content
   (B) disorder of thought form
   (C) an obsession
   (D) derealization
   (E) a formal thought disorder

6. From what specific type of delusion is this patient suffering?

(A) thought insertion

(B) somatic

(C) thought broadcasting

(D) paranoid

(E) idea of reference

Questions 7 and 8

A 27-year-old man complains that he has felt "down in the dumps" for months and is feeling guilty because he has been having an extramarital affair. In recent weeks, he has started to believe that his wife is poisoning his food and the rest of his family is involved in an elaborate plot to drive him from the house.

7. Assuming his thinking is delusional, how would his delusions be best characterized?

(A) ego-syntonic

(B) bizarre

(C) somatic

(D) mood-congruent

(E) mood-incongruent

8. What sort of diagnosis would these delusions most likely accompany?

(A) schizophrenia

(B) mania

(C) major depressive disorder (MDD)

(D) dysthymia

(E) adjustment disorder

Questions 9 and 10

A 45-year-old patient tells her doctor that after hearing that her husband died, she could not remember leaving her office and going home. In every other respect, her memory is intact.

9. This is an example of

(A) continuous amnesia

(B) retrograde amnesia

(C) localized amnesia

(D) generalized amnesia

(E) selective amnesia

10. The most likely diagnosis is

(A) dissociative amnesia

(B) dissociative fugue

(C) depersonalization disorder

(D) posttraumatic stress disorder (PTSD)

(E) adjustment disorder

11. When asked about his level of education, a 48-year-old man with a history of schizophrenia describes his high school grounds, friends he had at the time, clubs he joined, and his high school graduation. He concludes by saying, "And that was the end of my schooling." His answer demonstrates

(A) loosening of associations

(B) circumstantiality

(C) tangentiality

(D) pressured speech

(E) perseveration

12. When an examiner asks a patient to count backwards by seven, starting at 100 (referred to as "serial sevens"), what is principally being tested?

(A) recent memory

(B) remote memory

(C) concentration

(D) fund of knowledge

(E) mathematics skills

13. A 34-year-old man reveals to his doctor that he derives sexual satisfaction from rubbing up against women while on crowded subway trains. Which of the paraphilias is this an example of?

(A) exhibitionism

(B) fetishism

(C) pedophilia

(D) voyeurism

(E) frotteurism

14. A psychiatry consult is called on a patient who, in a variety of ways, is making the nursing staff angry at him. He became enraged during this hospitalization when he was told that he has a terminal illness. What defense mechanism is being demonstrated?

    (A) denial
    (B) sublimation
    (C) intellectualization
    (D) projective identification
    (E) reaction formation

15. The patient who is late for work because she spends all morning checking whether she turned off the gas burner demonstrates

    (A) paranoia
    (B) an obsession
    (C) a compulsion
    (D) hyperarousal
    (E) delusional thinking

16. A patient admitted to the dual-diagnosis unit of a psychiatric hospital most likely carries which diagnoses?

    (A) personality disorder and an Axis I diagnosis, such as PTSD
    (B) a psychiatric diagnosis and a medical diagnosis
    (C) two distinct psychiatric diagnoses
    (D) an active psychiatric diagnosis and a psychiatric diagnosis in remission
    (E) two psychiatric diagnoses, one of which relates to substance abuse

17. A patient who finds herself using increasing amounts of cocaine to achieve the same effect demonstrates

    (A) tolerance
    (B) dependence
    (C) addiction
    (D) withdrawal
    (E) abuse

18. In her psychiatrist's office, a patient suddenly lowers herself to the floor, begins flailing about wildly, then flings a garbage pail against the wall and runs out of the office. Immediately afterward, she returns. She is alert and oriented, yet does not remember the incident. What is the most likely diagnosis?

    (A) temporal lobe epilepsy
    (B) jacksonian seizure
    (C) tonic–clonic seizure
    (D) complex partial seizure
    (E) pseudoseizure

19. In a 29-year-old man being treated for depression, which of the following statements would most likely characterize his sleep patterns?

    (A) Depression has little impact on sleep.
    (B) Sleep latency decreases.
    (C) Early morning awakening is rare.
    (D) Rapid eye movement (REM) latency decreases.
    (E) REM sleep tends to be distributed to the latter half of the night.

20. A 45-year-old man is in the emergency department because of a diabetic foot ulcer. In gathering a history, the physician learns that this man lives alone and works nights as a security guard. He says he has no friends but that this does not bother him. He has never been hospitalized or received any psychiatric help. His affect is flat. While he answers questions and seems to trust the judgment of the doctors, he has little interest in the interview. He exhibits no signs or symptoms of psychosis or depression. What is the most likely diagnosis?

    (A) schizotypal personality disorder
    (B) schizoid personality disorder
    (C) paranoid personality disorder
    (D) MDD
    (E) schizophrenia

Questions 21 through 24

A 19-year-old man is admitted to a psychiatric hospital for the first time in his life and is discharged with a diagnosis of schizophrenia.

21. Which of the following statements best characterizes this patient?

    (A) His gender is a risk factor for schizophrenia.
    (B) His diagnosis came earlier than would be expected for a man.
    (C) It is unlikely that a stressful life event precipitated his recent admission.
    (D) He is equally likely to have a family history of schizophrenia as someone without schizophrenia.
    (E) He is at increased risk for suicide.

22. On Mental Status Examination (MSE), what negative symptom might be revealed?

    (A) echolalia
    (B) alogia
    (C) logorrhea
    (D) delusions
    (E) auditory hallucinations

23. When he returns to the hospital a month later for follow-up, the patient's speech is logical, and he is able to sit and talk with the interviewer, becoming relatively engaged in the examination. He says that he has been hearing voices since his discharge, and he believes his every word is being recorded by a tape recorder inside his mouth. What is the most likely type of schizophrenia in this patient?

    (A) paranoid
    (B) disorganized
    (C) catatonic
    (D) undifferentiated
    (E) residual

24. Which of the following types of schizophrenia has the best prognosis?

    (A) paranoid
    (B) disorganized
    (C) catatonic
    (D) undifferentiated
    (E) residual

25. A 33-year-old woman with a history of paranoid schizophrenia tells you she has been hearing voices. What is the most important information to obtain regarding her auditory hallucinations?

    (A) whether the voices come from inside or outside her head
    (B) how loud the voices are
    (C) how long she has been hearing voices
    (D) what the voices are saying
    (E) whether she recognizes the voices

Questions 26 and 27

A 40-year-old woman with a history of psychotic depression resistant to many trials of antidepressant medication is being considered for electroconvulsive therapy (ECT).

26. Which of the following is a reasonable statement to tell the patient in helping her decide on ECT?

    (A) ECT is physically uncomfortable.
    (B) ECT will likely enhance response to antidepressant treatment.
    (C) In some subtypes of depression, ECT is considered first-line treatment.
    (D) ECT has little effect on blood pressure.
    (E) Disruption in memory is uncommon.

27. Which of the following conditions is an absolute contraindication to ECT?

    (A) pregnancy
    (B) degenerative joint disease
    (C) hypertension
    (D) recent myocardial infarction
    (E) psychotic depression

Questions 28 and 29

A Vietnam War veteran describes a sensation in which, during battles, he felt as if time were moving slowly and sounds were muted and distant.

28. This is an example of

   (A) dissociative amnesia
   (B) depersonalization
   (C) derealization
   (D) dissociative identity disorder
   (E) dissociative fugue

29. Which of the following is most likely to include a phenomenon such as this?

   (A) complex partial seizures
   (B) MDD
   (C) general anxiety disorder
   (D) delusional disorder
   (E) visual hallucinations

30. Which of the following statements best characterizes a patient with hypomania?

   (A) It is highly unlikely that he or she has found any success in life.
   (B) Medications are contraindicated.
   (C) He or she may have a comorbid diagnosis of bipolar I disorder.
   (D) It is unlikely that this person will go on to develop mania.
   (E) Hypomania is to mania as dysthymia is to depression.

31. A 23-year-old patient with schizophrenia, who was recently started on a neuroleptic, complains that he cannot sit still and feels constantly restless. The nursing staff has noted that he often paces. This is known as

   (A) parkinsonism
   (B) dystonia
   (C) tremor
   (D) tardive dyskinesia
   (E) akathisia

Questions 32 and 33

A 38-year-old man complains that for the past 2 years he has required several naps over the course of the day; he finds the naps quite refreshing, but sees his doctor because lately, as he is waking up, he feels momentarily "paralyzed."

32. What is the most likely diagnosis?

   (A) cataplexy
   (B) hypnagogic hallucinations
   (C) idiopathic hypersomnolence
   (D) narcolepsy
   (E) advanced sleep wave syndrome

33. Which statement regarding this condition is true?

   (A) Medications are contraindicated.
   (B) Fatal accidents resulting from this condition are highly unlikely.
   (C) It is related to an abnormality in REM sleep.
   (D) Onset is usually in the fifth or sixth decade of life.
   (E) Genetic predisposition is unlikely.

34. Which of the following statements regarding the stages of sleep and the associated waves on an electroencephalogram (EEG) is true?

   (A) Stage 1 sleep is characterized by K complexes and sleep spindles.
   (B) Stage 2 is characterized by relatively low-voltage theta waves.
   (C) Delta waves predominate in Stage 2.
   (D) EEG tracing in REM sleep resembles that of an awake person.
   (E) The length of each successive REM period shortens as the night progresses.

35. Which of the following statements best characterizes a 34-year-old man being treated with systematic desensitization is true?

- (A) Reciprocal inhibition is key to his treatment.
- (B) Allowing this patient to use his imagination is far more effective than exposing him to the actual situation that engenders anxiety.
- (C) Psychoanalytic theory is the most important underpinning of this treatment.
- (D) It is likely that he is in treatment for depression.
- (E) He is being confronted directly with the feared situation and will eventually grow immune to the anxiety it produces.

36. A 65-year-old woman is admitted to the hospital for cellulitis, and you are asked to evaluate her because the intern on duty suspects that she is in delirium tremens. Which of the following statements should you keep in mind while evaluating her?

- (A) Delirium tremens is expected to occur two or more weeks after the last drink.
- (B) Her symptoms might be confused by a comorbid diagnosis of dementia.
- (C) Auditory hallucinations are common.
- (D) It will be important to look for signs of autonomic instability.
- (E) Up to half of patients in alcohol withdrawal will experience delirium tremens.

37. A 39-year-old woman presents to the outpatient mental health clinic at the request of her oncologist 3 weeks after being diagnosed with metastatic breast cancer. The patient denies strong feelings in relation to the diagnosis but talks a great deal about the epidemiology of breast cancer and the available treatment options. This patient is using which of the following defense mechanisms?

- (A) sublimation
- (B) dissociation
- (C) intellectualization
- (D) rationalization
- (E) self-observation

38. A 35-year-old woman presents with episodic anxiety and complains of the occasional feeling that she has heard or perceived things prior to actually hearing them. She expresses her concern that she is "going crazy." You assure her that this can occur in anxiety disorders and is called

- (A) déjà vu
- (B) jamais vu
- (C) déjà entendu
- (D) folie à deux
- (E) la belle indifférence

39. After he is severely reprimanded by his employer, a man goes home and is extremely nasty to his wife. His behavior is an example of

- (A) sublimation
- (B) dissociation
- (C) displacement
- (D) rationalization
- (E) conversion

40. A 28-year-old heterosexual man says that he enjoys dressing in his wife's clothing for sexual excitement. He is comfortable with his gender and sexual orientation but is disturbed by his sexual arousal while wearing women's clothing. This behavior is best termed

- (A) transsexualism
- (B) voyeurism
- (C) hermaphroditism
- (D) exhibitionism
- (E) transvestic fetishism

41. A 26-year-old man with narcolepsy explains that he has episodes of brief paralysis without any loss of consciousness or other deficits. These attacks are usually precipitated by laughter or anger. This patient is describing the phenomenon known as

(A) hypersomnia

(B) cataplexy

(C) hypnagogic hallucinations

(D) hypnopompic hallucinations

(E) catalepsy

42. A 19-year-old man is diagnosed with schizophreniform disorder and is given an intramuscular injection of haloperidol. Later, the patient is found arching forward. On physical exam, stiffness of the neck and back muscles are noted. This dystonia is best described as

(A) opisthotonos

(B) torticollis

(C) laryngospasm

(D) oculogyric crisis

(E) pleurothotonos

43. A 22-year-old man is brought to the emergency department 2 weeks after a motor vehicle accident in which he suffered significant head trauma. The parents are concerned because, although the patient recognizes them on the telephone and responds appropriately, when he is with them face to face he believes them to be imposters who have replaced his real parents. He agrees that these people look like his real parents but is convinced that they are indeed imposters. This delusion is known as

(A) cacodemonomania

(B) doppelganger

(C) folie à deux

(D) Capgras' syndrome

(E) delusion of reference

44. A 50-year-old woman is admitted to the hospital after complaining that she is dead. She believes that her flesh is rotting and that she is able to smell the rancid odor. This delusion is known as

(A) Cotard's syndrome

(B) Capgras' syndrome

(C) Fregoli's syndrome

(D) cacodemonomania

(E) koro

45. A 36-year-old man presents to the emergency department after being found without clothing in the street. He has multiple excoriations all over his body and states that bugs are crawling all over him. His toxicology screen is positive for cocaine. This particular tactile hallucination is known as

(A) hypnagogia

(B) hypnopompia

(C) haptia

(D) formication

(E) synesthesia

46. A 21-year-old man is noted to be restless and constantly moving. He states that he feels as if he has to be moving all the time and feels uncomfortable if he sits still. This sensation is known as

(A) akathisia

(B) akinesia

(C) tardive dyskinesia

(D) dystonia

(E) rabbit syndrome

Questions 47 and 48

A 21-year-old woman who was diagnosed with panic disorder comes to the outpatient mental health clinic with increased frequency of panic attacks and complaining of feeling as if her surrounding environment is unreal and strange. As a result of the increasing frequency of her attacks and this new symptom, she has been unwilling to leave her apartment for several weeks.

47. The feeling of a surreal environment is described as

(A) depersonalization

(B) derealization

(C) hypermnesia

(D) dereism

(E) paresthesia

48. The fact that she is unable to leave her apartment suggests that her panic disorder is complicated by

(A) agoraphobia
(B) social phobia
(C) phobophobia
(D) myxophobia
(E) panphobia

Questions 49 and 50

A 60-year-old man with alcoholism is brought to the emergency department by his family after they notice a decline in memory. Upon evaluation, the patient's remote memory is intact as verified by the family, but his recent recall is severely impaired. The patient provides verbose but erroneous answers in response to questions testing recent recall.

49. This patient's memory distortion is most likely which form of memory disorder?

(A) anterograde amnesia
(B) retrograde amnesia
(C) dissociative amnesia
(D) prosopagnosia
(E) astereognosis

50. The patient's answers in response to recent memory testing are best termed

(A) clang associations
(B) flight of ideas
(C) hypermnesia
(D) logorrhea
(E) confabulation

Questions 51 and 52

A 66-year-old college professor is being seen for a regular checkup. On exam, the patient is noted to demonstrate flat speech with no melodic intonation. In addition, although demonstrating proper word choice and grammar, the patient's answers are extensive with unnecessary detail, but do reach a point.

51. When describing the lack of emotional component of this patient's speech, which of the following terms should be used?

(A) aprosody
(B) stuttering
(C) scanning
(D) aphasia
(E) dysphagia

52. To describe the patient's thought process in relation to the verbose, highly detailed answer, which of the following terms should be used?

(A) flight of ideas
(B) tangential
(C) circumstantial
(D) loosening of associations
(E) derailment

53. An otherwise healthy 5-year-old boy is brought for evaluation after repeated passage of feces into his clothing for the past 6 months. The stools are noted to be small, soft, and poorly formed. He is not on any medications. The term that best defines this disorder is

(A) encopresis
(B) eneuresis
(C) pica
(D) incoherence
(E) logorrhea

54. An 86-year-old woman in the intensive care unit awakes at night and mistakes her IV pole for a family member coming for a visit. She calls the nurses to ask them to have the visitor leave until morning. Which term best describes the perceptual problem?

(A) illusion
(B) gustatory hallucination
(C) micropsia
(D) macropsia
(E) palinopsia

55. A psychiatrist discovers that she is frustrated and easily angered with one of her patients for no obvious reason. While talking to a colleague, she admits that the patient reminds her of her abusive father. The clinician's reaction is best termed

(A) transference
(B) countertransference
(C) reaction formation
(D) displacement
(E) projection

56. An anxious 23-year-old Asian male university student presents to student health services claiming that his penis is shrinking into his abdomen. Despite reassurances from the staff and the physician he remains convinced of this belief. This patient is likely demonstrating a specific delusion known as

(A) koro
(B) kuru
(C) taijin kyofusho
(D) zar
(E) Capgras' syndrome

57. A 36-year-old woman was placed on alprazolam (Xanax) 3 years ago for panic disorder. After watching a news report on television, she became frightened about addiction. She abruptly stopped the medication and during the next 3 days experienced increased anxiety attacks, but claims that she is now doing better. She denied any tremor, sweating, increased heart rate, or uneasiness except in relation to the panic attacks. This phenomenon is best labeled

(A) recurrence
(B) rebound
(C) withdrawal
(D) dystonic reaction
(E) akathisia

Questions 58 and 59

A 39-year-old college professor presents with a fear of public speaking that is affecting his job. Next semester, he is scheduled to teach an introductory chemistry course with more than 300 students. He denies any other complaints.

58. The type of disorder from which he is suffering is best termed

(A) social phobia
(B) agoraphobia
(C) phobophobia
(D) myxophobia
(E) panphobia

59. In formulating a treatment plan, you decide that, in addition to a beta blocker, you will gradually allow the patient to use visual imagery of disturbing situations associated with public speaking. This technique is called

(A) flooding
(B) implosion
(C) systematic desensitization
(D) projection
(E) displacement

Questions 60 through 63

A 36-year-old man is started on bupropion (Zyban/Wellbutrin) for depression. He returns 2 weeks later and states that he feels that his mood has improved slightly and that he has more energy. He has also noticed that his sexual desires have become insatiable. He notes a dramatic increase in his sexual energy and is masturbating frequently despite having intercourse up to two times per day with his wife.

60. The term used to indicate sexual energy is

(A) libido
(B) affect
(C) fugue
(D) gender identity
(E) gender role

61. The best term to describe this patient's insatiable sexual desire is

(A) hypervigilance
(B) hypermnesia
(C) satyriasis
(D) sexual sadism
(E) sexual masochism

62. The patient was switched to fluoxetine (Prozac) after the bupropion was stopped. One week later, he calls complaining of an inability to sleep. He is able to fall asleep but awakens within 2 hours and is unable to return to sleep. The patient is started on trazodone (Desyrel) for this problem. Three days later, he calls complaining of a painful erection that he cannot get rid of even after several hours. The particular sleeping difficulty described by the patient is called

    (A) terminal insomnia
    (B) catalepsy
    (C) cataplexy
    (D) narcolepsy
    (E) initial insomnia

63. The condition that the patient describes following the initiation of trazodone is called

    (A) parapraxis
    (B) priapism
    (C) nymphomania
    (D) satyriasis
    (E) libido

Questions 64 and 65

While interviewing a 78-year-old woman, you discover that, although she is able to recognize objects, she fails to provide an accurate name for many of them. When the patient is shown a pen, the response given is "that thing that you write with," and when shown a watch she replies "the time teller."

64. The patient's answers are examples of

    (A) clang association
    (B) circumlocution
    (C) neologism
    (D) confabulation
    (E) apraxia

65. This demonstrates a particular type of language disorder termed

    (A) alexia
    (B) apraxia
    (C) anomia

    (D) paralinguistic components of speech
    (E) prosopagnosia

66. A 36-year-old woman complains of depression. She reports a decrease in sleep, weight, and libido. She also complains of recent constipation. The changes in the patient's sleep, weight, libido, and bowel habits are all

    (A) neurovegetative signs
    (B) word salad
    (C) conversion
    (D) catatonia
    (E) neologisms

67. At a charity dinner honoring a newly crowned pageant winner, the speaker makes an embarrassing error during the introduction. In reference to some charity work that the winner had been involved in working with paraplegics, he said, "I am especially proud of her fondness and work with nipples . . . I mean cripples." This embarrassing situation could be an example of

    (A) parapraxis
    (B) echopraxia
    (C) copropraxia
    (D) bruxism
    (E) clang association

68. On a patient's first visit to his psychiatrist, the psychiatrist asks about family history and other medical illnesses, and performs a detailed physical and neurological examination. This psychiatrist is operating mainly under which paradigm?

    (A) dynamic
    (B) psychoanalytic
    (C) forensic
    (D) social
    (E) biological

69. During his session, a patient receives mainly empathetic reassurances from his psychiatrist. This best exemplifies which type of psychotherapy?

(A) existential

(B) dynamic

(C) biological

(D) supportive

(E) cognitive–behavioral

70. A 13-year-old girl is seen by her psychiatrist 1 year after an automobile accident. She demonstrates intact language ability and complex motor skills. She has no abnormalities in the perception of stimuli that are identifiable, but she has lost the ability to read since the accident. What deficit is she demonstrating?

(A) anomia

(B) aphasia

(C) alexia

(D) apraxia

(E) agnosia

71. A 35-year-old man complains that his partner enjoys sexual activity only when inflicting pain on him. He is disturbed and frustrated by this. This type of paraphilia exhibited by his partner is known as

(A) sexual masochism

(B) sexual sadism

(C) exhibitionism

(D) frotteurism

(E) transvestic fetishism

72. A 21-year-old man was arrested after he was found outside of a window masturbating. He admitted to having been watching the young girl inside over a period of several months. This patient demonstrates which paraphilia?

(A) transsexualism

(B) hermaphroditism

(C) voyeurism

(D) exhibitionism

(E) transvestic fetishism

DIRECTIONS (Questions 73 through 95): Each group of items in this section consists of lettered headings followed by a set of numbered words or phrases. For each numbered word or phrase, select the ONE lettered heading that is most closely associated with it. Each lettered heading may be selected once, more than once, or not at all.

Questions 73 through 76

Use the list below to identify the proper term for each question.

(A) inhalants

(B) withdrawal

(C) tolerance

(D) abuse

(E) dependence

(F) formication

(G) intoxication

(H) hallucinogens

(I) posthallucinogen perception disorder

(J) amotivational syndrome

73. A 45-year-old man presents to the emergency department in delirium tremens. He complains of bugs crawling on his skin.

74. A 14-year-old boy is brought to you by his mother. She states that he has no motivation and is failing in school. The boy admitted to his mother that he has been smoking marijuana. To what class of substances does marijuana belong?

75. A 21-year-old man presents to the emergency department after "huffing gas." The patient claims that he feels disconnected from reality and is frightened. After about 20 minutes, these effects diminish. Petroleum fumes are in what group of substances?

76. A 54-year-old man states that he continues to use alcohol despite having lost his family and job. He often drives his car while intoxicated and recently was arrested in a barroom brawl. The fact that this patient continues to drink alcohol, despite adverse effects, indicates that he has which substance problem?

Questions 77 through 80

Match each term with its definition.

   (A) lability
   (B) irritability
   (C) dyscalculia
   (D) verbigeration
   (E) dysarthria
   (F) gustation
   (G) glossolalia
   (H) hypochondriasis

77. Ability to speak a new language suddenly

78. Repetitive and meaningless talking

79. Difficulty with articulation

80. Taste sensation

Questions 81 through 85

Five responses to the question "Why did you go to medical school?" are given below. Match the response with the appropriate disorder of thought process or component of thought process disorder.

   (A) circumstantiality
   (B) tangentiality
   (C) flight of ideas
   (D) loosening of associations
   (E) clanging
   (F) derailment

81. I don't even need to make money. Money makes the world go 'round, 'round the mulberry bush the monkey chased the weasel. Weasels make good politicians you know.

82. People are in need wherever you go, and I've been to a lot of places. It is amazing how much traveling I have actually done. I do suffer a bad case of wanderlust.

83. Medical school in pools with spools of thread till you're dead, Fred.

84. Religions are the most important of all thought. Why do you bleed your school colors? I just wanted some publicity for my movie.

85. Well, medical school was actually something my parents . . . I am so worried about the state of the world today.

Questions 86 through 95

Use the following terms to match the correct response to the questions below.

   (A) galactorrhea
   (B) agranulocytosis
   (C) blepharospasm
   (D) opisthotonos
   (E) torticollis
   (F) rabbit syndrome
   (G) neuroleptic malignant syndrome
   (H) obstructive jaundice
   (I) gynecomastia
   (J) pigmented retinopathy
   (K) orthostatic hypotension
   (L) pseudoparkinsonism
   (M) akathisia
   (N) tardive dyskinesia
   (O) constipation
   (P) retrograde ejaculation

86. A 27-year-old man with paranoid schizophrenia notices the development of breasts, a decreased libido, and not ejaculating with orgasm. He is being treated with thioridazine (Mellaril). The development of breasts is due to the blockade of dopamine receptors in the tuberoinfundibular tract. What is this condition called?

87. Which term describes the inability to ejaculate that is most commonly associated with thioridazine?

88. A 22-year-old African-American man on clozapine (Clozaril) for 3 months reports a sore throat and fever. A complete blood count (CBC) is obtained with a white blood count of 1,000/mm^3 with 1% granulocytes. What is this potentially fatal side effect called?

89. A 43-year-old man with schizophrenia is on haloperidol (Haldol). He is noted to have a flexed posture, festinating gait, resting tremor, and bradykinesia. This patient is suffering

from what neurological side effect caused by D2 blockade of the nigrostriatal pathway?

90. The patient in question 89 was continued on haloperidol despite his side effects and after several years developed choreic movements of the trunk and limbs, along with lip smacking and tongue movements. What is this side effect called?

91. A 21-year-old man with psychosis was started on haloperidol at high doses. Eight days into his treatment, he developed fever, generalized rigidity, diaphoresis, and altered mental status. What is this potentially fatal reaction called?

92. A 26-year-old man being treated with high-dose thioridazine (Mellaril) is found on ophthalmologic exam to have peppery pigmentation of the retina. Despite discontinuation of the medication, the pigmentation continues and the patient eventually suffers total blindness. What is this complication called?

93. A 22-year-old man complains of severe restlessness and agitation after starting on a neuroleptic. He complains that he cannot sit still and paces constantly. What is this condition called?

94. A 26-year-old patient with schizophrenia is started on chlorpromazine (Thorazine). After 1 week, he complains of flulike symptoms. A complete blood count is obtained and is normal. After another week, the patient develops a yellowish color to his skin and sclera. Which term describes the side effect this patient is suffering?

95. A 45-year-old patient with schizophrenia is started on a high dose of chlorpromazine (Thorazine). The next day, he complains of being light-headed every time he stands. On examination, he is noted to have a significant decrease in blood pressure and an increase in heart rate. You speculate that this is secondary to the alpha-1-adrenergic blockade. What is this complication called?

Answers and Explanations

1. **(D)** Fixed interval, fixed ratio, variable interval, and variable ratio refer to schedules of reinforcement. In each case, some behavior is increased in response to a rewarding response to that behavior. The gambler at the slot machine is rewarded on a variable schedule, after some random number of tries (variable ratio). The interval schedules require the participant to wait either a static amount of time (fixed interval) or a varying amount of time (variable interval) before reward is possible. The variable schedules have longer extinction times; that is, the behavior persists longer in the absence of reward (the behavior is difficult to extinguish).

2. **(A)** Behaviorists would say some people have difficulty discontinuing slot machine use because it rewards its plays on a variable schedule and the behavior does not easily extinguish. Habituation refers to a decreasing response to a repeated stimulus. Classical conditioning involves pairing a neutral stimulus (e.g., a bell) with a nonneutral stimulus (e.g., an electric shock) and demonstrating that the neutral stimulus can evoke the same response as the nonneutral stimulus. Because Pavlov came up with the idea of classical conditioning, it is often referred to as pavlovian conditioning.

3. **(E)** The neurovegetative signs of depression are associated with somatic disturbances. Systems commonly affected are appetite, sleep, motor, and sexual function. Alterations—either increases or decreases—in any of these functions can help to make a diagnosis of depression.

4. **(E)** With antidepressant treatment, the neurovegetative symptoms tend to respond first. This is why it is a common wisdom in psychiatry that the person who begins to recover from depression may be at greater risk for suicide than when he is at the height of his depression. As he starts to function better physiologically, he may be more capable of carrying out a suicidal impulse.

5. **(A)** This patient demonstrates a disorder of thought content. Thought content refers to the particular ideas that are on a patient's mind. In this case, the patient's thought is delusional, that is, reveals a fixed, false belief. Suicidal ideation is another example of thought content. Thought form refers to the flow and sequencing of ideas, usually inferred from the manner in which one speaks. Circumstantiality, loose associations, and thought blocking are examples of disorders of thought form. An obsession is a recurrent intrusive thought, feeling, or action that is unpleasant and provokes anxiety. Derealization refers to a feeling of unreality in which the environment is experienced as unreal and flat, dull, or strange. Patients with disorders of thought form are said to have a formal thought disorder.

6. **(E)** The specific delusion referred to here is an idea of reference. The patient interprets an event as relating to him, even though it clearly does not. Thought insertion is a delusion in which the patient believes thoughts from some external entity are placed in his mind. Somatic delusions refer to a delusion about the patient's body; for example, a com-

mon belief is that one's body parts are diseased. Thought broadcasting is the belief that one's thoughts can be heard or somehow known by others, without direct communication. Paranoia often colors many delusions and involves the belief that other people, agencies, or forces mean harm or danger to the patient. Any of the above delusions may include elements of paranoia.

7. **(D)** Mood-congruent delusions are compatible and consistent with the state of mind of the patient. In this case, the patient feels guilty and presumably believes he deserves punishment. His delusions express these thoughts. If he described delusions of grandiosity, that would be an example of a mood-incongruent delusion. Bizarre delusions describe a circumstance that is virtually impossible to be true, for example, a schizophrenic patient believing a computer chip is implanted in his brain. The delusions in this question, however unlikely, are in some sense conceivable. Somatic delusions focus on bodily functions and integrity. Ego-syntonic delusions are experienced by the sufferer as acceptable; for example, the manic patient believing he is the greatest actor in the world. This patient's delusions are ego-dystonic, that is, experienced as unacceptable and unpleasant. Often, the nature of the delusion and its relation to mood state provide clues to a diagnosis. Delusions arising out of a severe depression, as in this case, are frequently mood-congruent.

8. **(C)** The delusions of schizophrenic patients can be bizarre and are often unrelated to mood state. Mania produces delusions that are grandiose, usually related to a sense of inflated self-esteem. The presence of delusions would rule out dysthymia and adjustment disorder, as these affective illnesses do not reach an intensity that would include delusional thinking.

9. **(C)** The choices in this question describe different patterns of amnesia. Localized amnesia refers to memory loss surrounding a discrete period of time, typically occurring after a traumatic event; in this case, the patient's amnesia results from learning of her husband's death. Selective amnesia involves the inability to recall certain aspects of an event, though other memories of the event may be intact. Rarely, a patient may forget his or her entire preceding life (generalized amnesia) or forget all events following a trauma, except for the immediate past (continuous amnesia). Retrograde amnesia is any amnesia for events that come before a traumatic event.

10. **(A)** The diagnosis in this case is dissociative amnesia, which typically results in the setting of some emotional or physical trauma. Dissociative fugue involves sudden, unexplained travel away from one's home, also accompanied with amnesic symptoms. Depersonalization disorder is a persistent or recurrent dreamlike state, in which one feels detached or outside of his or her own body or mind. PTSD is unlikely, as this patient did not witness a life-threatening or horrific event. Adjustment disorder is usually not diagnosed in the presence of bereavement.

11. **(B)** Circumstantiality involves a circuitous, overinclusive answer that only eventually gets to the point, as the patient demonstrates in this example. Loosening of associations is a response composed of a series of disconnected ideas. Tangentiality occurs when the patient strays off the point entirely, never returning to the original intention of the answer. Pressured speech is a continuous, usually rapid, uninterruptable stream of ideas that may make sense but is often hard to follow. This patient's speech may be pressured, but the question gives no clues to this. Pointless repetition of a word, a phrase, or an idea is perseveration. Generally, the speech of a schizophrenic patient may demonstrate any of these characteristics; his diagnosis provides no clue to the answer.

12. **(C)** Concentration refers to the ability to sustain focus on a cognitive task. Performing serial sevens and spelling "world" backwards are tests of concentration. While a certain facility with the remaining choices is necessary

to perform each task (no cognitive function is tested in absolute isolation), the serial sevens test provides a window on a patient's concentration. Remote memory involves the recall of events long past, for example, information from a patient's childhood. Recent memory is recall of events occurring in the last several minutes. Fund of knowledge is a test of information the patient readily has available to him; knowledge of current events is often used to assess this. The mental status exam will often contain tests of mathematics skills, but testing mathematics skills is not the purpose of the serial sevens test. Any test of cognitive function must take into account the patient's cultural, educational, and social background.

13. **(E)** Paraphilias encompass a wide variety of maladaptive sexual behaviors and fantasies. Frotteurism is the syndrome of recurrent, intense sexual fantasies and behaviors involving touching or rubbing against a nonconsenting adult. Exhibitionism involves revealing one's genitals to unsuspecting strangers. Pedophilia is sexual fantasies and behaviors involving children. Voyeurism involves secretly watching someone involved in disrobing, nudity, or sexual behavior. Fetishism is a sexual attraction to an inanimate object.

14. **(D)** In projective identification, the patient attributes unacceptable thoughts or feelings to those around him; the patient also recognizes the feeling in himself. The unacceptable feeling in this case is the patient's anger resulting from his terminal diagnosis. It is common that the unacceptable feelings are experienced by the objects of the projective identification—in this case, the nurses, who have become angry with the patient. The remaining defense mechanisms may each play a role here, but we are given no direct clues to this. Denial occurs when a patient selectively ignores an unacceptable feeling or fact, as may occur in an alcoholic who refuses to believe he has a problem. Intellectualization occurs when a patient "explains away" through intellectual reasoning the emotional impact of some feature of his life. Sublima-

tion is the channeling of unacceptable impulses into socially acceptable activities. Reaction formation is the endorsement of some opposite view of an unacceptable feeling or impulse.

15. **(C)** A compulsion is a repetitive act carried out to stave off some unwanted event—in this case, a gas leak. Compulsions are typically uncontrollable and experienced by the patient as unwanted, unpleasant, and often irrational. An obsession is a repetitive, unwanted idea or image that is experienced as intrusive. Compulsions are often performed to release the mounting anxiety associated with obsessions, as in this case. Paranoia refers to a heightened suspiciousness of other people. Hyperarousal is a state of heightened vigilance, and may include a startle response; this is seen often in PTSD. Delusions are fixed, false beliefs. Patients suffering from obsessive behavior usually have some insight into the irrationality of their obsession, so their "belief" does not rise to the level of a delusion.

16. **(E)** Dual diagnosis is common in psychiatric patients, and refers to any patient with a substance abuse disorder (e.g., alcohol dependence) in addition to any other psychiatric diagnosis that does not, by definition, necessarily include any substance abuse (e.g., MDD). It is always of paramount importance to know if a psychiatric patient is dually diagnosed, because typically each diagnosis has a tremendous impact on the other diagnosis. Frequently, it is difficult to understand or treat the disorders as separate entities. There is no particular terminology describing the other choices listed.

17. **(A)** The need for increasing amounts of a drug to achieve the same effect, or a diminishing effect achieved through the use of the same amount of a drug, describes tolerance. Withdrawal is a syndrome of behavioral, emotional, and physiological signs and symptoms that occur in a setting of the discontinuation of a drug. Dependence and abuse both require more history and clinical

information than is offered in this question. Dependence on a drug requires that its use causes significant impairment, anguish, or devastation to the individual and, despite this, the patient continues using. The presence of withdrawal on discontinuation and tolerance frequently help make a diagnosis of substance dependence. Abuse is similar, in that use causes significant problems for the patient, but use of the drug is generally more infrequent than is found in dependence, and consequently does not involve tolerance and withdrawal symptoms.

18. **(E)** A pseudoseizure is a psychogenically induced behavior that resembles epileptic activity. While the syndrome may in some cases be motivated by secondary gain (as in malingering), it most often occurs in reaction to stress or in a setting of personality disorder, severe affective disorders, or conversion reactions. The other choices, which each represent true epileptic seizures, rarely, if ever, include purposeful, complex activity as is seen in this case. Often, patients with pseudoseizures have a concurrent seizure disorder, and it is quite difficult to sort out the true seizures from the pseudoseizures. Diagnosing pseudoseizure often requires demonstrating a normal EEG at the time of the pseudoseizure. The prognosis for pseudoseizures is quite poor.

19. **(D)** Abnormal sleep patterns are common in depression and may be the chief complaint of the depressed patient. Classically, increased sleep latency (difficulty falling asleep), early morning awakening, and increased wakefulness are seen. REM (rapid eye movement) sleep tends to be redistributed, so that most of it occurs in the first half of the night. REM latency (the period of time between falling asleep and starting REM sleep) decreases.

20. **(B)** Patients with schizoid personality disorder will typically be socially isolated and be distinctly inept at forming and carrying on interpersonal relationships. They often come to the attention of physicians as a result of

some other issue, as seen in this case. Their apparent apathy and indifference may resemble the negative symptoms of schizophrenia, and indeed, that is in the differential here; but it would be difficult to make a diagnosis of schizophrenia without evidence of psychosis. This patient lacks the actively odd and peculiar mannerisms or eccentric way of thinking seen in schizotypal personality disorder. He exhibits none of the mistrust and suspiciousness seen in paranoid personality disorder. While he may be depressed, we are given no direct evidence of this.

21. **(E)** As many as 10% of patients with schizophrenia will die from suicide; the suicide rate in the general population is significantly lower. Overall, the ratio of males to females with schizophrenia is about 1:1. However, it has been demonstrated that the age of onset in men, 15 to 25 years, is lower than in women, usually 25 to 35 years. While schizophrenia is not caused by stressful life events, it is in the setting of stress that symptoms often emerge, leading to hospitalization. Any admission to a psychiatric hospital should include a careful search for precipitating events. Schizophrenia cannot be entirely attributed to genetics, but a family history of schizophrenia is linked to increased risk for developing the disease.

22. **(B)** Positive symptoms represent the presence of a behavior or emotion that is normally absent; negative symptoms are the absence of a behavior or emotion normally present. Logorrhea, excessive but coherent and logical speech, is a positive symptom, while alogia, absence of speech, is a negative symptom. Each of the remaining choices are positive symptoms. Echolalia describes a behavior in which a patient repeats back exactly what is spoken to him.

23. **(A)** Schizophrenia is commonly classified according to types, which try to capture descriptively the symptoms that predominate the clinical picture. In the paranoid type, the patient is preoccupied with delusions, typi-

cally persecutory in nature, and often has auditory hallucinations. Speech and behavior appear relatively organized. The disorganized type is characterized by disorganized speech and behavior as well as flat or inappropriate affect. In catatonic type, motor activity is retarded to the point of immobility, or excessive, yet purposeless and unrelated to external events. A diagnosis of undifferentiated type means that the patient meets criteria for schizophrenia, but does not meet criteria for paranoid, disorganized, or catatonic types. The residual type describes an absence of positive symptoms and a preponderance of negative symptoms.

24. **(A)** Of all the types of schizophrenia (see answer to question 23), the paranoid type carries the best prognosis.

25. **(D)** The most important aspect of voices heard by a patient with schizophrenia is the nature of what the voices are saying. Command auditory hallucinations telling a patient to harm or kill herself or someone else is almost always a psychiatric emergency, and the patient will require hospitalization to be safe or to keep someone else safe. The only possible exception is the case in which an experienced clinician knows the patient well and believes the situation to be safe; even then, hospitalization is probably necessary. All of the other choices in this question speak to important characteristics of auditory hallucinations and should be evaluated, but the presence of command auditory hallucinations requires immediate attention.

26. **(C)** ECT is widely used in the treatment of severe depression in patients whose illnesses have been refractory to antidepressant medications. It can be considered a first-line agent in psychotic depressions and patients who, for whatever reason, cannot tolerate or benefit from antidepressant medication. In today's practice, ECT is administered under conditions of complete anesthesia and blockade of the neuromuscular junction; other than the starting of intravenous lines, it is not considered physically uncomfortable. Many

patients who undergo ECT will have had histories of depression refractory to medication, and there is no evidence to suggest that ECT will change their response to antidepressant medications. Immediately after ECT, many patients have a vagal response and experience a decrease in blood pressure and pulse; shortly thereafter, a sympathetic surge often increases blood pressure and pulse.

27. **(D)** ECT has relatively few contraindications and in some cases is preferred for its rapid onset of action. However, because of the cardiovascular effects of ECT, a history of a recent myocardial infarction (within the past 6 months) is an absolute contraindication. Another contraindication is the presence of a clinically significant intracranial space-occupying lesion, because of the risk of brain stem herniation. Otherwise, ECT has relatively few contraindications and may even be performed in pregnancy. The most common complaints patients will have following ECT are impairments in both anterograde and retrograde memory. While most memory problems will resolve, some may persist indefinitely.

28. **(C)** Derealization is a feeling of unreality or sense of alteration of the external world. It often accompanies depersonalization, a similar feeling, except that depersonalization applies to an unreal feeling about one's self and his body. Dissociative amnesia is a memory loss, usually in a setting of physical or emotional trauma. Dissociative identity disorder, previously known as multiple personality disorder, is diagnosed in the rare patient who manifests more than one distinct, complex personality. Dissociative fugue, a darling of tabloid news programs, is the sudden, inexplicable, and complete loss of one's identity and memory, often accompanied by travel away from one's home or work and the assumption of a new identity elsewhere.

29. **(A)** While derealization may be found to some extent in a great many psychiatric illnesses, including MDD, general anxiety disorder, and delusion disorder, it is common in complex partial seizures. A visual hallucina-

tion would not be characterized as derealization.

30. **(E)** Hypomania is a kinder, gentler mania. The hypomanic patient is activated and full of energy, but manages to act in a reasonable manner. In contrast, bipolar I patients in full-blown mania often come to the attention of psychiatrists because they have in some way infringed on the rights of others. Many people with hypomania will enjoy success in business and other endeavors. If the patient is in some way impaired because of hypomania, a mood stabilizer can be tried. The presence of bipolar I disorder, a disabling and long-term illness involving at least one episode of mania, would preclude the diagnosis of bipolar II disorder, in which episodes of hypomania and major depression have occurred. The patient with hypomania is far more likely than the general population to develop full-blown mania. As stated, hypomania is a milder mania, just as dysthymia is a milder form of depression.

31. **(E)** A subjective feeling of restlessness and a need to constantly move about and pace is known as akathisia, a common side effect of neuroleptic medication that can occur soon after such medications are started. The other choices listed are also neuroleptic side effects. Parkinsonism refers to symptoms evoked by neuroleptics that are commonly seen in Parkinson's disease. Parkinsonian symptoms include tremor (a 3- to 6-cycle-per-second motion), akinesia (or bradykinesia), and rigidity. Dystonias are uncontrolled muscle contractions. Tardive dyskinesia is a rhythmic, involuntary movement of the tongue, jaw, trunk, or extremities appearing weeks to months after the initiation of neuroleptic therapy.

32. **(D)** Narcolepsy is characterized by persistent daytime hypersomnolence that is temporarily relieved by brief naps. Narcolepsy is often accompanied by phenomena commonly associated with REM sleep, including hypnagogic hallucinations (vivid dreams occurring just as someone is falling asleep or waking up),

cataplexy (a sudden dramatic loss of muscle tone, usually following an intense emotional reaction), and sleep paralysis (a loss of voluntary muscle tone at the beginning or end of sleep, seen in this case). Idiopathic hypersomnolence is also characterized by persistent sleepiness, but can be distinguished from narcolepsy by the fact that the naps accompanying it are often long and unrefreshing.

33. **(C)** As stated in answer 32, disturbances in REM sleep phenomena seem to be the central feature of narcolepsy. Cataplexy and excessive drowsiness may indeed lead to automobile accidents and other fatal mishaps. For this reason, in significant cases, pharmacological treatment is indicated. The treatment of choice is stimulants, for example, methylphenidate or dextroamphetamine. Age of onset is usually around the second decade of life. Genetically, a high association has been found between narcolepsy and the HLA-DR2 antigen.

34. **(D)** During REM sleep, as during wakefulness, the characteristic EEG pattern is that of low-voltage, mixed-frequency waves. Stage 1, the first stage of sleep, is characterized by theta waves. Stage 2 is characterized by sleep spindles and K complexes. Stages 3 and 4 are characterized by delta waves. The sleep cycle consists of shifting from non-REM (stages 1 to 4) to REM sleep. The entire cycle (non-REM and REM) lasts about 90 minutes and repeats itself throughout the night. As the night progresses, the REM part of the cycle becomes longer and longer.

35. **(A)** In systematic desensitization, one response to some situation stimulus is substituted for another response. This is known as reciprocal inhibition. Most commonly, the former response is anxiety—usually enough to interfere with someone's ability to lead a fulfilling life—and the latter response is relaxation. This is accomplished by gradually exposing the patient to increasingly greater approximations of some situation that causes great concern—say air travel—and pairing that experience with a more pleasant response. The most effective way to conduct

systematic desensitization is to gradually expose the patient to the very situations that cause him extreme concern, not some imagined facsimile. Systematic desensitization arises from the teaching of the behaviorists, who postulate that the behaviors are learned; the behaviorists are less concerned that some unconscious process might be at play as psychoanalytic theory proposes. The most common application of systematic desensitization is helping a patient deal with a phobia. Depression is more readily treated pharmacologically and/or with psychotherapy.

36. **(D)** Delirium tremens, an acute confusional state induced by severe alcoholic withdrawal, will occur in 3 to 5% of patients withdrawing from alcohol. Although it may be seen in patients with dementia, as well as in those without, any delirium, including delirium tremens, differs from dementia in that one finds a relatively acute onset. The patient with dementia, by history, will have evidenced a slow (months to years) decline, whereas the patient in an alcohol withdrawal delirium is expected to manifest symptoms in a matter of days, if not hours. While auditory hallucinations are possible, visual hallucinations (e.g., little scary creatures lurking about the room) are far more common. Delirium tremens usually occurs 3 days to a week after the patient's last drink. Autonomic instability, particularly fever and elevated pulse and blood pressure, are common signs of alcohol withdrawal and often provide a key clue to the fact that the patient is in withdrawal and in need of emergent treatment, namely, administration of benzodiazepines.

37. **(C)** Intellectualization is the utilization of abstract thinking to deal with or cover internal or external stressors; in this case, the unacceptable feelings of having cancer. Sublimation is a defense mechanism employed to deal with unacceptable feelings or desires by channeling them into socially acceptable behaviors. Like sublimation, rationalization is a defense against undesired motivations, but in this case the motivations are concealed by elaborate and reassuring explanations that avoid the actual underlying motives. Dissociation is a defense mechanism that deals with stressors with a breakdown of the usual integration of memory, behavior, and perception. Self-observation is a defense mechanism involving the reflection of one's own thoughts and behavior with appropriate responses.

38. **(C)** Déjà entendu is the feeling that one is hearing something one has heard before. It is usually associated with anxiety states or fatigue. Déjà vu is a similar experience but refers to the sensation that something has been seen before. Jamais vu is the opposite of déjà vu in that it refers to something that should be familiar but seems quite unfamiliar. Folie à deux is a shared delusion aroused in one person by the influence of another. La belle indifference is the indifference shown toward a deficit or loss of function classically seen in a conversion disorder.

39. **(C)** The man is naturally angry, anxious, and sensitive at being reprimanded by his employer. He has found it difficult to express his feelings toward the disturbing person, the employer. Instead of suppressing or repressing the anger, or sublimating his tension in more forceful work, he displaces his anger onto a safer target, his wife. This is an example of displacement.

40. **(E)** Transvestic fetishism is a paraphilia that involves dressing in clothing of the opposite sex. It is often present in heterosexual men and differs from transsexualism in that the person is usually comfortable and content with their gender. It is, however, possible to see these disorders concomitantly. Voyeurism and exhibitionism are also paraphilias and involve, respectively, watching others without their knowledge and exposing one's genitalia to an unsuspecting audience. Hermaphroditism is not a paraphilia but is a rare disorder in which one possesses the sexual characteristics of both sexes.

41. **(B)** Narcolepsy is a sleep disorder characterized by the tetrad of excessive daytime somnolence (hypersomnia), cataplexy (transient loss of motor tone associated with strong emotions), sleep paralysis (total or partial paralysis in sleep–wake transition), and hypnagogic hallucinations (vivid dreamlike hallucinations occurring in the wake–sleep transition). Hypnopomic hallucinations occur in the sleep–wake transition. Catalepsy is a state of immobility sometimes seen in catatonic states.

42. **(A)** All of these are types of dystonic reactions that are induced by the use of neuroleptics. Opisthotonos, also known as arc de cercle, is a spasm of the neck and back that causes the patient to arch forward. Torticollis is a spasm of the neck muscles that usually brings the neck to one side or another but can also pull forward or backward. Pleurothotonos, also known as Pisa syndrome, is a leaning posture induced by the spasm of the torso muscles. Oculogyric crisis is simply the spasm of the extraocular muscles. The most alarming of these dystonias is laryngospasm, which is the spasm of the muscles controlling the tongue and the throat. This can lead to respiratory distress.

43. **(D)** Capgras' syndrome is the delusional idea that imposters have replaced once familiar persons. This belief is held despite the acknowledgment that the people appear exactly the same. Doppelganger is the belief in the existence of an identical counterpart. Cacodemonomania is the delusion of being poisoned by an evil spirit. Folie à deux is a delusion shared by more than one person, and delusion of reference is the ascribing of personal meaning or messages that are not intended. Koro is a traumatic fear that the penis is shrinking into the body cavity.

44. **(A)** Cotard's syndrome is a delusion that nothing exists (nihilism) or the person herself does not exist. The person may feel that her body has disintegrated or that she is dead. Occasionally, the belief may be so vivid that it can even be associated with the sensation of a rancid or rotting odor, which is quite un-

pleasant for the patient. It can be seen in schizophrenia or severe bipolar disorder. It can also be early evidence of Alzheimer's disease. Capgras' syndrome and Fregoli's syndrome are both delusions but are opposite in content. Capgras' syndrome is the belief that an imposter has replaced a familiar person, whereas Fregoli's syndrome is the delusion that a person is taking the form of a number of people or creatures. Cacodemonomania is the delusion that one is poisoned by an evil spirit.

45. **(D)** Formication is a particular type of tactile hallucination in which one has the sensation of bugs crawling on or under the skin. It can be seen in cocaine intoxication and in major alcohol withdrawal. Haptic hallucination is another tactile hallucination in which one feels as if he is being touched, for example, by a phantom. Hypnagogic and hypnopompic hallucinations are not tactile hallucinations but are hallucinations experienced in the transition state from wakefulness to sleep and from sleep to wakefulness, respectively. Synesthesia is a secondary sensation following an actual perception (e.g., the sensation of a color associated with taste). Synesthesia usually is secondary to neurological disease or hallucinogen use, most notably LSD.

46. **(A)** All of the choices are possible side effects, either short term or long term, of neuroleptics. Akathisia is the subjective sensation of motor and mental restlessness. Akinesia is a dysfunction of slowed or absent movement that can be associated with pseudoparkinsonism in the setting of neuroleptics. A dystonia, like akathisia and akinesia, can occur acutely and involve muscle rigidity and spasticity. Tardive dyskinesia is a late-onset neurological effect of neuroleptics and can include tongue and lip movements and choreic movement of the trunk or limbs. Rabbit syndrome is also a late-onset side effect that involves fine, rhythmic movements of the lips.

47. **(B)** Both depersonalization and derealization can be seen in anxiety disorders. Derealization is the sense that one's surroundings are strange or unreal, while depersonalization is

the feeling that one's identity is lost, or the feeling of being unreal or strange. Dereism is simply mental activity not in accordance with reality. Hypermnesia is an abnormal recall of details. Paresthesia is an abnormal sensation such as tingling or prickling.

48. **(A)** Each of these terms, as is suggested by the common suffix, is a fear or phobia. Agoraphobia is Greek for "fear of the marketplace" and is an anxiety that occurs when one is in a situation that might be difficult or embarrassing to escape or in which help might not be readily available. This can limit one to a small, familiar territory such as one's home. Social phobia is an anxiety disorder that involves an irrational fear of public situations such as public speaking. Phobophobia, myxophobia, and panphobia are all types of simple phobias and are fear of fear itself, fear of slime, and fear of everything, respectively.

49. **(A)** This patient may be suffering from Wernicke–Korsakoff syndrome, a complication of long-term alcoholism. Anterograde amnesia is the loss of immediate or short-term memory. Patients are unable to form new memories. Retrograde amnesia is the loss of remote or previously formed memories. Dissociative amnesia is the loss of memory without the loss of ability to form new memories. It is usually associated with emotional trauma and is not due to drugs or a medical condition. Prosopagnosia is the inability to remember faces despite being able to recognize that they are faces. Astereognosis is the inability to recognize an object by touch despite the tactile sensations being intact.

50. **(E)** Confabulation is the fluent fabrication of fictitious responses in compensation of memory disturbance. Clang associations are the use of words based on sound and not with reference to the meaning. Flight of ideas is another form of speech in which one shifts rapidly from one idea to another, but the relationship between the themes can sometimes be followed. Hypermnesia is the ability to recall detailed material that is not usually available to recall. Logorrhea is uncontrollable or

excessive talking, sometimes seen in manic episodes.

51. **(A)** All of these terms are used to describe speech. Prosody is used to describe the melody, rhythm, or intonation of speech that carries its emotional quality. The lack of this type of emotionally varied speech is called aprosodic speech. Stuttering is the disturbance of the fluidity of speech, as in repeating sounds or syllables or using broken words. Scanning speech is irregular pauses between syllables, which also breaks the fluidity but does not cause the repeating of sounds or syllables. Aphasia is the inability to communicate by speech or language. Dysphagia is difficulty in swallowing.

52. **(C)** Circumstantial speech is the overuse of detailed information, providing extraneous detail in a digressive manner to convey an idea. Tangential speech quickly moves off topic but can be followed, and the patient never arrives at the point that is trying to be made. Flight of ideas is like tangential speech, but the changes in ideas or topics are more frequent and more abrupt; like tangential speech, the connections are still recognizable. In loosening of associations, the logical connections between ideas are completely lost; although proper grammar and words may be used, the speech is not logical or goal-directed. Derailment refers to the abrupt interruption of an idea and then resuming after a period of time (a few seconds) to a new topic. This is usually without the patient's being aware of the switch in material.

53. **(A)** Encopresis and enuresis are elimination disorders, each with specific diagnostic criteria that deal with the passage of feces in inappropriate places and the voiding of urine into bed or clothes, respectively. Pica is the ingestion of substances with no nutritional value that cannot be attributed to developmental stage or another disorder. Incoherence refers to looseness of thought that makes no apparent sense. Logorrhea is excessive speech.

54. (A) An illusion is a misperception of an actual stimulus, while a hallucination is the perception in the absence of a stimulus. Micropsia and macropsia are the misperceptions of objects being smaller or larger than they really are. Palinopsia is the persistence of the visual image after the stimulus has been removed.

55. (B) Transference, in strict terms, is the patient's reexperiencing of past experiences in the setting of psychoanalytic psychotherapy. Countertransference is the analyst's (or therapist's) response to this. These terms have come to mean the transferring of emotions and feelings that one has from one's past to the other person—in the case of transference, the feelings are experienced in the patient and relate to how they feel about their therapist. In the case of countertransference, the feelings are experienced in the analyst or therapist and reflect how they feel about the patient. Reaction formation, displacement, and projection are all defense mechanisms used by the ego to keep potentially anxiety-provoking feelings out of awareness. Reaction formation is the formation of thoughts that are opposite to the anxiety-provoking feelings. Displacement is the transferring of a feeling toward an object that is less threatening, as in the family pet or one's spouse or children. Projection is the false attribution of one's own unacceptable feelings to another.

56. (A) Koro, zar, and taijin kyofusho are all examples of culture-bound delusions. Koro is the worry that the penis is shrinking into the abdomen and is found in South and East Asia. Zar is the delusional possession by a spirit, and taijin kyofusho is the belief that one's body is offensive to others. Kuru is a slowly progressive neurological disease leading to death, thought to be caused by an agent similar to Creutzfeldt–Jakob. Capgras' syndrome is the delusional idea that imposters have replaced once familiar persons.

57. (B) Rebound is a return of symptoms that are brief and transient and is frequently associated with the abrupt discontinuation of benzodiazepines. Recurrence is the long-term return of the original symptoms. Withdrawal is characterized by a specific set of signs and symptoms specific to a particular substance. These are not necessarily similar to the original symptoms that were being treated by the medication. Akathisia is the subjective sensation of motor and mental restlessness. A dystonic reaction is an increase in muscle rigidity and spasticity that is usually associated with the use of neuroleptics.

58. (A) Social phobia is an anxiety disorder that involves an irrational fear of public situations. Agoraphobia is an anxiety that occurs when one is in a situation that might be difficult or embarrassing to escape or in which help might not be readily available. Patients suffering from agoraphobia commonly try to avoid movie theaters and malls. Phobophobia, myxophobia, and panphobia are all types of simple phobias and are fear of fear itself, fear of slime, and fear of everything, respectively.

59. (C) Systematic desensitization is a type of behavior therapy in which a person is exposed to a hierarchy of increasingly anxiety-provoking situations. These can be imagined or real situations, and when coupled with relaxation techniques, the process is called reciprocal inhibition. Implosion is a type of therapy in which the patient is exposed to an imagined situation that is the cause of the anxiety. Another type of behavior therapy that is incorporated under the heading implosive therapy is flooding, which is an exposure to the actual situation that produces anxiety. Displacement and projection are types of defense mechanisms. Displacement is the transferring of a feeling toward an object that is less threatening, as in the family pet or one's spouse or children. Projection is the false attribution of one's own unacceptable feelings to another.

60. (A) Libido refers to sexual energy. Affect is the outward expression of one's internal state. Gender identity is the inner perception of how one views one's gender as being either male or female. Gender role is the external expression of one's gender identity. Fugue is characterized by memory loss and wandering.

61. (C) Satyriasis is a man's insatiable need for sexual gratification. Hypervigilance is a term often used in anxiety disorders and is simply an increased awareness of internal or external stimuli. Hypermnesia is the ability to recall detailed material that is not usually available to recall. Sexual sadism and sexual masochism are deriving sexual pleasure from causing or receiving mental or physical abuse, respectively.

62. (A) Insomnia, or the inability to sleep, can be categorized as initial (the inability to fall asleep, often associated with anxiety), or terminal (early wakening, commonly seen in depression). Narcolepsy is a sleep disorder characterized by the tetrad of hypersomnia, cataplexy (the transient loss of motor tone associated with strong emotions), sleep paralysis, and hypnagogic hallucinations. Catalepsy is a state of immobility sometimes seen in catatonic states.

63. (B) Priapism is a painful prolonged erection that can be seen as an uncommon side effect of trazodone in men. Parapraxis is a slip of the tongue, also known as a freudian slip. Nymphomania is insatiable sexual desire in a woman, and satyriasis is its male counterpart. Libido is the term for sexual energy.

64. (B) Circumlocution is the substitution of a word or description for a word that cannot be recalled or spoken. Confabulation is the fluent fabrication of fictitious responses in compensation of memory disturbance. Clang association is the use of words based on sound and not with reference to the meaning. A neologism is a novel word that is used by a patient, and apraxia is the inability to perform previously learned motor skills.

65. (C) Anomia is an inability to name objects outside of an aphasia. Alexia is the inability to read. Apraxia is the inability to perform previously learned motor skills. Paralinguistic components of speech refer to nonverbal communications such as facial expression and body movements. Prosopagnosia refers to the inability to recognize faces despite perception of all the components.

66. (A) Neurovegetative signs are physiological aspects of depression such as changes in sleep, bowel habits, and weight. Conversion symptoms are physical manifestations of underlying unconscious motivation or drives. Catatonia is a state of stupor, negativism, and rigidity. A neologism is a novel word that is used by a patient, and apraxia is the inability to perform previously learned motor skills. Word salad is an incoherent mix of words and phrases.

67. (A) A parapraxis, or freudian slip, is a slip of the tongue that can reveal repressed or unconscious motives or drives. Copropraxia and echopraxia are both terms used in relation to movements and are specifically used in reference to obscene gestures and repeating another's movements, respectively. Bruxism is the grinding of the teeth and is often a symptom of anxiety. A clang association is the use of words based on sound and not with reference to the meaning.

68. (E) Dynamic and psychoanalytic psychiatry utilize psychoanalytic principles originated by Sigmund Freud in order to render subconscious material available to the conscious mind. Forensic psychiatry focuses on the legal aspects of psychiatry. Social psychiatry emphasizes the cultural and sociological aspects of the study of psychiatry. Biological psychiatry is a branch of psychiatry that specifically focuses on the genetic and the pharmacological aspects of psychiatry.

69. (D) Supportive psychotherapy attempts to fortify psychological defenses by providing empathetic reassurance as opposed to probing into a patient's psychological conflicts. Dynamic psychotherapy probes such conflicts to bring unconscious material into consciousness. Existential psychotherapy, as the

name implies, is based on existential philosophy and emphasizes personal feeling and experience over rational thinking. Biological psychiatry is a branch of psychiatry that specifically focuses on the genetic and the pharmacological aspects of psychiatry. Cognitive–behavioral therapy, used often in mood and anxiety disorders, is a mix of behavioral therapy and cognitive psychology.

70. **(C)** Anomia is the specific inability to name objects even though the object is recognizable and can be described by the patient. Aphasia is more global and is an abnormality in either the expression or the comprehension of language. Agnosia is the inability to recognize objects, but as in anomia, the object can be perceived by the patient's intact senses. Apraxia is an inability to perform learned motor skills despite normal strength and coordination. Alexia is the inability to read.

71. **(B)** Sexual sadism and sexual masochism are, respectively, the derivation of sexual pleasure from causing or receiving mental or physical abuse. Exhibitionism is exposure of the genitalia in public to an unwilling participant and usually occurs in males. Transvestic fetishism is arousal by cross-dressing. Frotteurism, the rubbing of genitals against another to achieve arousal and orgasm, is usually seen in men and is usually performed in crowded places.

72. **(C)** Voyeurism is deriving sexual pleasure from watching another person or persons involved in the act of undressing or other sexually oriented activity. Transvestic fetishism involves being dressed in clothing of the opposite sex for sexual excitement. It is often present in heterosexual men and differs from transsexualism in that the person is usually comfortable and content with his gender identity. It is, however, possible to see these disorders concomitantly. Exhibitionism is another paraphilia and involves exposing one's genitalia to an unsuspecting audience. Hermaphroditism is not a paraphilia but is a rare disorder in which one possesses the sexual characteristics of both sexes.

73–76. **(73-F, 74-H, 75-A, 76-D)** Intoxication is represented by behavioral, cognitive, or perceptual changes taken in relationship to drug ingestion. Withdrawal is a set of signs and symptoms, physical and psychic, that are associated with drug cessation. Tolerance is the need for higher doses of a drug needed for intoxication. Abuse is drug use in spite of adverse consequences related to the substance. Dependence is a physical or psychological need to continue taking a drug. Inhalants are volatile substances that have rapid-onset intoxicating effects. Formication is the feeling of bugs crawling on the skin. Amotivational syndrome is a lack of drive or motivation usually associated with drug use, especially marijuana. Hallucinogens are a group of drugs administered by various routes that cause perceptual changes. Posthallucinogen perception disorder is also known as a flashback. It is characterized by a distressing return of perceptual changes without the ingestion of hallucinogens.

77–80. **(77-G, 78-D, 79-E, 80-F)** Lability refers to rapid fluctuations in affect, often between states of elation and sadness. Irritability refers to being easily brought to anger. Dyscalculia is difficulty with simple arithmetic. Verbigeration is repetitive and meaningless talking. Dysarthria is difficulty with articulation. Gustation is taste sensation. Glossolalia is the ability to speak a new language suddenly. Hypochondriasis is the misinterpretation of bodily symptoms, leading one to erroneously believe he or she has a physical illness.

81–85. **(81-C, 82-B, 83-E, 84-D, 85-F)** Thought process disorders can be identified by the nature of the response. A circumstantial thought finally reaches a point but after much unnecessary detail and digressions. It can be seen in disorders such as obsessive–compulsive disorder but can also be normal in some people. A tangential thought differs from a circumstantial thought in that it never comes to a point, but like circumstantial thought it remains logically connected and can be followed. Flight of ideas represents a change of direction every sentence or two, again with identifiable connections or associations tying them together. It is often a symptom of manic behavior and reflects underlying racing thoughts. Loosening of associations is characterized by the lack of logical connections between ideas, but sentence structure remains intact. Another component of thought disorders, clanging or clang associations, is word choice based on sound and not meaning or semantics.

In question 81, in the first sentence, the thoughts can be connected, but do not reach a point. In question 82, the thoughts are more goal-directed than in question 81, and this sentence is more consistent with tangentiality. In question 83, clanging is easily identified by word choice based on similar sounds rather than semantics. Associations between ideas are lost in question 84. Question 85 is a representation of thought blocking with derailment. The patient stops in one thought, pauses, and then resumes with an unrelated thought.

86–95. (86-I, 87-P, 88-B, 89-L, 90-N, 91-G, 92-J, 93-M, 94-H, 95-K) Antipsychotics, also known as neuroleptics, can cause a wide variety of side effects. These side effects can be broken down into some of the following categories for an easier approach.

The dopaminergic side effects include those that are due to the blockade of the natural dopamine inhibition of prolactin release from the anterior pituitary causing galactorrhea (lactation) and gynecomastia (breast development). The dopaminergic side effects also include those that arise from the dopamine blockade in the basal ganglia causing extrapyramidal and other side effects such as blepharospasm (spasm of the eyelids), opisthotonos (spasm of the neck and back causing an arched posture), and torticollis (spasm of the sternocleidomastoid). The blockade of D2 receptors in the basal ganglia

can also cause pseudoparkinsonism disorder resembling Parkinson's disease, characterized by muscle rigidity and a short festinating gait, and tardive dyskinesia, a disorder of abnormal involuntary movements caused by prolonged use of neuroleptics. Akathisia (subjective or observable restlessness) and rabbit syndrome (rapid movement of the lips) are also highly distressing side effects related to the dopaminergic system.

Another side effect that can be caused, especially by high-potency neuroleptics such as haloperidol, is neuroleptic malignant syndrome. This is characterized by hyperthermia, change in mental status, and increased muscle tone. It can lead to renal failure following dehydration and a rise in muscle breakdown products (creatine kinase levels are typically elevated), pulmonary complications, and death.

Clozapine and chlorpromazine can both cause agranulocytosis, a dangerous side effect that sometimes produces symptoms of sore throat and fever. The drug must be stopped immediately. Constipation is a complicating side effect of some antipsychotics with anticholinergic effects. This troublesome side effect can often be relieved with use of a laxative. Orthostatic hypotension, a drop in blood pressure while standing, is a side effect from alpha-1-adrenergic blockade. This is especially troublesome with chlorpromazine and clozapine and is best handled by raising doses slowly. Obstructive jaundice is rare and occurs mainly with chlorpromazine. Symptoms are fever, nausea, malaise, and pruritus. Pigmented retinopathy is observed with uses of high doses of thioridazine and is best detected with a good ophthalmologic exam.

Another side effect that can decrease compliance with antipsychotics is retrograde ejaculation. Orgasm may be achieved, but ejaculation is abnormal, with retrograde propulsion of the semen.

CHAPTER 2

Psychological Testing
Questions

Brian Greenlee, MD, and Elizabeth Walter, MD

DIRECTIONS (Questions 96 through 124): Each of the numbered items or incomplete statements in this section is followed by answers or by completions of the statement. Select the ONE lettered answer or completion that is BEST in each case.

96. You are asked to evaluate a 68-year-old man on the inpatient medicine service for increasing confusion. The patient was admitted 2 days earlier for pneumonia. After performing a mental status evaluation, you suspect delirium. The patient dropped out of school in the seventh grade. The best test to assess this patient's ability to maintain and focus attention is

    (A) serial sevens
    (B) counting by twos to 20
    (C) serial threes
    (D) the Random Letter Test
    (E) simple calculations

Questions 97 and 98

A 34-year-old woman suffering from severe depression and chronic renal failure is a candidate for electroconvulsive therapy (ECT).

97. Which test listed below can be used to monitor the patient's depressive symptoms with the greatest reliability and validity?

    (A) Thematic Apperception Test
    (B) Rorschach Test
    (C) Halstead–Reitan Neuropsychological Battery
    (D) Draw-a-Person Test
    (E) Beck Depression Inventory

98. The most useful test to assess for memory impairments in the setting of ECT is the

    (A) Brown–Patterson Task
    (B) Beck Depression Inventory
    (C) State-Trait Anxiety Inventory
    (D) Bulimia Test–Revised
    (E) Eating Disorder Inventory-2 (EDI-2)

Questions 99 through 102

You admit an 83-year-old widowed white woman for further evaluation because she is no longer able to care for herself at home. She has lost 30 pounds in the past year, has poor hygiene, and admits to increasing forgetfulness.

99. A commonly administered screening test to evaluate for dementia is the

    (A) Geriatric Rating Scale
    (B) Glasgow Coma Scale
    (C) Folstein Mini-Mental Status Examination (MMSE)
    (D) Mental Status Examination (MSE)
    (E) Blessed Rating Scale

100. Factors influencing the score on this test include

    (A) geographic location
    (B) education
    (C) gender
    (D) wealth
    (E) criminal history

101. Another psychiatric diagnosis that may mimic dementia is

(A) panic disorder

(B) depression

(C) posttraumatic stress disorder (PTSD)

(D) generalized anxiety disorder

(E) obsessive–compulsive disorder

102. An advantage of the Folstein MMSE is

(A) its high 24-hour retest reliability

(B) it is simple and quick to administer

(C) it is cost effective

(D) B and C

(E) all of the above

Questions 103 and 104

A 28-year-old single African-American man with a long history of schizophrenia and prominent thought disorganization asks you if there are psychological tests that would demonstrate which part of his brain "isn't working." While you explain that no test can indicate exactly which part of his brain is different from those without schizophrenia, you suggest a certain test to assess his ability to organize and correctly process information.

103. The neuropsychological test you recommend is the

(A) MMSE

(B) Wisconsin Card Sorting Test (WCST)

(C) Bender–Gestalt Test

(D) Luria–Nebraska Neuropsychological Battery

(E) Draw-a-Person Test

104. This test assesses

(A) executive functions of the brain

(B) attentional state

(C) the ability to draw

(D) orientation

(E) memory

Questions 105 and 106

While reading a medical journal, you find an article about a new screening test that predicts a patient's risk for suicide. The authors have shown that high scores on their screening test correlates with an increased risk for completed suicide. Nine months later, another group repeats the study and demonstrates that male patients consistently scored higher on the screening test than females. Furthermore, the authors of the second article state that when gender is taken into account, the previously reported correlation between the screening test and increase in suicide rate vanishes. The authors of the second study conclude that this limits the usefulness of the screening test to predict a patient's risk of suicide.

105. The authors of the initial article regarding the screening test suggested that their test was useful because of its

(A) internal reliability

(B) test–retest reliability

(C) content validity

(D) predictive validity

(E) discriminative validity

106. The authors of the second paper faulted the usefulness of this screening tool because of its lack of

(A) internal reliability

(B) test–retest reliability

(C) content validity

(D) predictive validity

(E) discriminative validity

Questions 107 through 109

A patient is administered a test that consists of viewing a set of 10 inkblots sequentially. The responses to the inkblots are noted by the examiner in relationship to the content of the perception, the area of the blot that forms the basis of the response, and the aspects of the area that are used to form the response.

107. The test being administered is the

(A) Thematic Apperception Test (TAT)

(B) Rorschach Test

(C) Sentence Completion Test

(D) Draw-a-Person Test

(E) Minnesota Multiphasic Personality Inventory (MMPI)

108. This type of projective test is best classified as

(A) self-expression

(B) constructions

(C) completions

(D) associations

(E) choice of ordering

109. To score and interpret this test using a data-based system one would rely on the

(A) Exner Comprehensive System

(B) Five-Factor Model

(C) Eysenck Personality Questionnaire

(D) California Personality Inventory

(E) MMPI-2

110. You are asked to perform a Folstein MMSE on a recently admitted patient. Which of the following items is a component of the Folstein MMSE?

(A) affect

(B) perception

(C) language

(D) thought process

(E) insight

111. Which of the following is a limitation of the Folstein MMSE?

(A) It is high-tech.

(B) It is time consuming.

(C) It has low specificity.

(D) It has low sensitivity.

(E) It is costly.

112. An 89-year-old married African-American woman is admitted to the medical service with a diagnosis of "failure to thrive." The team following her has asked you to assess her. In their notes, they observe that the patient is not oriented to time. To evaluate orientation, you perform the

(A) Spatial Orientation Memory Test

(B) Fargo Map Test

(C) Stroop Test

(D) WCST

(E) Temporal Orientation Test

Questions 113 through 116

A 25-year-old single African-American woman who carries the diagnosis of dependent personality disorder is referred for psychological testing. Your first consideration is whether to perform a set of projective or objective tests.

113. You decide to perform projective tests because

(A) they provide numerical scores

(B) they ask specific questions with itemized responses

(C) they are unstructured and allow for a variety of responses from the examinee

(D) statistical analysis is easily undertaken on the data

(E) you want to determine how the patient feels about you

114. Examples of projective testing include the

(A) Tilt-Table Test

(B) California Personality Inventory

(C) Sentence Completion Test

(D) MMPI-2

(E) The Luria–Nebraska Neuropsychological Battery

115. The Rorschach Test involves

(A) colored inkblots

(B) asking the patient to redraw inkblots

(C) evaluation of response only if the entire inkblot is used for the response

(D) multiple-choice questions

(E) a quantitative scale

116. After performing a battery of projective tests, you chose to continue testing with the MMPI-2. You chose this test because

(A) it is the most widely used test in the evaluation of personality structure

(B) it can be scored by nonprofessionals

(C) it is a specific type of projective test

(D) the patient is single

(E) it is designed to evaluate attitudes about test taking at the time the test is administered

Questions 117 through 121

A 22-year-old college student is referred for neuropsychological testing to evaluate worsening academic performance since a bicycle accident 1 month earlier during which he struck his head and lost consciousness for a few minutes. Other than difficulty concentrating and problems with memory, he denies any other complaints. He reports that 2 years ago he was involved in a research study and took a series of "intelligence tests." The patient's full-scale performance and verbal intelligence quotient (IQ) are listed in his medical records.

117. Which of the following tests is used to determine an adult patient's IQ?

(A) MMPI-2

(B) Draw-a-Person Test

(C) Wechsler Adult Intelligence Scale—Revised (WAIS-R)

(D) Wechsler Intelligence Scale for Children (WISC)

(E) Wechsler Memory Test (WMT)

118. The IQ is calculated by which of the following formulas?

(A) performance IQ/verbal IQ × 100

(B) mental age/full-scale IQ × 100

(C) chronological age/performance IQ × 100

(D) mental age/chronological age × 100

(E) actual IQ/theoretic IQ × 100

119. An IQ of 120 is considered

(A) normal

(B) bright normal

(C) superior

(D) very superior

(E) borderline

120. Full-scale IQ measures current functional ability and is most likely to predict

(A) future earning potential

(B) academic achievement

(C) level of social functioning

(D) future employment

(E) your children's IQ

121. Differences between full-scale IQ, performance IQ, and verbal IQ are

(A) helpful in evaluating neuropsychological dysfunction

(B) not helpful in evaluating neuropsychological dysfunction

(C) integral in assessing the location of the lesion

(D) reflective of culture differences

(E) reflective of social skills

Questions 122 and 123

A 72-year-old man is suspected to have suffered a stroke in his right parietal region.

122. The test most likely to show abnormalities is the

(A) WMT

(B) WCST

(C) MMPI-2

(D) Rey–Osterrieth Test

(E) Rorschach Test

123. This test assesses

(A) visual nonverbal memory

(B) verbal memory

(C) tactile memory

(D) long-term procedural memory

(E) long-term implicit memory

124. A 70-year-old man with multiple medical problems is suspected to have had a stroke, affecting his ability to speak. The test most likely to adequately describe the nature of the difficulty is the

(A) Stroop Test
(B) Boston Diagnostic Aphasia Exam
(C) Folstein MMSE
(D) Bender–Gestalt Test
(E) Sentence Completion Test

DIRECTIONS (Questions 125 through 132): Each group of items in this section consists of lettered headings followed by a set of numbered words or phrases. For each numbered word or phrase, select the ONE lettered heading that is most closely associated with it. Each lettered heading may be selected once, more than once, or not at all.

Question 125 through 132

Match the clinical presentation with the appropriate neuropsychological test.

(A) MMPI-2
(B) WISC
(C) Rey–Osterrieth Test
(D) Beck Depression Inventory
(E) Blessed Rating Scale
(F) WAIS-R
(G) Boston Diagnostic Aphasia Examination
(H) Rorschach Test
(I) Folstein MMSE
(J) Bender–Gestalt Test
(K) WCST
(L) Wada Test

125. A 40-year-old woman who scores a 26/30 on the Folstein MMSE gave many answers of, "I don't know, I'm too tired to answer." You want to assess for the possibility of depression.

126. A 65-year-old man has difficulty organizing, sequencing, and planning activities but no impairment in memory.

127. The family of an 80-year-old man with mild dementia has asked you to evaluate his ability to continue to live in his current environment. You would like to ask his family and friends their assessment of how he has been doing.

128. A 16-year-old boy with a family history of mental retardation presents with long-standing poor school performance and aggressive behavior toward peers.

129. A 37-year-old man has a history of avoiding social situations, no close friends, and a preference for being alone. He has been described by others as unemotional and detached. You would like to evaluate this patient with a projective test.

130. You would like to quickly assess for dementia in a 75-year-old woman admitted to the emergency department for failure to thrive.

131. A 45-year-old woman has a long history of unstable relationships, self-injurious behavior, and affective instability. She does not meet criteria for an Axis I disorder.

132. You are asked to preoperatively evaluate hemispheric dominance in an 18-year-old left-handed woman with a history of seizure disorder who is about to undergo surgery to remove a seizure focus in the left hemisphere.

Answers and Explanations

96. (D) In this instance, the Random Letter Test, which relies on concentration, cooperation, and the ability to hear, is the test of choice. The other tests rely not only on attention but also on calculation abilities and educational level. The Random Letter Test consists of telling a patient a letter and then in a monotone listing a random string of letters. The patient responds by raising a finger to indicate when he or she hears the key letter.

97. (E) The Beck Depression Inventory is a widely used test that allows clinicians to follow the severity of previously diagnosed depression. The Thematic Apperception Test, the Rorschach Test, and the Draw-a-Person Test are all types of projective testing. Projective tests, although useful clinical tools, often suffer on reliability and validity. Projective tests require a person who is skilled at this type of evaluation and often do not have rigorous empirical data and group comparison. The evaluation of depression in relation to the Halstead–Reitan Test is limited by the fact that many depressed patients fail to show deficits on such classic neuropsychological batteries. In addition, these tests, even when demonstrating deficits in cognitive domains such as attention and learning, still have very limited usefulness in evaluating the severity of the depression.

98. (A) The Brown–Patterson Task is a test specifically designed to evaluate short-term memory, a capacity that can be affected during ECT. The Bulimia Test–Revised and the EDI-2 are both useful for the evaluation of bulimia and eating disorders, respectively.

The State-Trait Anxiety Inventory and the Beck Depression Inventory are used to evaluate anxiety disorders and depression, respectively.

99. (C) The Folstein MMSE is a frequently used screening assessment for dementia. It is a 30-point scale with deductions for incorrect answers. The Glasgow Coma Scale is an easy-to-perform instrument to evaluate the level of consciousness. There are three general categories that the examiner tests: eye opening, verbal response, and best motor response. Each category receives a number for patient response. Overall scores range from 3 to 15, with lower scores reflecting more severely impaired consciousness. The Geriatric Rating Scale is a rating scale for nonprofessional staff to evaluate patients' abilities to perform their activities of daily living and interact with others. It may be most helpful in evaluation of the moderately to severely demented individual. The Blessed Rating Scale is a tool that typically asks friends or relatives of the patient to assess the ability of the patient to function in his or her current environment. An MSE is the formal psychiatric exam that includes appearance of the patient, assessment of mood and affect, the presence of psychosis, and evaluation of insight and judgment. It is not a substitute for the Folstein MMSE.

100. (B) Both age and level of education may be associated with lower scores on this instrument without the presence of dementia. Gender, wealth, geographic location, and the presence of a criminal history do not affect the score.

101. **(B)** When evaluating the total score for dementia, it is critical to consider that depression (also known as pseudodementia) may produce similar scores. The other choices would not decrease the Folstein MMSE score.

102. **(E)** The advantages of using this screening tool are that it is simple, low cost, quick to administer, and has high 24-hour retest reliability.

103. **(B)** In the WCST, examinees are asked to sort cards depicting various pictures and symbols according to a variety of different criteria that change over time without the subject knowing. The WCST assesses a person's ability to switch sets, reason abstractly, and solve problems. These capacities are also known as "executive functions" and are thought to be localized in the frontal lobes. Current research regarding the psychopathology of schizophrenia suggests that there are abnormalities in the frontal lobes, specifically in the dorsolateral prefrontal cortex, that are reflected in poor performance on the WCST. People with schizophrenia perform more poorly on the WCST than people without schizophrenia; however, individuals with damage to their frontal lobes from a variety of causes also show executive function deficits. The Draw-a-Person Test requires the examinee to draw a person. It was initially devised to test intelligence in children, but is now used primarily as a screening test for brain damage. The Luria–Nebraska Neuropsychological Battery is a comprehensive set of neuropsychological tests used to assess specific cortical areas and aids in assessment of hemispheric dominance. The MMSE is a commonly used scale to assess the possibility of dementia. The Bender–Gestalt Test involves copying figures, which helps determine if organic brain disease is present.

104. **(A)** See answer 103.

105. **(D)** Because the screening test seemed to indicate which patients are at a higher risk for completed suicide, it would have utility based on its predictive validity. Content validity is a test's ability to cover the conceptual domain that the test intends to measure. Conceptual domain is usually established by a large group of experts through a wide review of the literature. It is unclear in this case as to whether suicide or depression, critical aspects of this test's conceptual domain, was adequately addressed. Discriminative validity is the measure of a test's ability to differentiate between issues that are theoretically unrelated. Reliability is a test's ability to provide reproducible results. Test–retest reliability measures a test's reproducibility over a short period of time in a person whose state is assumed not to have fluctuated. Internal reliability evaluates whether the questions within the test are measuring the same thing. Reliability may be a problem with this test, but it is not a concern in determining the test's usefulness.

106. **(E)** In this case, the authors of the second study show that the test fails to discriminate suicide risk when gender is removed. Knowing that males are at an increased risk for successful suicide attempts may decrease the test's usefulness. See answer 105 for definitions of other choices.

107. **(B)** The Rorschach Test was developed in 1921 by Hermann Rorschach. It consists of showing a subject a set of 10 inkblot stimuli in a sequential manner while noting (1) the responses in relationship to the content of the perception, (2) the area of the blot that forms the basis of the response, and (3) the aspects of the area that are used to form the response.

The TAT, the Sentence Completion Test, and the Draw-a-Person Test are similar to the Rorschach in that they are also projective tests. The TAT was developed in the 1930s by Henry Murray and consists of 20 cards featuring ambiguous situations. The subject is asked to develop a narrative based on the scene. In the Sentence Completion Test, the answer is evaluated for its relationship with the stimulus and for content, among other criteria. The Draw-a-Person Test is evaluated in relationship to detail, size of various parts in relationship to one another, and the size of the overall picture. The MMPI-2 consists of true/false questions designed to assess personality characteristics. The MMPI-2 is the most widely used and highly standardized test of personality structure.

108. **(D)** In 1961, Lindzey proposed a method of classifying projective tests based on the type of activity. The Rorschach is classified in the category of associations. Another test in this category is the Word Association Test. The construction category requires the subject to construct content based on a stimulus such as a story in the TAT. The self-expression category consists of tests such as the Draw-a-Person Test in which the subject produces a response without a stimulus. Tests such as the Sentence Completion Test fall into a category of completions, in which a person completes an uncompleted stimulus. The last category is the choice of ordering in which patients place objects in a rank order with respect to preference.

109. **(A)** One data-based system used to score and interpret the Rorschach is the Exner Comprehensive System. It is limited in its validity and requires highly trained examiners. All of the other choices are types of personality assessment not associated with the Rorschach. The Eysenck Personality Questionnaire constructs questions designed to assess aspects of personality predicted to exist by theoretical constructs. The MMPI-2 is the most widely used and highly standardized test of personality. The California Personality Inventory is similar to the MMPI but is used in counseling situations, rather than with pathologic populations.

110. **(C)** Although affect, perception, thought process, and insight are all components of a full mental status examination, they are not formally represented on the Folstein MMSE. The Folstein MMSE consists of the following subsections: orientation, registration, attention and recall, and language.

111. **(D)** The MMSE is a brief, rapid, and inexpensive evaluation of cognitive functioning. The test is quite specific, in that a low score is highly correlated with cognitive impairment; however, the test has a low sensitivity, particularly in patients with a higher level of education. A good score does not always assure a lack of cognitive impairment. This is one reason why correlation with the rest of the exam and with collateral information is essential.

112. **(E)** The Temporal Orientation Test asks the patient to identify the appropriate day, month, day of the week, and current time. Deviation from the correct response is differentially scored in each category. Total score and the data incorrectly identified separate the patients into two groups: patients with brain damage and patients without brain damage. The Temporal Orientation Test is also sensitive to cognitive abnormalities in dementing illnesses. The Spatial Orientation Memory Test evaluates the ability to immediately recall the orientation of figures and is used to evaluate immediate memory. The Stroop Test has a number of different formats, but the general concept is that it takes longer to correctly identify a color than to read words and longer yet to correctly identify a word (e.g., name of a color) when that word is in a color different from that word. This test seems to be primarily an assessment of ability to concentrate. The Fargo Map Test assesses recent and remote spatial memory and visuospatial orientation by using maps of the United States and different regions within it. Patients are asked to identify certain areas. Education level and age influence the score on this test. The WCST is used to evaluate executive functioning of the brain.

113. **(C)** Objective tests usually involve questions with lists of possible responses. These tests provide numerical scores on which statistical analyses are easily performed. Examples include the United States Medical Licensing Exams (USMLE). Conversely, projective tests

usually involve stimuli, to which there are a variety of responses, without a single correct answer. Many of these tests, including the Rorschach Test, the TAT, the Sentence Completion Test, and the Draw-a-Person Test, require specific training in giving the test and interpreting the results. Projective tests do not necessarily tell the interviewer how the patient feels about him or her.

114. **(C)** The Tilt-Table Test is used to determine cardiovascular status. The MMPI-2 is the most widely used and highly standardized test of personality structure. The California Personality Inventory is similar to the MMPI but is used in counseling situations, rather than with pathologic populations. In the Sentence Completion Test, the only projective test among the choices, the answer is evaluated for its relationship with the stimulus and for content, among other criteria. The Luria–Nebraska Neuropsychological Battery is a comprehensive set of tests used to evaluate specific cortical areas in dysfunction and aids in assessment of hemispheric dominance.

115. **(A)** The Rorschach Test involves a series of colored and black and white inkblots to which the patients draw associations. Responses are recorded verbatim. Later in the test, the examiner further evaluates responses based on which parts (or all) of the inkblot were used in the response. Accurate interpretation of response requires much training. This test has been used to assist in psychodynamic formulations.

116. **(A)** The MMPI and now the MMPI-2 are objective tests that have been used for over 50 years in the assessment of personality structure. They consist of more than 500 statements, which are condensed into 10 clinical scales. Additionally, questions are asked at the time of the exam to evaluate attitudes when taking the test. These questions help provide information about the validity of the exam. Interpretation of the results requires an experienced evaluator. Together with the clinical history, this test provides valuable information about personality structure. Its accuracy does not depend on the patient's marital status, and the results do not reflect how the examinee feels about test taking.

117. **(C)** The Wechsler Adult Intelligence Scale was initially published in 1955 and since that time has undergone a series of revisions until the current scale, the WAIS-R. The test is composed of 11 different subtests—six verbal and five performance—that allow for the calculation of the full-scale IQ, performance IQ, and verbal IQ. The WAIS-R has high reliability, which means that in normal subjects, retesting does not lead to significantly different evaluations. This means that it can be used to follow people over time. A test that has high validity means that it accurately measures the variable that it purports to measure. The MMPI-2 is a test used for assessment of personality structure, while the Draw-a-Person Test is used to evaluate for organic brain disease. The WMT was designed to evaluate a variety of aspects of memory function in adults. None of these tests are useful in the determination of IQ.

118. **(D)** The IQ is calculated by dividing the mental age by the chronological age and multiplying this by 100.

119. **(C)** IQs are divided into groups: 90 to 109 is considered average or normal, 110 to 119 is bright normal, 120 to 129 is superior, and 130 and above is very superior. Borderline intellectual functioning is a term no longer in use, but it referred to an IQ between 71 and 84.

120. **(B)** The full-scale IQ is a useful predictor of academic achievement. It cannot predict any of the other choices listed.

121. **(B)** The battery of WAIS-R tests are good for measuring IQ and for identifying neuropsychological dysfunction. Full-scale IQ, performance IQ, and verbal IQ have only limited value in predicting neuropsychological dysfunction and neurologic localization. While gross IQ scores sometimes reflect cultural differences, differences between subscores do

not. Differences between IQ subscales do not directly predict an individual's social skills.

122. **(D)** The Rey–Osterrieth Test is a complex figure that the patient is asked to copy while looking at the figure. The figure is then taken away and the patient is asked to draw the picture from immediate memory. The patient is again asked to draw the figure 5 minutes and 30 minutes after the figure has been removed. The tasks assess visual nonverbal memory. People with right parietal lesions usually show abnormalities in copying the figure correctly by neglecting the items in the left visual field. Conversely, a patient with a right temporal lobectomy may have no difficulty in copying the figure, but show marked abnormalities in drawing the item from memory. The WMT, WCST, MMPI-2, and the Rorschach Test would not be as useful in assessing a right parietal lesion as the Rey–Osterrieth figure.

123. **(A)** See answer 122.

124. **(B)** The Boston Diagnostic Aphasia Exam is a comprehensive set of tests given by a skilled interviewer to evaluate aphasic disorders and to help define further interventions to improve speech. The Stroop Test aids in the evaluation of concentration. The Folstein MMSE is used for rapid assessment of dementia and delirium. The Bender–Gestalt Test is a constructional test for evaluation of brain damage and has some ability to differentiate the location of the lesion. The Sentence Completion Test is a projective test used to describe personality structure.

125. **(D)** The Beck Depression Inventory is a 21-item test with three responses per item that is an easily used screening tool to evaluate for depression. As it would be unusual for an individual so young to have a dementia and because many of the answers reflect a lack of interest, the Beck Depression Inventory in conjunction with the Folstein MMSE may help distinguish depression from dementia.

126. **(K)** The WCST assesses executive functions of the brain such as organizational abilities, mental flexibility, and the ability to abstract and reason. These capacities are believed to be located in the frontal lobes. Damage to the frontal lobes can lead to abnormalities on this test.

127. **(E)** The Blessed Rating Scale is a tool that asks friends or family of the patient to assess the ability of the patient to function in his or her usual environment.

128. **(F)** An assessment of IQ is indicated to rule out mental retardation and help better understand the individual's level of intellectual level of functioning. IQ assessment will also aid the school in developing an individualized study program for this student. Because the patient is older than 15, the WAIS-R would be used.

129. **(H)** The Rorschach Test is a projective test that may be used to assess personality structure. The patient has characteristics of schizoid personality disorder, which may be better elucidated with further skilled assessment in the context of the clinical history.

130. **(I)** The Folstein MMSE is a quick, easily administered test that allows for immediate assessment of dementia. Scores of less than 24 are suggestive of a dementia.

131. **(A)** The MMPI-2 is an objective test consisting of several hundred true–false questions used to assess an individual's personality. It is the most widely used and highly standardized test of personality.

132. **(L)** The Wada Test is used to evaluate hemispheric language dominance prior to surgical amelioration of seizure focus. While most right-handed individuals show left hemispheric dominance for language, left-handed individuals may be either right or left dominant. The test consists of injecting sodium amytal into the carotid artery and observing

the transient effects on speech. Injection into the left carotid artery will anesthetize the left side of the brain, and people with left hemispheric language dominance will show interrupted speech.

The Rey–Osterreith figure is sensitive to deficits in copying and lack of attention to detail in people with right-sided parietal lobe lesions. The appropriate test to evaluate IQ would be the WISC. The Boston Diagnostic Aphasia Examination is a series of tests given by an experienced clinician to evaluate and make treatment recommendations for individuals with aphasia. The Bender–Gestalt Test involves copying figures, which helps determine if organic brain disease is present.

CHAPTER 3

Child and Adolescent Psychiatry
Questions

Julie E. Peters, MD

DIRECTIONS (Questions 133 through 226): Each of the numbered items or incomplete statements in this section is followed by answers or by completions of the statement. Select the ONE lettered answer or completion that is BEST in each case.

Questions 133 through 135

A 17-year-old boy with a history of major depressive disorder (MDD) comes to your office for a routine visit. When you walk into the examining room, you notice that the boy is sitting slumped forward with his head bent down. He does not make eye contact and says nothing. You suspect that he is having a recurrence of depressive symptoms and are concerned about his risk for suicide.

133. Which of the following statements or questions is most likely to be helpful?

    (A) "Are you feeling depressed?"

    (B) "You're looking down. Tell me what's going on."

    (C) "I can see you don't want to talk. Should I talk with your mother instead?"

    (D) "Hey buddy, what's going on?"

    (E) "How's school?"

134. Which of the following statements regarding depression and suicide in adolescents is true?

    (A) Rates of suicidal behavior are similar in adolescent girls and boys.

    (B) More girls than boys commit suicide.

    (C) Suicide is a considerable risk in depressed adolescents and should be specifically addressed during an interview.

    (D) A prior suicide attempt does not increase an adolescent's risk of a subsequent one.

    (E) The adolescent suicide rate has remained stable during the past few decades.

135. Which of the following is the most common method by which adolescents commit suicide?

    (A) drug overdose

    (B) stabbing or cutting

    (C) jumping from buildings

    (D) hanging

    (E) firearms

Questions 136 through 139

A mother brings her 7-year-old son to you because she is worried about him. She tells you that he sits up in bed in the middle of the night and screams. She says he is inconsolable but eventually falls back to sleep. She starts crying as she tells you she can't sleep after these episodes and is exhausted at work during the day.

136. Which of the following initial responses is most appropriate?

    (A) "I can see this is very upsetting for you."

    (B) "I know you're upset, but this problem will get better."

    (C) "I can see you're upset, but you're really overreacting."

    (D) "Tell me why you can't fall back to sleep after your son does."

    (E) "Are you worried that this is your fault?"

137. Which of the following questions is likely to confirm the diagnosis?

(A) "Does your son wet his bed?"

(B) "Does your son go to sleep late?"

(C) "Does your son watch scary movies?"

(D) "Does your son make jerking movements in his sleep?"

(E) "Does your son wake up and remember a nightmare?"

138. During what stage of sleep do these episodes most likely occur?

(A) stage 1

(B) stage 2

(C) stages 3–4

(D) rapid eye movement (REM) stage

(E) any stage

139. Which of the following *Diagnostic and Statistical Manual of Mental Disorders,* 4th Edition, Text Revision (DSM-IV-TR) sleep disorders is most likely to be treated pharmacologically?

(A) nightmare disorder

(B) sleep terror disorder

(C) sleepwalking disorder

(D) circadian rhythm sleep disorder

(E) narcolepsy

Questions 140 through 142

A 17-year-old girl with a history of asthma presents for a physical examination prior to entering college. You note that she appears sad. Upon further questioning, you learn that she has felt depressed for the past 6 months since breaking up with her boyfriend of 2 years. She says she feels tired all the time and comes home from school every day, lies on the couch, and sleeps or watches television. She reports that she quit the senior celebration committee, no longer "hangs out" with her friends, cannot imagine things will improve, and is considering not going to college. In addition, she has been binge eating and abusing laxatives. Her physical and laboratory examinations are normal. You diagnose her with major depressive disorder (MDD), single episode, and bulimia nervosa, purging type.

140. Which of the following is the most appropriate pharmacologic agent to use to treat this girl's MDD?

(A) carbamazepine (Tegretol)

(B) imipramine (Tofranil)

(C) lithium

(D) olanzapine (Zyprexa)

(E) sertraline (Zoloft)

141. Which of the following types of psychotherapy is most effective for the treatment of bulimia nervosa in adolescents?

(A) cognitive–behavioral therapy

(B) family therapy

(C) psychoanalytic psychotherapy

(D) psychodynamic psychotherapy

(E) group therapy

142. When interviewing this girl, you ask about drug use and specifically name several substances. Which of the following is this girl most likely to be using?

(A) cannabis

(B) cocaine

(C) lysergic acid diethylamide (LSD)

(D) phencyclidine (PCP)

(E) heroin

Questions 143 and 144

A 6-year-old boy is brought to the clinic by his parents at the request of the boy's teachers. The teachers report that he is quiet in class. When he does talk, he frequently makes errors with verb tense. His parents recall that his speech was delayed. On examination, the boy is friendly and cooperative. His speech is clear, but he uses simple sentences with a limited vocabulary. Otherwise, he has a normal physical, and laboratory examinations are normal.

143. Which of the following DSM-IV-TR diagnoses is most appropriate?

(A) disorder of written expression

(B) expressive language disorder

(C) phonological disorder

(D) stuttering

(E) developmental coordination disorder

144. Which of the following would be most helpful in confirming the diagnosis?

(A) intelligence quotient (IQ) test

(B) Children's Assessment Scale (CAS)

(C) Diagnostic Interview for Children and Adolescents (DICA)

(D) Diagnostic Interview Schedule for Children (DISC)

(E) Schedule for Affective Disorders and Schizophrenia for School-Age Children (K-SADS)

Questions 145 and 146

A 6-month-old girl is brought in by her grandmother for a routine visit. The physical examination is normal except that the baby has not gained weight as expected. Prior to this visit, the baby had been gaining weight appropriately. The grandmother reports that the baby likes to eat and is generally happy and playful. On further questioning, the grandmother describes chaotic mealtimes at home and says that the baby drools more than usual.

145. Which of the following DSM-IV-TR eating disorders is the most likely diagnosis?

(A) anorexia nervosa

(B) bulimia nervosa

(C) pica

(D) rumination disorder

(E) feeding disorder of infancy or early childhood

146. Which of the following tests would be most helpful in making the diagnosis?

(A) serum lead level

(B) calculation of the percentage of expected weight that the child's weight is

(C) 24-hour video monitoring

(D) complete blood count (CBC)

(E) esophageal pH measurement

Questions 147 through 149

An 8-year-old boy is referred to you by a school nurse because he has been complaining of stomachaches every morning in school. Upon interviewing the boy's mother, you learn that he does not like to go to school, insists on coming home immediately after school each day, and sleeps in his parents' bed at night. The mother denies other complaints.

147. Which of the following is the most likely diagnosis?

(A) social phobia

(B) posttraumatic stress disorder (PTSD)

(C) separation anxiety disorder

(D) reactive attachment disorder of early childhood

(E) specific phobia

148. Which of the following statements is true regarding this boy's disorder?

(A) It is seen almost exclusively in boys.

(B) It is primarily seen in unusually intelligent and sensitive children.

(C) Physical complaints, such as stomachaches, are uncommon.

(D) Diagnosis requires the presence of symptoms for at least 6 months.

(E) Diagnosis requires onset of symptoms prior to age 18.

149. This boy's stomachaches are an example of which of the following?

(A) coprolalia

(B) anhedonia

(C) reaction formation

(D) coprophagia

(E) somatization

Questions 150 and 151

A 5-year-old boy is brought to the pediatric emergency department because he is frantically trying to run away from lions that he says are chasing him. He says that when he sees the lions he has to jump out of their way or else they will attack him.

150. Which of the following disorders is the most likely diagnosis?

   (A) schizophrenia
   (B) panic disorder
   (C) autistic disorder
   (D) moderate mental retardation
   (E) substance-induced psychotic disorder

151. Which of the following is the most common psychiatric emergency in the child and adolescent population?

   (A) psychotic behavior
   (B) assaultive behavior
   (C) suicidal behavior
   (D) homicidal behavior
   (E) sexually inappropriate behavior

Questions 152 through 154

A 15-year-old girl with a history of separation anxiety disorder presents complaining of distress over her habit of biting her fingernails. Since starting high school 6 months earlier, the girl says that her nail biting has been "out of control" and that she is extremely embarrassed about how her fingers look. All her fingers bleed every day, and they throb constantly. The girl reports that high school is stressful and that her grades are suffering because her nail biting interferes with her ability to do her homework. She denies obsessional thoughts or compulsions. Physical and laboratory examinations are normal, with the exception of the girl's hands. Her fingers show signs of extreme nail biting and there are abrasions on the back of her right hand.

152. Which of the following is the most appropriate Axis I diagnosis?

   (A) obsessive–compulsive disorder (OCD)
   (B) stereotypic movement disorder

   (C) attention deficit–hyperactivity disorder (ADHD)
   (D) chronic motor tic disorder
   (E) MDD

153. Which of the following is true of the girl's academic difficulties related to her nail biting?

   (A) They are part of the diagnostic criteria for her Axis I diagnosis and therefore do not need to be coded elsewhere.
   (B) They should be coded on Axis II.
   (C) They should be coded on Axis III.
   (D) They should be coded on Axis IV.
   (E) They should be coded on Axis V.

154. Which of the following responses is most appropriate to use in order to determine the etiology of the abrasions on the dorsum of the girl's right hand?

   (A) "Tell me about the scratches on your hand."
   (B) "Do you scratch yourself in addition to biting your nails?"
   (C) "How did the scratches happen?"
   (D) "I see you have scratches on your hand. Do you have a cat?"
   (E) "Sometimes I see girls who make themselves throw up. Have you ever done that?"

Questions 155 and 156

An 8-year-old boy with a history of MDD treated with fluoxetine (Prozac) is brought to the pediatric emergency department after running into the street in front of a car on the way home from school. The boy says that he wants to be dead and refuses to say more. The boy was not hit by the car, and physical and laboratory examinations were normal.

155. Which of the following symptoms of MDD is seen more commonly in children than in adolescents?

   (A) hypersomnia
   (B) hopelessness
   (C) psychomotor agitation

(D) weight change

(E) drug abuse

156. Which of the following is the most common method by which children attempt suicide?

(A) substance ingestion

(B) stabbing or cutting

(C) jumping from buildings

(D) hanging

(E) firearms

Questions 157 and 158

An 11-year-old boy with enuresis presents to the clinic for routine follow-up. His bedwetting has not responded to behavioral interventions, so you initiate treatment with intranasal desmopressin (DDAVP). You complete a full physical and laboratory examination.

157. During this visit, you would be most likely to identify which of the following signs and symptoms as an adverse effect of DDAVP?

(A) sedation

(B) hypotension

(C) liver toxicity

(D) tremor

(E) headache

158. Which of the following laboratory abnormalities are you most likely to identify in association with DDAVP?

(A) hyponatremia

(B) hypocalcemia

(C) hypokalemia

(D) hypomagnesemia

(E) hypophosphatemia

Questions 159 and 160

A 9-year-old boy with a history of panic disorder treated with cognitive–behavioral therapy is brought to your office by his mother because he has been irritable and depressed. On physical examination, the boy appears depressed but otherwise has a normal examination. Laboratory examination is normal. After a thorough history and mental status examination, you diagnose the boy

with MDD and decide to initiate treatment with fluoxetine (Prozac).

159. What is the approximate comorbidity of childhood anxiety disorders and MDD?

(A) 10%

(B) 25%

(C) 33%

(D) 50%

(E) 75%

160. You inform the boy and his mother of possible adverse effects of fluoxetine. Which of the following is the most common adverse effect of fluoxetine?

(A) hypotension

(B) nausea

(C) liver toxicity

(D) weight gain

(E) sedation

Questions 161 through 163

A 3-year-old girl with moderate mental retardation is brought to the clinic by her mother because she has been complaining that her arm hurts. On physical examination, the girl has several bruises on her thorax and a tender right forearm. On laboratory examination, you discover a normocytic, normochromic anemia and basophilic stippling. On x-ray, you find signs of multiple fractures of different ages and increased density at the metaphyseal plate of the growing long bones.

161. Which of the following diagnoses is most likely?

(A) pica

(B) anorexia nervosa

(C) encopresis

(D) schizophrenia

(E) bulimia nervosa

162. Which of the following is the most appropriate treatment?

- (A) edetate calcium disodium (CaEDTA)
- (B) flumazenil (Romazicon)
- (C) naloxone (Narcan)
- (D) deferoxamine (Desferal)
- (E) acetylcysteine (Mucomyst)

163. Which of the following is the most likely cause of this girl's bruises?

- (A) thrombocytopenia
- (B) developmental coordination disorder
- (C) malnutrition
- (D) physical abuse
- (E) hepatic failure

Questions 164 and 165

A 24-month-old girl is brought to the clinic by her mother for a routine visit. The mother tells you that the girl has not spoken her first clear word yet, at times seems not to understand what people say to her, and does not play with her 3-year-old brother. The mother also tells you that her daughter seems clumsy and has started to make odd repetitive movements with her hands. According to the girl's chart, she had a normal head circumference at birth, at 6 months, and at 12 months, and had seemed to be developing normally. On physical examination, you note that the rate of head growth has slowed.

164. Which of the following pervasive developmental disorders is the most appropriate diagnosis?

- (A) autistic disorder
- (B) Rett's disorder
- (C) childhood disintegrative disorder
- (D) Asperger's disorder
- (E) pervasive developmental disorder not otherwise specified

165. Which of the following statements best describes this girl's disorder?

- (A) It is seen exclusively in girls.
- (B) There is usually an Axis II diagnosis.

- (C) There are no clear characteristic chromosomal abnormalities associated with the disorder.
- (D) There are familial clusters of the disorder.
- (E) It is the most common of the pervasive developmental disorders.

Questions 166 through 168

A 12-year-old boy is referred by the court for evaluation. He skips school, stays out late at night, and verbally abuses his parents. He has run away from home on three separate occasions, prompting his parents to call the police.

166. Which of the following is the most appropriate diagnosis?

- (A) mental retardation
- (B) conduct disorder
- (C) oppositional defiant disorder
- (D) ADHD
- (E) disruptive behavior disorder not otherwise specified

167. This adolescent is most likely to have an additional Axis I diagnosis from which of the following DSM-IV-TR diagnostic categories?

- (A) substance-related disorders
- (B) schizophrenia and other psychotic disorders
- (C) anxiety disorders
- (D) eating disorders
- (E) somatoform disorders

168. Which of the following personality disorders is this boy most likely to develop?

- (A) antisocial personality disorder
- (B) paranoid personality disorder
- (C) schizoid personality disorder
- (D) schizotypal personality disorder
- (E) avoidant personality disorder

Questions 169 and 170

A 10-year-old girl who has recently been diagnosed with diabetes mellitus type 1 is referred to you by her pediatrician for an evaluation. You notice that she seems sad. After interviewing the girl and her parents, you determine that she meets DSM-IV-TR criteria for adjustment disorder with depressed mood.

169. Which of the following criteria for the diagnosis of adjustment disorder distinguishes it from MDD?

(A) Symptoms develop following an identifiable stressor.

(B) Symptoms develop within 3 months of the onset of the stressor.

(C) Symptoms do not persist for more than 6 months following termination of the stressor.

(D) Symptoms cause marked distress or significant impairment in functioning.

(E) Symptoms do not represent bereavement.

170. Approximately what percentage of children who are diagnosed with diabetes mellitus type 1 develop adjustment disorder following their medical diagnosis?

(A) 1%

(B) 5%

(C) 10%

(D) 33%

(E) 75%

Questions 171 through 174

A 9-month-old girl is brought to the clinic by her foster mother for a routine examination. The girl's biological mother was infected with human immunodeficiency virus (HIV), was enrolled in a methadone maintenance program, and was using cocaine. The baby girl's HIV test is negative, but you are concerned about the possibility of developmental delays due to the mother's cocaine use.

171. At which of the following ages does a child normally speak his or her first word?

(A) 4 months

(B) 6 months

(C) 9 months

(D) 11 months

(E) 15 months

172. At what age does a child normally start holding up his or her head?

(A) 4 months

(B) 6 months

(C) 9 months

(D) 11 months

(E) 15 months

173. At what age is a child normally able to sit for a brief period?

(A) 4 months

(B) 6 months

(C) 9 months

(D) 11 months

(E) 15 months

174. You learn that this girl has a 2-year-old brother who is infected with HIV. Which of the following is the best place for HIV-infected children under the age of 3 who cannot be cared for by their family?

(A) a hospital

(B) a group home

(C) a foster home

(D) a nursing home

(E) a hospice

Questions 175 and 176

A 9-year-old boy is referred to you for evaluation for increasingly disruptive behavior in school. The teachers report that at any time, without warning, the boy will make a disruptive sound or shout out in class. They describe him as polite and neat but "restless and jumpy."

175. Which of the following is the most likely diagnosis?

(A) oppositional defiant disorder

(B) conduct disorder

(C) separation anxiety disorder

(D) panic disorder

(E) Tourette's disorder

176. Which of the following medications is most likely to be effective in the treatment of this boy's disorder?

(A) bupropion (Wellbutrin)

(B) paroxetine (Paxil)

(C) venlafaxine (Effexor)

(D) risperidone (Risperdal)

(E) clonidine (Catapres)

Questions 177 through 179

A 7-year-old boy with leukemia is referred to you because of concerns for his mood. His parents report that he fluctuates between appearing depressed and acting angry. At times he plays quietly in his room, but at other times he displays angry outbursts, often hitting his 4-year-old brother.

177. Which of the following methods would be the most useful way to interview this child?

(A) Sit quietly and allow the child to talk.

(B) Encourage the child to talk about whatever is on his mind.

(C) Provide toys and allow the child to play.

(D) Use the Diagnostic Interview Schedule for Children (DISC).

(E) Ask the child specific questions about how he feels about his disease.

178. Which of the following is true for children with a medical illness and a psychiatric illness?

(A) The psychiatric illness does not need to be treated until the medical illness is resolved.

(B) The psychiatric illness should not be treated pharmacologically in the setting of a medical illness.

(C) The psychiatric illness should be treated by the same physician who is treating the medical illness.

(D) The psychiatric illness should be treated aggressively in the setting of a medical illness.

(E) Psychotherapy is unlikely to be effective in the setting of a medical illness.

179. Hospitalization at what age places a child at greatest risk for developing difficulties in adaptive functioning later in life?

(A) birth to 6 months

(B) 1 to 3 years

(C) 5 to 8 years

(D) 9 to 12 years

(E) 13 to 16 years

Questions 180 through 183

An 8-year-old boy presents to your office for a routine visit. One month earlier you diagnosed him with Tourette's disorder and prescribed medication. He and his parents report that the medication has been helpful.

180. Which of the following is the most common initial symptom of Tourette's disorder?

(A) eye tics such as blinking

(B) facial tics such as grimacing or licking

(C) vocal tics, such as throat clearing or grunting

(D) whole-body tics, such as body rocking or pelvic thrusting

(E) self-abusive tics such as hitting

181. Which of the following is true regarding the DSM-IV-TR diagnosis of Tourette's disorder?

(A) Motor and vocal tics must occur concurrently.

(B) Onset must be before the age of 21.

(C) Tics much be present every day consecutively for at least 1 year.

(D) Vocal tics must improve production of words.

(E) Multiple motor tics must occur.

182. What is the approximate concordance rate for Tourette's disorder among monozygotic twins?

(A) 10%

(B) 30%

(C) 50%

(D) 75%

(E) 90%

183. Which of the following classes of medications is most effective in the treatment of Tourette's disorder?

(A) stimulants

(B) selective serotonin reuptake inhibitors (SSRIs)

(C) monoamine oxidase inhibitors (MAOIs)

(D) dopamine-2 (D_2) antagonists

(E) benzodiazepines

Questions 184 through 187

After you complete a routine physical examination of a healthy 11-year-old girl, the girl's mother asks to talk with you in private. She tells you that her daughter was given an IQ test in school, and that she scored a 68. The mother is extremely upset and wonders if it is her fault that her daughter is "dumb." She says she lies awake at night worrying and wonders why her daughter would have done so poorly on the test.

184. Which of the following statements is the most appropriate initial response?

(A) "There's no need to be upset about this."

(B) "Your IQ is probably similar to your daughter's."

(C) "Maybe your daughter just had a bad test day."

(D) "Tell me what IQ means to you."

(E) "Look at it this way, it could be worse."

185. The girl's IQ of 68 corresponds to which of the following DSM-IV-TR diagnoses?

(A) mild mental retardation

(B) moderate mental retardation

(C) severe mental retardation

(D) profound mental retardation

(E) mental retardation, severity unspecified

186. Which of the following is the most common predisposing factor for mental retardation?

(A) heredity

(B) pregnancy and perinatal problems

(C) early alterations in embryonic development

(D) general medical conditions acquired during infancy and childhood

(E) environmental influences and mental disorders other than mental retardation

187. According to DSM-IV-TR, mental retardation is coded on which of the following axes?

(A) Axis I

(B) Axis II

(C) Axis III

(D) Axis IV

(E) Axis V

Questions 188 and 189

An 8-year-old boy with a family history of tic disorders is referred to you for an evaluation of behavioral difficulties in school. His teachers report that he is unable to sit still, constantly fidgets, and is unable to complete classwork because he is so easily distracted. The boy's mother reports that he has always had a lot of energy. She says that preparing to leave for school in the morning is extremely difficult due to her son's disorganization and forgetfulness. Otherwise, she has no complaints. She denies that her son produces any repetitive movements or sounds.

188. Which of the following is the most likely diagnosis?

(A) dementia

(B) conduct disorder

(C) oppositional defiant disorder

(D) ADHD

(E) disruptive behavior disorder not otherwise specified

189. Which of the following classes of medications is most likely to unmask an underlying predisposition to developing tics?

(A) stimulants

(B) SSRIs

(C) MAOIs

(D) D_2 antagonists

(E) benzodiazepines

Questions 190 and 191

A 6-year-old boy is referred to you by his school to evaluate his difficulty with reading. It is suspected that he suffers from a reading disorder, but a subtle impairment in vision or hearing must be ruled out as a causative or contributing factor.

190. Learning disorders are most commonly associated with which of the following disorders?

    (A) ADHD
    (B) bipolar disorder
    (C) Tourette's disorder
    (D) Asperger's disorder
    (E) schizophrenia

191. Which of the following percentages approximates those children and adolescents with learning disorders who drop out of school?

    (A) 5%
    (B) 10%
    (C) 25%
    (D) 40%
    (E) 66%

Questions 192 through 194

An 8-year-old child is referred to you for an evaluation of bedwetting. Several behavioral interventions have been attempted, including eliminating fluid intake in the evening, scheduled awakenings at night to use the bathroom, and a urine alarm (a bell and pad). These techniques have been unsuccessful, and the child continues to urinate in bed every night.

192. A child with enuresis is most likely to be which of the following?

    (A) an otherwise normal boy
    (B) an otherwise normal girl
    (C) a child with mental retardation
    (D) a child with autistic disorder
    (E) a child with OCD

193. Which of the following statements is true?

    (A) Diurnal enuresis is more common than nocturnal enuresis.

    (B) Enuresis often occurs during nightmares.
    (C) The occurrence of enuresis is associated with being hungry.
    (D) Enuresis occurs more frequently on the weekends and on vacations than during the school week.
    (E) Children with enuresis often have a family history of the disorder.

194. Which of the following medications is most appropriate for you to prescribe to treat the enuresis?

    (A) methylphenidate (Ritalin)
    (B) paroxetine (Paxil)
    (C) trazodone (Desyrel)
    (D) imipramine (Tofranil)
    (E) benztropine (Cogentin)

Questions 195 through 198

A 10-year-old boy is referred to you because his pediatrician suspects that he may have ADHD. After a thorough history, physical examination, and laboratory investigation, you make the diagnosis of ADHD. After discussing the adverse effects of medications, you prescribe methylphenidate (Ritalin) to be taken in the morning and at lunch on school days.

195. Which of the following represents the prevalence of ADHD among school-age children in the United States?

    (A) less than 1%
    (B) 1 to 2%
    (C) 3 to 5%
    (D) 8 to 10%
    (E) 12 to 15%

196. Which of the following is a common adverse effect of methylphenidate?

    (A) tremor
    (B) hypotension
    (C) weight gain
    (D) insomnia
    (E) liver toxicity

197. Stimulants such as methylphenidate effectively treat symptoms of ADHD in what percentage of patients?

(A) 10%

(B) 25%

(C) 33%

(D) 50%

(E) 70%

198. How often does childhood ADHD persist into adulthood?

(A) 10%

(B) 25%

(C) 33%

(D) 50%

(E) 70%

Questions 199 and 200

During a routine office visit, the mother of a 22-month-old girl tells you that she is concerned about her daughter's behavior. Since the birth of her son 4 months earlier, the mother states that her daughter is more irritable and angry. The mother is especially concerned that her daughter is aggressive and violent toward the baby.

199. Which of the following statements is the most appropriate response to this mother?

(A) "If you simply ignore your daughter's behavior, it will pass."

(B) "Your daughter's behavior is normal for her age."

(C) "Every day, schedule some time for you and your daughter to spend together without the baby."

(D) "Explain to your daughter that the baby needs more attention that she does right now."

(E) "Your daughter must be precocious since the terrible twos are starting early."

200. At 22 months of age, this girl should be able to do which of the following?

(A) copy a circle

(B) copy a square

(C) identify her left hand

(D) tell her age and sex

(E) ride a tricycle

Questions 201 and 202

A 4-year-old boy is referred to you for evaluation because he has not started walking. He appears healthy and well cared for. He readily comes with you to the examining room. In your office, he notices a wind-up toy and immediately becomes engrossed in winding it up, watching it move around until it winds down, and winding it up again. After about 10 minutes, you attempt to take the toy from him, and he becomes extremely upset, making an insistent, piercing cry.

201. Which of the following is the most likely diagnosis?

(A) oppositional defiant disorder

(B) conduct disorder

(C) separation anxiety disorder

(D) autistic disorder

(E) selective mutism

202. Which of the following qualities is associated with a more favorable prognosis for children similar to this boy?

(A) easily toilet trained

(B) organized in play

(C) interested in mechanical toys

(D) able to converse

(E) able to dance to a beat

Questions 203 through 205

A 17-year-old girl comes to your office for a routine visit. She states that she feels fine and offers no complaints. On physical examination, you find that her weight is 92 pounds and her height is 5 feet 5 inches. One year earlier, her weight had been 126 pounds, and her height was 5 feet 5 inches. After further discussion, you learn that this girl is terrified of gaining weight and thinks that she looks fat and needs to lose more weight. She reports that she has not menstruated in the past 6 months.

203. Which of the following laboratory abnormalities are you most likely to discover?

(A) hypercholesterolemia

(B) increased thyroid-stimulating hormone (TSH)

(C) hypocarotenemia

(D) leukocytosis

(E) hyperkalemia

204. Which of the following findings is most consistent with this girl's disorder?

(A) sinus tachycardia

(B) increased resting energy expenditure

(C) elevated serum estrogen levels in females

(D) elevated serum testosterone levels in males

(E) increased ventricular–brain ratio on brain imaging

205. Which of the following regimens is most likely to be successful in the treatment of this girl's disorder?

(A) individual psychotherapy

(B) family therapy

(C) fluoxetine (Prozac)

(D) fluoxetine and individual psychotherapy

(E) fluoxetine and family therapy

Questions 206 and 207

An 8-month-old boy is brought to the clinic by his mother. She complains that her son has been experiencing screaming and crying fits when she leaves him with a babysitter. She says that in the past he did not object to being left with a babysitter, and asks you why he becomes so upset now and what she can do about it.

206. Which of the following statements is the most appropriate response?

(A) "This behavior is characteristic of autistic children."

(B) "It is possible that your son has separation anxiety disorder."

(C) "This behavior suggests that you're not spending enough time with your son."

(D) "It sounds as though your son is overly attached to you."

(E) "This behavior is normal at your son's age and will pass with time."

207. Which of the following statements is true regarding attachment by an infant to a caretaker?

(A) Attachment is prevented by mental illness in the caretaker.

(B) Attachment requires consistent interaction with the caretaker.

(C) Attachment is prevented by physical abuse from the caretaker.

(D) Attachment usually does not occur if the infant is blind.

(E) Attachment requires contact beginning in the perinatal period.

Questions 208 and 209

A 14-year-old boy is referred to you due to extreme difficulties in school. He has been held back a grade and is still not passing. During the course of your evaluation, you learn that the boy hears voices telling him that he is stupid and to leave the classroom. Afraid to disobey, he goes to the bathroom frequently. He has difficulty falling asleep at night because the voices keep him awake. In addition, you learn that the boy believes others can read his thoughts. The physical and laboratory examinations are normal.

208. You suspect that the boy may be suffering from schizophrenia. Which of the following subtypes of schizophrenia is most probable?

(A) paranoid type

(B) disorganized type

(C) catatonic type

(D) undifferentiated type

(E) residual type

209. Which of the following is the worst prognostic feature of schizophrenia with onset in childhood?

(A) affective symptoms

(B) acute onset

(C) onset before the age of 10

(D) good premorbid adjustment

(E) well-differentiated symptoms

Questions 210 and 211

A 9-year-old girl with a family history of bipolar disorder is referred to you by her school due to disruptive behavior in class that has been worsening over the past 3 months. Her teachers report that her energy level is high.

210. Which of the following would be most helpful in distinguishing between mania and ADHD in children?

(A) pressured speech

(B) distractibility

(C) motoric overactivity

(D) low self-esteem

(E) impulsivity

211. Which of the following disorders is more common among girls than among boys?

(A) ADHD

(B) conduct disorder

(C) Rett's disorder

(D) Tourette's disorder

(E) Asperger's disorder

Questions 212 and 213

A 6-year-old boy is brought to your office by his mother for evaluation of an upper respiratory infection. The mother mentions that her son has started sucking on his thumb again. In addition, she mentions that the boy's grandmother died recently and asks how children view death.

212. At what age can a child normally appreciate that death is irreversible?

(A) 2 years

(B) 3 years

(C) 5 years

(D) 7 years

(E) 12 years

213. Which of the following defense mechanisms is the boy employing when he starts sucking his thumb?

(A) repression

(B) acting out

(C) denial

(D) regression

(E) blocking

Questions 214 and 215

A 12-year-old boy with Tourette's disorder comes to your office for a routine visit. Two weeks earlier, you had prescribed clonidine (Catapres) for his illness. The boy reports that his tics have subsided slightly since starting the clonidine, but complains about the medicine.

214. This boy is likely experiencing which of the following as an adverse effect of clonidine?

(A) sedation

(B) light-headedness due to hypotension

(C) dry mouth

(D) tremor

(E) nausea

215. If this boy's 7-year-old brother were to have ADHD, which of the following classes of medications would be the most appropriate choice for him?

(A) a stimulant such as methylphenidate (Ritalin)

(B) a tricyclic antidepressant (TCA) such as desipramine (Norpramin)

(C) an SSRI such as fluoxetine (Prozac)

(D) an MAOI such as phenelzine (Nardil)

(E) a neuroleptic such as haloperidol (Haldol)

216. A 6-year-old boy is brought to the emergency department by his mother, who reports that he was playing on some steps in front of the house when he slipped and fell. She tells you that she is concerned that he might have broken his arm. An x-ray of the boy's arm shows a fracture of the ulna, as well as signs of several old fractures of varying ages. Which of the following is the most appropriate action?

(A) Refer the boy to an orthopedist for further evaluation.

(B) Tell the mother that you notice that the boy has had multiple broken bones and recommend that she limit the boy's sports activities.

(C) Set the current broken bone in a cast and recommend that the boy see his pediatrician for follow-up care.

(D) Recommend calcium supplements and a multiple vitamin daily.

(E) Tell the boy that you notice that he has had multiple broken bones and ask him how each of these fractures happened.

217. The mother of one of your 4-year-old patients calls and asks you for advice. She says that her son has been stealing toys from other children at school and bringing them home with him. Which of the following suggestions is most appropriate?

(A) The mother should return the toys herself and buy her son similar toys.

(B) The mother should tell her son that if he stops stealing, she will give him a reward each week.

(C) The mother should point out to her son that he is stealing and punish him for it.

(D) The mother should help her son return the toys.

(E) The mother should ignore the entire situation because her son's behavior is part of a developmental phase that will pass.

218. A 14-year-old girl presents to her pediatrician complaining that she has been "freaking out." The girl describes episodes of palpitations, shaking, gasping for air, and feeling like she is going to die. These feelings intensify for a few minutes and resolve spontaneously. These episodes have occurred at various times, in various situations, and the girl is worried that she is "going crazy." Which of the following is the most appropriate treatment?

(A) valproate (Depakote)

(B) risperidone (Risperdal)

(C) clozapine (Clozaril)

(D) sertraline (Zoloft)

(E) carbamazepine (Tegretol)

219. A 5-year-old girl with asthma is seen by her pediatrician for a routine visit. After returning home from the clinic, the girl asks her friend to "play doctor." This behavior is a manifestation of which of the following phenomena?

(A) reaction formation

(B) identification

(C) displacement

(D) rationalization

(E) dissociation

220. A 4-year-old boy whose mother had rubella during her pregnancy is brought to the clinic for a routine visit. The physical and laboratory examinations are normal. The highest risk of physical and/or mental defects in the fetus as a result of maternal rubella infection occurs during which month of the pregnancy?

(A) first

(B) third

(C) fifth

(D) seventh

(E) ninth

221. A 10-year-old girl with a history of asthma is brought to the clinic after a recent increase in asthma symptoms. During the visit, you learn that she is being beaten by her mother's boyfriend. Under which of the following circumstances does the law require mandatory reporting of suspected child abuse by a physician who evaluates a child?

(A) in all cases

(B) only when the physician believes it is in a child's best interests

(C) only when consent of a parent or guardian is obtained

(D) only in cases in which the child shows behavioral manifestations of abuse

(E) only when the physician has examined all children in the family

222. A 4-year-old boy is referred to you because he will not speak in preschool. Over the course of about 2 months, he gradually stops talking. Initially his mother reports that he objected to going to preschool, but no longer complains. She states that at times, her son is quiet and stays in his room, but that she has not noticed a significant change in his speech or behavior. Which of the following is the most likely diagnosis?

(A) selective mutism

(B) MDD

(C) separation anxiety disorder

(D) social phobia

(E) dysthymic disorder

223. A 2-year-old boy is referred to you for evaluation due to the suspicion that the child is the victim of physical abuse secondary to Munchausen syndrome by proxy. Which of the following family members is most frequently the perpetrator who fabricates the presenting illness?

(A) the brother

(B) the sister

(C) the father

(D) the mother

(E) the uncle

Questions 224 through 226

A frustrated mother brings her 14-year-old son to a child psychiatrist after he is expelled from three high schools in one year. She reports the boy has tried twice to set his school on fire, has slashed school bus tires, and has broken into the principal's office to steal athletic trophies. In addition, he has been suspended numerous times for getting into fights with other students. She shudders and tearfully relates that she recently caught him singeing one of the family cats with a cigarette butt.

224. What is the son's most likely diagnosis?

(A) schizophrenia

(B) antisocial personality disorder

(C) conduct disorder

(D) attention deficit disorder

(E) oppositional defiant disorder

225. Diagnosis of this disorder requires the presence of what personality disorder?

(A) schizotypal

(B) borderline

(C) obsessive–compulsive

(D) antisocial

(E) histrionic

226. In addition, the disorder in question 225 may demonstrate comorbidity with which of the following?

(A) major depression

(B) learning disabilities

(C) substance abuse

(D) mental retardation

(E) all of the above

DIRECTIONS (Questions 227 through 234): Each set of items in this section consists of a list of lettered headings followed by several numbered words or phrases. For each numbered word or phrase, select the ONE lettered option that is most closely associated with it. Each lettered option may be selected once, more than once, or not at all.

Questions 227 through 230

    (A) Rett's disorder

    (B) bulimia nervosa

    (C) stereotypic movement disorder

    (D) social phobia

    (E) separation anxiety

    (F) pica

    (G) enuresis

    (H) conduct disorder

    (I) panic disorder

    (J) Asperger's disorder

227. A 7-year-old boy with *Toxocara* and visceral larva migrans

228. A 17-year-old girl with hypokalemia

229. A 6-year-old boy with rectal bleeding and anemia

230. A 15-year-old boy with a urine toxicology screen positive for cocaine

Questions 231 through 234

    (A) OCD

    (B) pica

    (C) hypochondriasis

    (D) Tourette's disorder

    (E) panic disorder

    (F) bulimia nervosa

    (G) anorexia nervosa

    (H) Asperger's disorder

    (I) pyromania

    (J) trichotillomania

231. A 14-year-old girl with episodes of palpitations, chest pain, shortness of breath, and diaphoresis who has a normal physical and laboratory examination

232. A 10-year-old girl with physical findings that include hypotension, bradycardia, and lanugo hair

233. An 8-year-old boy with erythematous, chapped hands and an otherwise normal physical and laboratory examination

234. A 13-year-old girl with a bald patch on the back of her head and an otherwise normal physical and laboratory examination

Answers and Explanations

133. **(B)** The use of direct but open-ended statements, such as "You look down. Tell me what's going on," is most likely to be helpful. By commenting on how the boy looks, you convey to him that you understand at least somewhat how he feels. It is extremely important for patients to feel as though their physicians understand them. Using an upbeat statement, such as "Hey buddy, what's going on?" suggests that you are ignoring how the boy looks and feels. Questions such as "Are you feeling depressed?" or "How's school?" are not open-ended and are unlikely to yield much information. When treating a child or adolescent, it is critical to hear how he or she feels, in addition to obtaining information from parents and teachers. Children or adolescents may tell a physician things that they feel they cannot tell their parents. A response such as "I can see you don't want to talk. Should I talk with your mother instead?" will not be helpful and may even be experienced as rejection.

134. **(C)** Suicide is a considerable risk in depressed adolescents and should be specifically addressed during an interview with a patient who appears depressed or agitated or has a history of a suicide attempt. Surveys of adolescents in the general community have estimated that approximately 9% of adolescents have attempted suicide at least once in their lives. Among adolescents with known psychiatric disorders, the rate is much higher. More girls than boys demonstrate suicidal behavior, but nearly five times more teenage boys successfully commit suicide than do teenage girls, due to the more frequent use of guns and violent methods used by boys. History of a prior suicide attempt is an important risk factor for suicide in all ages; the majority of those who successfully complete suicide have attempted suicide in the past. The adolescent suicide rate has increased substantially during the past few decades.

135. **(E)** The use of firearms is the most common method by which adolescents die by suicide. Drug overdose is the most common method of suicide attempts, but accounts for fewer completed suicides. Stabbing, cutting, jumping from buildings, and hanging are other methods frequently employed.

136. **(A)** A simple, nonjudgmental statement, such as "I can see this is very upsetting for you," will convey to the mother that you are concerned about her and that, at least on some level, you understand her and sympathize with her suffering. This form of sentence also acts as an open-ended question that is most likely to elicit the most important information most efficiently. The mother may be most troubled by something other than her son's episodes and her daytime sleepiness. Specifically directed statements, such as "Tell me why you can't fall back to sleep after your son does," or leading questions, such as "Are you worried that this is your fault?" are less likely to be helpful in gaining this information than an open-ended statement or question. Usually, any statement containing "but" is inappropriate as the initial response to a person who is describing a problem to you. Statements such as "I know you're upset, but this problem will get better" or "I can see you're upset, but you're really overreacting" may indicate that you do not take the problem seriously or that you are minimizing how the person feels. Such an approach may prevent you from obtaining further important information.

137. **(E)** This boy's episodes are most consistent with sleep terror disorder, in which patients repeatedly awaken abruptly from sleep with a panicky scream, show intense fear and signs of autonomic arousal, are unresponsive to others and to comforting during the episode, and remember no detailed dream nor anything else about the episode. Asking a question such as "Does your son wake up and remember a nightmare?" will enable you to distinguish between sleep terror disorder and nightmare disorder. A person with nightmare disorder awakens and has detailed recall of an extremely frightening dream. Wetting the bed (enuresis), going to sleep late, watching scary movies, and making jerky movements during sleep are unrelated to the diagnosis of sleep terror disorder.

138. **(C)** Episodes of sleep terror, as well as of sleepwalking, occur during deep sleep (stages 3–4). Sleep terror does not occur during stage 1 or 2 of sleep or during REM sleep.

139. **(E)** Narcolepsy that significantly interferes with functioning may be treated with stimulants, such as methylphenidate (Ritalin) or magnesium pemoline (Cylert). Nightmare disorder, sleep terror disorder, sleepwalking disorder, and circadian rhythm sleep disorder are less likely to require pharmacologic intervention.

140. **(E)** A selective serotonin reuptake inhibitor (SSRI) such as sertraline is the first-line agent for MDD in children and adolescents. Tricyclics (TCAs) such as imipramine cause more adverse effects than SSRIs typically do, and an overdose is much more likely to be lethal. Mood stabilizers such as carbamazepine and lithium are used for bipolar disorder and as adjuncts to the treatment of MDD that is refractory to antidepressant medications alone.

Antipsychotics such as olanzapine are usually reserved for use as adjuncts when psychosis develops.

141. **(A)** Bulimia nervosa is most effectively treated with cognitive–behavioral therapy. Family therapy, psychoanalytic psychotherapy, and group therapy may be used as adjuncts to cognitive–behavioral therapy, but are not as effective in changing the behaviors associated with bulimia nervosa.

142. **(A)** Cannabis is the most common illicit substance used by adolescents, and can cause or contribute to feelings of depression. Cocaine, LSD, PCP, and heroin are less frequently used. In order to obtain accurate information from adolescents, it is critical to name specific substances when asking about drug use.

143. **(B)** This boy most likely suffers from expressive language disorder. The typical symptoms of this disorder include having a markedly limited vocabulary, making errors in tense, and having difficulty recalling words or producing sentences with developmentally appropriate length or complexity. In addition, the boy's difficulties are interfering with academic functioning. There is no indication that this boy has difficulty with written expression, so a diagnosis of disorder of written expression would be inappropriate. This boy does not suffer from phonological disorder, because his speech is clear and he has not failed to develop expected speech sounds. Similarly, he is not suffering from stuttering, a DSM-IV-TR communications disorders diagnosis, because there is no disturbance in the fluency and time patterning of his speech. There is no indication that he has difficulty with motor coordination, so a diagnosis of developmental coordination disorder would be inappropriate.

144. **(A)** An IQ test would be most helpful in confirming the diagnosis of expressive language disorder because a diagnosis of mental retardation must be ruled out. The CAS, DICA, DISC, and K-SADS are semistructured interviews that aid primarily in the assessment of

mood disorders, anxiety disorders, disruptive behavior disorders, and eating disorders.

145. **(D)** The most likely diagnosis is rumination disorder, in which there is repeated regurgitation and rechewing of food for a period of at least 1 month following a period of normal functioning. Rumination disorder is often seen in infants who have a variety of caretakers in an unstable environment. The drooling exhibited by this baby is most likely the milk or food that has been regurgitated. Lack of appropriate weight gain is typical when the baby does not reswallow the food. This baby is not suffering from anorexia nervosa because she likes to eat and does not display fears of becoming overweight. Similarly, she is not suffering from bulimia nervosa because she does not display episodes of binge eating with compensatory behavior, such as self-induced vomiting or misuse of laxatives. A diagnosis of pica would require that the baby persistently eat nonnutritive substances such as dirt, plaster, hair, bugs, or pebbles. A diagnosis of feeding disorder of infancy or early childhood is not appropriate because the baby's disturbance is better accounted for by a diagnosis of rumination disorder.

146. **(E)** In order to confirm the diagnosis of rumination disorder, an associated gastrointestinal or other general medical condition, such as esophageal reflux, must be ruled out. Esophageal pH measurement indicates if acidic gastric contents move into the esophagus during periods when the infant is not eating or actively regurgitating, as occurs in esophageal reflux. Measurement of the serum lead level is appropriate when pica is suspected, because old paints may contain lead, which can cause significant neurologic problems when ingested. Calculating the percentage of expected weight represented by the infant's current weight would be required for a diagnosis of anorexia nervosa (85% or less) but is not a criterion for rumination disorder. Twenty-four-hour video monitoring would greatly aid in assessing the baby's behavior and the context in which the disturbance occurs, but would not rule out a gastrointesti-

nal condition as the cause of this problem. Results of a CBC would not be helpful in determining the diagnosis.

147. **(C)** This boy's behavior and symptoms are most consistent with separation anxiety disorder, characterized by developmentally inappropriate and excessive anxiety concerning separation from the home or from those to whom the individual is attached. Consistent with this diagnosis, the boy does not like to go to school, comes home immediately after school, sleeps in his parents' bed at night, and has repeated physical symptoms when at school. The boy does not suffer from social phobia disorder because he does not have marked and persistent fear of a social or performance situation with exposure causing intense anxiety, expressed as a tantrum or a panic attack. The boy is not suffering from PTSD because there is no evidence of a traumatic event that is persistently reexperienced and has caused symptoms of increased arousal and avoidance of associated stimuli. For a diagnosis of reactive attachment disorder of infancy or early childhood, the boy would need to have suffered markedly disturbed social relatedness, in most contexts, beginning before the age of 5. Finally, a diagnosis of specific phobia would require the display of marked and persistent fear cued by the presence of anticipation of a specific object or situation, expressed as a tantrum or panic attack.

148. **(E)** Diagnosis of separation anxiety disorder requires onset of symptoms prior to the age of 18. Onset is considered early if symptoms begin before age 6. Separation anxiety disorder is seen in both boys and girls; intelligent and sensitive children are not particularly prone to it. It can occur whenever there is a significantly emotional separation from a gratifying relationship. Physical complaints, such as headaches, stomachaches, nausea, or vomiting, are common when separation from the major attachment figure occurs or is anticipated. Diagnosis of separation anxiety disorder requires the presence of symptoms for at least 4 weeks.

149. **(E)** Somatization is a defense mechanism in which emotional concerns are manifested as physical symptoms. Coprolalia is the repetitive speaking of obscene words, seen in severe cases of Tourette's disorder. Anhedonia is the lack of interest or pleasure in activities that were once enjoyable, seen in MDD. Reaction formation is a defense mechanism in which an unacceptable impulse is transformed into its opposite. Coprophagia is the eating of feces.

150. **(E)** Substance-induced psychotic disorder is the most common cause of florid visual hallucinations in a child. The child may have ingested prescription drugs, illicit drugs, over-the-counter medications, or a household agent. Schizophrenia rarely presents in young children. When it does, it is much more likely to present with auditory hallucinations than with visual hallucinations. Hallucinations do not occur in panic disorder, autistic disorder, nor mental retardation.

151. **(C)** Suicidal behavior is the most common psychiatric emergency in children and adolescents. Psychotic behavior, particularly assaultive behavior, and homicidal behavior are less common emergencies. Sexually inappropriate behavior alone is rarely an emergency.

152. **(B)** This girl's symptoms are most consistent with stereotypic movement disorder, in which there is a repetitive, seemingly driven, and nonfunctional motor behavior that markedly interferes with normal activities or results in self-inflicted bodily injury requiring medical attention. Common behaviors include hand shaking or waving, body rocking, head banging, mouthing of objects, self-biting, picking at skin or bodily orifices, or hitting one's own body. In the case of this girl, the repetitive behavior of nail biting does not have the ritual quality seen in OCD or the sudden, rapid, involuntary nature of motor tics seen in chronic motor tic disorder. The girl's inability to complete her homework is due to her nail biting rather than to inattention, hyperactivity, or impulsiveness

seen in ADHD. The history does not suggest a diagnosis of MDD as the girl does not seem to feel depressed, hopeless, or worthless, and does not express loss of interest or pleasure in activities.

153. **(D)** This girl's academic difficulties related to her nail biting should be coded on Axis IV along with any other psychological and environmental problems that may affect the diagnosis, treatment, and prognosis of her Axis I disorder (or are a significantly distressing effect of her Axis I disorder). The fact that the girl's behavior is interfering with normal activities (e.g., homework) is part of the diagnostic criteria for her Axis I diagnosis, but the stress of falling grades requires coding on Axis IV. Mental retardation and personality disorders are coded on Axis II. Medical (physical) disorders are coded on axis III. The Global Assessment of Functioning (GAF), the clinician's judgment of the individual's overall level of functioning, is coded on Axis V.

154. **(A)** A direct but open-ended statement such as "Tell me about the scratches on your hand" is most likely to be helpful in this situation. It is not a secret that the abrasions are there, but the patient has not mentioned them. Usually, a patient will appreciate a direct question rather than wonder if you ignored or did not notice something obvious. Questions such as "Do you scratch yourself in addition to biting your nails?" or "Do you have a cat?" are not open-ended; they require "yes" or "no" answers and are unlikely to yield new information. "How did the scratches happen?" may sound accusatory; patients will be more likely to offer information if you seem nonjudgmental. Signs of bulimia nervosa include erosion of tooth enamel caused by acidic vomitus and abrasions on the dorsum of the hand due to scraping by the upper teeth as the individual pushes the hand to the back of the throat to induce vomiting. If this girl does not volunteer information that confirms to you that she is not inducing vomiting, you should use a reassuring statement such as "Sometimes I

see girls who make themselves throw up. Have you ever done that?"

155. **(C)** Psychomotor agitation is more commonly seen in children with MDD compared to adolescents with MDD. Children with MDD may appear more anxious and irritable than sad and depressed. Hypersomnia, hopelessness, weight change, and drug abuse are more commonly seen in adolescents with MDD compared to children with MDD.

156. **(A)** Substance ingestion is the most common method children use when attempting suicide. Other methods frequently used by children include stabbing, cutting, jumping from buildings, hanging, running in front of vehicles, and gas inhalation. Firearms are used less frequently than substance ingestion but are more often lethal. It is important to note that some suicide attempts may be mistaken for accidents, so it is important to directly ask children if they intended to hurt or kill themselves.

157. **(E)** Headaches and nausea are common adverse effects associated with the synthetic antidiuretic hormone DDAVP. Sedation, hypotension, liver toxicity, and tremor are not associated with desmopressin.

158. **(A)** DDAVP is effective in treating enuresis because it suppresses urine production for 7 to 10 hours following administration by intranasal spray. It lacks the pressor effects of antidiuretic hormone, but can cause a mild hyponatremia. Hypocalcemia, hypokalemia, hypomagnesemia, and hypophosphatemia are not side effects of the drug.

159. **(D)** The approximate comorbidity of childhood anxiety disorders (overanxious disorder, separation anxiety disorder, panic disorder) and MDD is 50%. The approximate comorbidity of childhood anxiety disorders and ADHD is 30%.

160. **(B)** The most common adverse effects of fluoxetine include gastrointestinal symptoms, insomnia, agitation, and headaches. In general, hypotension, liver toxicity, adverse weight gain, and sedation are not side effects associated with fluoxetine.

161. **(A)** Signs of lead toxicity include normocytic, normochromic anemia, basophilic stippling, and increased density at the metaphyseal plate of the growing long bones, also referred to as "lead lines" on x-ray. Eating chips of old paint, as seen in pica, is a common cause of lead toxicity in young children. Pica is often associated with mental retardation and with poor parental supervision. Anorexia nervosa can result in anemia if severe, but basophilic stippling, the bone abnormalities seen, and the history are not consistent with anorexia nervosa or with bulimia nervosa. There is no indication that this girl is repeatedly passing feces in inappropriate places, ruling out encopresis. Bizarre eating patterns can occur with psychotic disorders, but these are much less common than pica. In addition, the presentation of schizophrenia in a 3-year-old child is rare.

162. **(A)** CaEDTA is a chelating agent used to treat lead toxicity. Flumazenil is used to reverse the sedating effects of excess benzodiazepines, while naloxone is used to reverse the effects of excess opiates. Deferoxamine is a chelating agent used to treat iron toxicity. Acetylcysteine is used to treat acetaminophen toxicity.

163. **(D)** The girl's bruises are most likely the result of physical abuse, which is strongly suggested by the presence of multiple fractures of different ages. Thrombocytopenia and malnutrition are rare in the United States. In developmental coordination disorder, there is a delay in achieving major milestones and "clumsiness," but there is not typically a pattern of repeated injury. Hepatic failure is extremely rare in a 3-year-old child.

164. **(B)** This girl's history and presentation are consistent with Rett's disorder, which is characterized by normal prenatal and perinatal development, normal head circumference at birth, and normal psychomotor development

through the first 5 months of life. Between the ages of 5 months and 48 months, there is deceleration of head growth, loss of hand skills with development of stereotyped hand movements such as hand wringing, loss of social interaction (which may improve later), appearance of poorly coordinated gait or trunk movements, and severely impaired expressive and receptive language development with severe psychomotor retardation. Autistic disorder and pervasive developmental disorder not otherwise specified are not appropriate diagnoses because this girl's presentation is better accounted for by Rett's disorder. Children with childhood disintegrative disorder do not develop normally for at least 2 years after birth. Children with Asperger's disorder do not show delay in language development (e.g., single words are used by the age of 2).

165. **(A)** Rett's disorder is the only DSM-IV-TR disorder that is seen only in girls. Children with Rett's disorder commonly suffer from mental retardation, which is coded on Axis II. Although there are no clear characteristic laboratory findings associated with the disorder, there is a genetic test available. There are no known familial clusters of the disorder. Autistic disorder is the most common of the pervasive developmental disorders.

166. **(B)** Conduct disorder is the most appropriate diagnosis for this boy because he has repeatedly violated serious rules and is threatening and intimidating toward his parents. There is no indication that this boy's intelligence is limited, making mental retardation an inappropriate diagnosis. Oppositional defiant disorder is not appropriate, because his behavior surpasses the negativistic, angry behavior seen in this disorder. Similarly, his behavior is not characteristic of a simple ADHD because of his repeated and serious violations of rules. Disruptive behavior not otherwise specified is not the most appropriate diagnosis for this boy because he meets full criteria for conduct disorder.

167. **(A)** This boy is most likely to have a substance-related disorder in addition to conduct disorder. Children and adolescents with conduct disorder often have a substance-related disorder and/or ADHD. Schizophrenia and other psychotic disorders, anxiety disorders, eating disorders, and somatoform disorders are less frequently associated with conduct disorder.

168. **(A)** Children and adolescents who are diagnosed with conduct disorder are at increased risk for antisocial personality disorder as adults. Antisocial personality disorder is not diagnosed until after the age of 18, and one of the criteria is evidence of conduct disorder prior to the age of 15. Earlier onset of conduct disorder is associated with an increased risk of developing antisocial personality disorder. Conduct disorder is not as closely associated with paranoid personality disorder, schizoid personality disorder, schizotypal personality disorder, or avoidant personality disorder.

169. **(C)** By definition, symptoms of adjustment disorder do not last longer than 6 months after a stressor or the termination of its consequences. If depressive symptoms persist, MDD may be diagnosed. In both adjustment disorder and MDD, symptoms may develop following a stressor, may develop within 3 months of the onset of a stressor, must cause marked distress or significant impairment in functioning, and must not represent bereavement.

170. **(D)** Following a diagnosis of diabetes mellitus type I, approximately 33% of children develop symptoms of adjustment disorder.

171. **(D)** At the age of 11 months, a child normally speaks his or her first word. The range of ages considered normal is 8 to 18 months. Babbling begins around 6 months of age.

172. **(A)** At the age of 4 months, a child normally begins holding up his or her head.

173. **(B)** At the age of 6 months, a child is normally able to sit for brief periods.

174. (C) A foster home is the optimal place for young children with HIV. In a foster home, a child has the psychological benefit of belonging to a family and is more likely to receive adequate emotional support than in a group setting. In addition, the risk of opportunistic infections is higher in group settings, such as hospitals, group homes, nursing homes, and hospices, than in private home environments.

175. (E) Tourette's disorder is the most likely diagnosis because the boy's outbursts are consistent with vocal tics, and the report of "restless and jumpy" behavior is consistent with misinterpretation of motor tics. Tourette's disorder most commonly develops in grade school–age boys, and the voluntary tics may be misinterpreted as purposefully disruptive behavior. Of note, there is frequent comorbidity with ADHD. This boy does not suffer from oppositional defiant disorder or conduct disorder because he is polite and neat and does not display hostile, destructive, or angry behaviors. There is no evidence that this boy experiences distress and worry when separated from an important attachment figure, as in separation anxiety disorder. The outbursts are not typical of panic disorder, in which there are discrete panic attacks, periods of intense fear, or discomfort with physical manifestations such as palpitations and subjective difficulty breathing.

176. (E) Clonidine has become the first-line treatment for Tourette's disorder. It has a limited side effect profile and helps control symptoms of the two frequently associated comorbid disorders, ADHD and OCD. Tricyclic antidepressants have been shown to be effective in the treatment of Tourette's disorder, but other antidepressants such as bupropion, paroxetine, and venlafaxine are not known to be effective. High-potency antipsychotics such as haloperidol and pimozide were traditionally the first-line agents for Tourette's disorder. The newer atypical antipsychotics, such as risperidone, are not known to be effective in treating the disorder.

177. (C) A play interview, in which a child is provided with toys and allowed to play, is an effective and efficient way to interview a child. Even with encouragement, a child is unlikely to produce much spontaneous talk in the uncomfortable setting of sitting with a stranger evaluating her. Likewise, asking specific questions will not be as helpful as observing the child's play. Semistructured interviews are useful tools in combination with play interviews, but the DISC is unreliable in 6- to 9-year-old children.

178. (D) A psychiatric illness in a child or adolescent with a medical illness should be treated aggressively using the type of treatment most effective for the specific psychiatric illness. Effective treatment of a mental illness may positively affect a medical illness if improvement of psychiatric symptoms enables the child to more fully participate in treatment of the medical illness. In addition, emotional state is related to immune response. Appropriate pharmacologic treatment should be avoided only if there are specific contraindications based on the medical treatment the child is receiving. There is no need for the psychiatric illness to be treated by the same physician who is treating the medical illness. In general, the effectiveness of psychotherapy is related to the specific mental illness, not to the existence of, or lack of, a medical illness.

179. (B) Hospitalization of a child between the ages of 1 and 3 is associated with the greatest difficulties in later adaptive functioning. Developmental features associated with the 1- to 3-year age range makes this a particularly vulnerable period.

180. (A) Eye tics such as blinking and eye rolling are the most common initial symptoms in Tourette's disorder. Facial tics such as grimacing or licking movements and vocal tics such as throat clearing or grunting are the next most common initial symptoms. Whole-body tics, such as body rocking or pelvic thrusting, and self-abusive tics, such as hitting, may develop later.

181. **(E)** In Tourette's disorder, multiple motor tics and one or more vocal tics must be present at some time during the illness. The motor and vocal tics do not need to occur concurrently. Onset is before the age of 18. The average age of onset is 7. Tics must be present nearly every day or intermittently for at least 1 year, with no tic-free period longer than 3 consecutive months. Vocal tics include various sounds such as grunts, yelps, coughs, and throat clearing, as well as words.

182. **(C)** The concordance rate for Tourette's disorder among monozygotic twins is approximately 50%. The concordance rate increases to approximately 75% when the tic spectrum disorders, including chronic motor tic disorder, are considered.

183. **(D)** Traditionally, D_2 antagonists such as haloperidol and pimozide have been the treatment of choice for Tourette's disorder. Recently, the noradrenergic agents clonidine and guanfacine, as well as TCAs, have become more frequently used. Stimulants exacerbate tics. In general, MAOIs are not effective. SSRIs and benzodiazepines may be used as adjunctive therapies in Tourette's disorder.

184. **(D)** In order to understand why this mother is so troubled, it will be helpful to understand how she thinks about the IQ test. An open-ended statement such as "Tell me what IQ means to you" will be most helpful. Reassurances, such as "There's no need to be upset about this" or "Look at it this way, it could be worse," are inappropriate as an initial response if you do not fully understand why a person is upset. Furthermore, premature reassurances are likely to be interpreted as rejection or lack of interest. It is important to avoid potentially insulting statements, such as "Your IQ is probably similar to your daughter's," or potentially false statements, such as "Maybe your daughter just had a bad test day."

185. **(A)** An IQ of 68 corresponds to mild mental retardation. According to DSM-IV-TR, an IQ below 20 or 25 corresponds to profound mental retardation, 20–25 to 35–40 corresponds to severe mental retardation, 35–40 to 50–55 corresponds to moderate mental retardation, and 50–55 to approximately 70 corresponds to mild mental retardation. A diagnosis of mental retardation, severity unspecified, is made when there is a strong presumption of mental retardation but the person's intelligence is untestable by standard testing, such as in infants or in patients who are too impaired or uncooperative to complete testing.

186. **(C)** Early alterations in embryonic development, such as chromosomal changes (e.g., Down syndrome) and prenatal damage due to toxins (e.g., maternal alcohol consumption) are the most common predisposing factors for mental retardation, accounting for approximately 30% of cases. Heredity accounts for about 5%. Pregnancy and perinatal problems account for approximately 10%. General medical conditions acquired during infancy and childhood account for approximately 5%. Environmental influences and mental disorders other than mental retardation account for approximately 15 to 20%. There is no clear etiology in 30 to 40% of cases.

187. **(B)** Mental retardation is coded on Axis II. All psychiatric disorders except mental retardation and personality disorders are coded on Axis I. Medical (physical) disorders are coded on Axis III. Psychosocial and environmental problems of clinical significance are coded on Axis IV. The GAF, the clinician's judgment of the individual's overall level of functioning, is coded on Axis V.

188. **(D)** This boy's history is typical of ADHD, combined type. He is fidgety and distractible in school, as well as at home, and this is interfering with his ability to function. Forgetfulness due to distractibility is commonly seen in ADHD and is not a sign of dementia. This boy does not display excessive aggression, destruction of property, deceitfulness, theft, or serious violations of rules, as seen in conduct disorder. His behaviors are not negativistic, hostile, or defiant, so he does not suffer from oppositional defiant disorder. Disruptive behavior disorder not otherwise specified is a diagnosis reserved for cases in which there are conduct or oppositional defiant behaviors that do not meet the full criteria for conduct disorder or oppositional defiant disorder but cause significant impairment.

189. **(A)** Stimulant medications have been associated with an increased risk of developing tics. In general, if a child suffers from tics or has a family history of tics, stimulant medications should be avoided and a TCA should be used to treat ADHD if necessary. SSRIs, MAOIs, D_2 antagonists, and benzodiazepines are not known to exacerbate tics.

190. **(A)** Learning disorders are commonly associated with ADHD. Children with conduct disorder, oppositional defiant disorder, MDD, and dysthymic disorder are also at increased risk for learning disorders. Bipolar disorder, Tourette's disorder, Asperger's disorder, and schizophrenia are not commonly associated with learning disorders.

191. **(D)** Approximately 5% of students in public schools are identified as suffering from a learning disorder. Nearly 40% of those students drop out of school.

192. **(A)** Most commonly, enuresis occurs in otherwise normal boys. Enuresis is more common in boys than in girls. There is no increased prevalence of enuresis in children with mental retardation, autistic disorder, or OCD.

193. **(E)** Children with enuresis often have a family history of the disorder. Nocturnal enuresis is much more common than diurnal enuresis. Enuresis is not associated with nightmares or being hungry, and does not occur more frequently on weekends or on vacations. Although only a small percentage of children who wet their beds have an abnormality of the urinary tract, the occurrence of a defect must be ruled out.

194. **(D)** Imipramine, a TCA, is the standard agent used in the pharmacologic treatment of enuresis. Methylphenidate is commonly used in the treatment of attention deficit disorder, paroxetine is an SSRI, trazodone is an antidepressant most often used for insomnia, and benztropine is used to prevent extrapyramidal symptoms caused by neuroleptic use.

195. **(C)** The prevalence of ADHD is estimated at 3 to 5% in school-age children.

196. **(D)** The most common adverse effects of methylphenidate and other stimulant medications include insomnia, decreased appetite, weight loss, dysphoria, and irritability. Tremor, hypotension, weight gain, and liver toxicity are not common.

197. **(E)** Stimulant medications such as methylphenidate are effective in diminishing symptoms of ADHD in approximately 70% of patients.

198. **(D)** ADHD persists into adulthood in approximately 50% of cases.

199. **(C)** Since the birth of the baby, the parents have probably spent a lot of time tending to the new baby's needs and paying less attention to their daughter. The girl may feel rejected, jealous, and angry. The most helpful approach is for the mother to spend time alone with her daughter every day, giving her undivided attention and showing her that she is still loved and wanted. The girl is unlikely to be reassured by a single discussion about how the baby needs more attention than she does. Being consistently irritable, angry, and violent is not normal behavior at 20 months or at 24 months. The girl's behavior should not be ignored.

200. **(A)** A developmentally normal child can copy a circle at the age of 2. She can tell her age and gender and ride a tricycle at age 3. She can copy a square and can identify her left hand at age 5.

201. **(D)** This boy's behavior is characteristic of autistic disorder. He suffers from impaired social interactions and attachments, restricted interests and behaviors, and impaired communication. He does not object to going with a stranger to the examining room, does not interact with the physician, becomes preoccupied with a toy to an abnormal degree, and screams when the toy is taken away. He is not primarily negativistic and hostile as in oppositional defiant disorder. He is not aggressive, destructive, deceitful, or in violation of rules, as in conduct disorder. He does not become upset when separated from his mother, as in separation anxiety disorder.

202. **(D)** Children with autistic disorder have more favorable prognoses if they are able to converse meaningfully, rather than unable to interact positively with others. They are often easily toilet trained, often enjoy mechanical toys, are rigidly organized in their play, and may become preoccupied with the rhythm or beat of music. These characteristics are not associated with a good prognosis.

203. **(A)** Hypercholesterolemia is common in anorexia nervosa. Other findings associated with the starvation state are mild normocytic normochromic anemia and leukopenia. Hypercarotenemia, causing yellowing of the skin, may be seen if many carrots are eaten in an attempt to satisfy the appetite with a low-calorie food. TSH is not typically altered. If vomiting is induced, hypokalemia, hypochloremia, and metabolic alkalosis may be seen.

204. **(E)** During anorexia nervosa, the body is in a state of starvation and, as a result, most bodily functions are suppressed. The resting energy expenditure is decreased, there is a sinus bradycardia, serum estrogen levels are low in females, and serum testosterone levels are low in males. Brain imaging may show an increase in ventricular–brain ratios secondary to starvation.

205. **(D)** The most effective treatment of anorexia nervosa is the combination of pharmacologic and psychotherapeutic modalities, using fluoxetine and individual psychotherapy. Either pharmacologic treatment or psychotherapeutic treatment alone is not as effective as the combination of the two. For adolescents with anorexia nervosa, individual psychotherapy is more helpful than family therapy.

206. **(E)** Stranger anxiety occurs as part of normal child development and is evidence of the development of a strong bond of attachment. It does not suggest that a parent is inattentive; it usually appears by 7 to 8 months and generally resolves with time. Typically, stranger anxiety is stronger toward completely unknown persons than to those who are more familiar. Autistic children lack this developmental marker. Because stranger anxiety at this age is developmentally appropriate, this boy cannot be diagnosed with separation anxiety disorder and is not overly attached to his mother.

207. **(B)** Bonding is believed to begin in the immediate postdelivery period. However, the slow-growing attachment between an infant and his or her caretakers occurs with ongoing interaction over time and does not require contact in the perinatal period. Attachment occurs in the face of many obstacles, including sensory deficit, maltreatment, and physical disabilities on both sides.

208. **(A)** Schizophrenia, paranoid type, is the most likely diagnosis due to the frequency of the auditory hallucinations without prominent disorganization or inappropriate affect, as seen in disorganized type, or motor abnormalities, as seen in catatonic type. Criteria for paranoid type are met, so this is not an undifferentiated type. Hallucinations are not present in residual type.

209. **(C)** The very early onset of schizophrenia, before the age of 10, is rare and is associated with a poor outcome. A better outcome is associated with more affective symptoms, acute onset, older age at onset, good premorbid functioning, well-differentiated symptoms, and lack of a family history of schizophrenia.

210. **(D)** Children with ADHD often suffer from low self-esteem, while children with mania are more likely to be euphoric. Pressured speech, distractibility, motoric overactivity, and impulsivity are seen in children with both disorders.

211. **(C)** Rett's disorder occurs exclusively in girls. ADHD, conduct disorder, Tourette's disorder, and Asperger's disorder are seen more commonly in boys.

212. **(D)** Typically, children are 7 or 8 years old when they begin to understand the irreversibility of death. In order to understand that death is irreversible, a child must be aware of the continuity of time, be able to fantasize, and have a solid sense of his or her own individuality. Usually, this level of maturity is achieved between the ages of 6 and 10.

213. **(D)** This boy is displaying regression, a defense mechanism in which there is an attempt to return to an earlier developmental phase in order to avoid the tension and conflict at the present level of development (e.g., distress over the grandmother's death). Repression is a defense mechanism in which an idea or feeling is expelled or withheld from consciousness. Acting out is a defense mechanism in which an unconscious wish or impulse is expressed through action to avoid an accompanying affect. Denial is a defense mechanism in which the awareness of a painful aspect of reality is avoided by negating sensory data. Blocking is a defense mechanism in which a thought, impulse, or affect is transiently inhibited, causing tension or distress.

214. **(A)** Sedation is a frequent adverse effect of clonidine upon initiating treatment. With continued treatment, the sedation usually subsides. Dry mouth is a less common adverse effect. Hypotension is a rare adverse effect. In general, tremor and nausea are not seen.

215. **(B)** Stimulants are the most commonly used medication in the treatment of ADHD, but they can unmask tic disorders. TCAs are as effective as stimulants and are the first-line treatment for patients with ADHD and co-morbid tics. They are also used when there is a significant family history of the disorder. SSRIs may be used to augment treatment in some cases. MAOIs and neuroleptics are not used for ADHD.

216. **(E)** The finding of multiple fractures, especially when they are of different ages, is a red flag for physical abuse. Even though the boy may be scared to report what happened for fear of punishment, it is important to try to talk with him alone and find out as much information as possible. It is not appropriate to refer the boy to an orthopedist or his pediatrician prior to investigating the possibility of physical abuse. Recommending limited sports or extra vitamins does not address the question of whether the boy is safe at home.

217. **(D)** The most appropriate advice is that the mother should help her son return the toys. The boy is in a developmental period when his conscience is being established, and the parental model is important. The parent can show the child how to act responsibly by helping him return the toys himself. At the age of 4, a child cannot adequately grasp the abstract concept of stealing, so punishment would not be helpful. His sense of time is limited, so he cannot integrate the idea of a reward after a week.

218. **(D)** SSRIs such as sertraline are effective in the treatment of panic disorder. Mood stabilizers, such as valproate and carbamazepine, and antipsychotics, such as risperidone and clozapine, are not indicated for the treatment of panic disorder.

219. **(B)** Identification is the process of adopting other people's characteristics. Identification with a parent is important in personality formation. This girl's behavior may occur as an attempt to imitate the doctor because she admires her, or it may represent an effort to

cope with anxiety about the doctor because she fears her. Reaction formation is a defense mechanism in which an unacceptable impulse is transformed into its opposite. Displacement is a defense mechanism in which emotions are shifted from one idea or object to another that resembles the original but evokes less distress. Rationalization is a defense mechanism in which rational explanations are offered in an attempt to justify unacceptable attitudes, beliefs, or behaviors. Dissociation is a defense mechanism in which a person's character or sense of identity is temporarily but drastically modified in order to avoid emotional distress.

220. **(A)** When the mother is infected with rubella during the first month of the pregnancy, the risk of congenital defects is 50%. The risk of defects decreases inversely with the duration of pregnancy at the time of disease.

221. **(A)** In all jurisdictions in the United States, clinicians are required to report all cases of suspected child abuse. The law does not leave the issue to the clinician's discretion.

222. **(A)** This boy's history is most consistent with selective mutism. He does not speak at school but continues to talk at home. Consistent failure to speak in a specific social situation despite speaking in other situations is not characteristic of MDD, separation anxiety disorder, social phobia, or dysthymic disorder.

223. **(D)** The mother is most commonly the perpetrator of intentionally producing physical or psychological symptoms in her child in order to assume the sick role by proxy. The victim is usually a preschool child, and an Axis I diagnosis of physical abuse of a child may be appropriate.

224. **(C)** This patient does not exhibit the hallmark psychotic symptoms, such as hallucinations, prominent delusions, or disorganized thoughts or speech, necessary for a diagnosis of schizophrenia. A patient must be at least 18 years old to have a diagnosis of antisocial personality disorder, although symptoms must have been present since age 15. The persistent pattern of behavior that violates the basic rights of others makes a diagnosis of conduct disorder more appropriate than that of oppositional defiant disorder, which describes a milder, less offensive pattern of hostile/negativistic behavior of milder nature. This patient does not present with age-inappropriate difficulty with sustaining attention or concentration, forgetfulness, organizing tasks, or hyperactivity, thus making a diagnosis of ADHD unlikely.

225. **(D)** DSM-IV-TR criteria for antisocial personality disorder requires evidence of a conduct disorder before the age of 15. No other personality disorder requires a previous diagnosis of conduct disorder. In addition, there is no evidence of a reduced capacity for close relationships or eccentric behavior, making a diagnosis of schizotypal personality disorder unlikely. Recurrent suicidal behavior or an identity disturbance is a common finding in borderline personality disorder, and there is no evidence of excessive attention-seeking behavior, thus making histrionic personality disorder unlikely.

226. **(E)** All of the listed disorders have comorbidity with conduct disorder and must be considered in the diagnosis.

227. **(F)** When children with pica eat soil or feces, eggs of *Toxocara canis* or *cati* may be ingested, causing visceral larva migrans. The other disorders are not associated with behavior likely to include ingestion of parasite eggs.

228. **(B)** Bulimia nervosa is seen in 1 to 3% of adolescent girls and young women. In the purging type of disorder, repeated vomiting can produce fluid and electrolyte abnormalities, most frequently hypokalemia, hyponatremia, and hypochloremia. Metabolic alkalosis may occur as well. The other disorders are not associated with hypokalemia.

229. **(C)** One of the presentations of stereotypic movement disorder is self-inflicted bodily in-

jury that is severe enough to require medical attention. An individual's repetitive motor behavior may cause chronic rectal bleeding severe enough to lead to anemia. The other disorders are not associated with rectal bleeding.

230. **(H)** Adolescents with conduct disorder often abuse substances, including alcohol, marijuana, and cocaine. The other disorders are not as often associated with substance abuse.

Rett's disorder is characterized by normal prenatal and perinatal development, normal head circumference at birth, and normal psychomotor development through the first 5 months of life. Between the ages of 5 months and 48 months, there is deceleration of head growth, loss of hand skills with development of stereotyped hand movements such as hand wringing, loss of social interaction (which may improve later), appearance of poorly coordinated gait or trunk movements, and severely impaired expressive and receptive language development with severe psychomotor retardation. To date, Rett's disorder has been observed only in females. Patients suffering from social phobia demonstrate a marked and persistent fear of a social or performance situation with exposure causing intense anxiety, expressed as a tantrum or a panic attack. Separation anxiety disorder is characterized by developmentally inappropriate and excessive anxiety concerning separation from the home or from those to whom the individual is attached. Enuresis refers to bedwetting. In panic disorder, there are discrete panic attacks, periods of intense fear or discomfort with physical manifestations such as palpitations and subjective difficulty breathing. Asperger's disorder is a particular type of autism most commonly seen in boys.

231. **(E)** Palpitations, chest pain, shortness of breath, and diaphoresis commonly occur during panic attacks. These symptoms do not occur routinely in any of the other disorders.

232. **(G)** Hypotension, bradycardia, and lanugo hair are classic sequelae of starvation seen in anorexia nervosa. These signs are not associated with any of the other disorders.

233. **(A)** Chapped hands and other dermatologic problems are often present in OCD due to excessive washing with water or caustic cleaning agents. Chapped hands are not specifically associated with any of the other disorders.

234. **(J)** Trichotillomania usually occurs around ages 5 to 8 or age 13. The repeated pulling out of hair results in decreased or complete loss of hair in a specific area. The scalp, eyebrows, and eyelashes are the sites most commonly involved. Patches of baldness are not associated with any of the other disorders.

Pica is the eating of nonnutritional substances such as dirt or paint. Hypochondriasis is the preoccupation that one has a serious disease based on misinterpretation of symptoms, despite appropriate medical evaluation and reassurance. Eye tics such as blinking and eye rolling are the most common initial symptoms in Tourette's disorder. Facial tics such as grimacing or licking movements and vocal tics such as throat clearing or grunting are the next most common initial symptoms. Whole-body tics, such as body rocking or pelvic thrusting, and self-abusive tics, such as hitting, may develop later. Asperger's disorder is a pervasive developmental disorder characterized by impairments in social interactions and the development of stereotyped or repetitive patterns of behaviors without significant delay in language skills or cognitive function. Asperger's occurs more commonly in males and is commonly referred to as a "high functioning" autism. A DSM-IV-TR diagnosis of pyromania requires several criteria, including deliberate and purposeful fire setting and tension or affective arousal before the act, which is not better accounted for by conduct disorder, a manic episode, or antisocial personality disorder.

CHAPTER 4

Adult Psychopathology
Questions

R. Andrew Chambers, MD, and Blake Taggart, MD

DIRECTIONS (Questions 235 through 378): Each of the numbered items or incomplete statements in this section is followed by answers or by completions of the statement. Select the ONE lettered answer or completion that is BEST in each case.

Questions 235 through 238

A 22-year-old single white man is referred to you for a one-year history of strange behavior characterized by talking to the television, accusing local police of bugging his room, and carrying on conversations with himself. His mother also describes a 3- to 4-year history of progressive withdrawal from social activities. The patient dropped out of college in his final year, and since then has been living in his room at home. Attempts to hold a job as a busboy at a local restaurant and as a night janitor have abruptly ended after disputes with the employers.

235. How prevalent is this patient's illness in the general population?

(A) 0.1%
(B) 0.5%
(C) 1.0%
(D) 3.0%
(E) 5.0%

236. The monozygotic (identical) twin concordance for this patients illness is

(A) 10%
(B) 25%
(C) 50%
(D) 100%
(E) the same incidence as in the general population

237. Which substance would this patient be most likely to abuse?

(A) alcohol
(B) cannabis
(C) tobacco
(D) cocaine
(E) lysergic acid diethylamide (LSD)

238. In which brain region is this patient most likely to have abnormal findings on magnetic resonance imaging (MRI)?

(A) hippocampus
(B) occipital lobe
(C) parietal lobe
(D) cingulate gyrus
(E) basal ganglia

Questions 239 and 240

A patient reports to you that for the past week or two he has had the belief that his intestines and his heart have been removed. When asked about his lack of "getting out in the world," he responds, "What world? There is no world!"

239. This aspect of the patient's illness would best be referred to as

(A) schizoaffective disorder
(B) Capgras syndrome
(C) folie à deux
(D) Cotard syndrome
(E) major depression

240. If this patient consistently reported to you the belief that his mother and father have been replaced by "cyborg alien robots" that look identical to his parents, this would be most indicative of

(A) delusional disorder

(B) Capgras syndrome

(C) folie à deux

(D) Cotard syndrome

(E) simple schizophrenia (simple deteriorative disorder)

Questions 241 through 244

An 18-year-old woman without a history of psychiatric illness has recently started her freshman year of college. The woman is brought to a psychiatric emergency department after being found on the roof of her dormitory dressed only in her underwear, despite below freezing temperatures. The campus police who bring her in report that she appeared to be dancing in a disorganized and agitated fashion, speaking angrily to someone that was not apparent to them, and accused the policemen of being "Satan's horsemen" and "adulterers from the Court of King Herod." On psychiatric exam she reports to you that "Lucifer is telling me I'm an angel of death. He told me to flap my wings and soar to my death."

241. Which of the following personality disorders is the least similar to her Axis I diagnosis?

(A) schizotypal

(B) schizoid

(C) antisocial

(D) borderline

(E) paranoid

242. A careful history is obtained. Her roommates report that for the past 5 weeks the patient has been delusional, mostly with religious or persecutory content, and her thoughts seem disorganized. The most appropriate diagnosis at this time would be

(A) schizophreniform disorder

(B) schizophrenia, paranoid type

(C) psychotic disorder not otherwise specified

(D) brief psychotic disorder

(E) delusional disorder, paranoid type

243. Which of the following statements about schizophrenia is true?

(A) Schizophrenic patients are generally higher functioning in the community than mood disorder patients.

(B) Onset of the disorder seldom seems to have been precipitated by an environmental change or social stressor.

(C) Onset of the disorder has been linked in many cases to the use of psychoactive substances.

(D) Positive symptoms usually precede the development of negative symptoms.

(E) More than 50% of patients with schizophrenia are able to live productive lives.

244. In talking with this patient's family you would be most likely to gather a history of

(A) low intelligence

(B) head trauma

(C) progressive social withdrawal

(D) a neglectful mother

(E) physical or sexual abuse

Questions 245 through 251

In performing a mental status exam on a 26-year-old male graduate student, you make the following notes: The patient is poorly oriented to time and place, is dressed in pink bathroom slippers, and is wearing only a trench coat. He reports auditory hallucinations and fears that his classmates are conspiring to embarrass him in front of his teachers.

245. Which of the following would make a diagnosis of new onset/first-break schizophrenia unlikely?

(A) auditory hallucinations

(B) age 26 years

(C) inappropriate dress

(D) bizarre mannerisms

(E) poor orientation

246. His fears about his classmates represent what phenomenon?

(A) formication

(B) trichotillomania

(C) ideas of reference

(D) reaction formation

(E) hallucinations

247. This patient is most likely to exhibit which of the following?

(A) elective mutism

(B) tactile hallucinations

(C) catatonia

(D) flattened affect

(E) hyperactivity

248. Abnormalities in which of the following would be least likely to be correlated to the course of schizophrenia?

(A) dopaminergic system

(B) amygdala

(C) mesolimbic tract

(D) serotonergic system

(E) acetylcholine system

249. Which of the following is the best statement regarding schizophrenia?

(A) Auditory, visual, and tactile hallucinations are experienced with equal frequency.

(B) There is no increased incidence of schizotypal personality disorder in family members of affected individuals.

(C) It is frequently difficult to tell the difference between the flattened affect often seen in schizophrenia and the parkinsonian side effects of antipsychotic medicines.

(D) Nontwin siblings of schizophrenics have the same risk of developing schizophrenia as does the general population.

250. If, while you are performing a Mental Status Exam (MSE), the patient stands uncomfortably close to you as you talk to him, this would most likely be an example of

(A) formication

(B) flight of ideas

(C) circumstantiality

(D) ideas of reference

(E) loss of ego boundaries

251. If, in the course of this patient's chronic mental illness, he becomes jobless, homeless, and destitute, the history would exemplify which concept?

(A) stress-diathesis model

(B) drift hypothesis

(C) sometimes intolerable side effects of antipsychotic drugs

(D) socioeconomic burden of schizophrenia

(E) Bleuler's classical model of schizophrenia

252. A 36-year-old patient you have seen twice is brought to your walk-in department by family members. On previous occasions, he presented with delusions, hallucinations, and prominent negative symptoms. During the visit, he exhibits motoric, waxy flexibility and resistance to all instructions. He methodically repeats words and phrases and appears to crudely mimic your movements. The most likely diagnosis is

(A) elective mutism

(B) malingering

(C) schizophrenia, disorganized type

(D) schizophrenia, catatonic type

(E) drug-induced psychosis

253. A 49-year-old bank teller without a psychiatric history is referred to your office for the first time by her internist for an evaluation. For the past 2 months, she has been increasingly convinced that a well-known pop music star is in love with her and that they have had an ongoing affair. She is well groomed, and there is no evidence of thought disorder or hallucinations. Her husband reveals that she has been functioning well at work and in other social relationships. Which of the following is the most likely diagnosis?

(A) delusional disorder
(B) acute reactive psychosis
(C) prodromal schizophrenia
(D) paranoid personality disorder
(E) schizophreniform disorder

254. Which of the following is true regarding schizophrenia?

(A) There is an increased homicidal risk compared to the general population.
(B) There is an increased suicidal risk compared to the general population.
(C) There is not an increased risk to abuse substances compared to the general population.
(D) There is no increased risk for development of mood disorders compared with members of the general population.

255. Negative symptoms of schizophrenia

(A) include affective lability
(B) are more prominent than positive symptoms in the prodromal phase of the illness
(C) do not include autistic features
(D) usually become milder over the course of the illness
(E) are easily distinguished from depressive illness

256. Positive symptoms of schizophrenia

(A) include apathy and social withdrawal
(B) are more responsive to antipsychotic medications than are negative symptoms

(C) Remain stable over the course of the illness
(D) are easily distinguished from delirium
(E) include hallucinations

Questions 257 through 265

A 46-year-old divorced, middle-class, African-American woman is admitted to your inpatient psychiatric ward after a suicide attempt by overdosing on Tylenol. She has a history of multiple psychiatric hospitalizations with similar presentations. She has been unable to work due to her depression and has lost interest in activities she once enjoyed. Additionally, the patient reports a 2-week history of decreased sleep, difficulty concentrating, low energy, hopelessness, and a decreased appetite.

257. The symptom reported by this patient that is necessary to diagnose a major depressive episode is

(A) decreased sleep
(B) decreased energy
(C) loss of interest in activities
(D) suicidal thoughts
(E) hopelessness

258. Which of the following factors would influence you to recommend electroconvulsive therapy (ECT)?

(A) severe, melancholic depression and history of poor response to medications
(B) severe adverse reactions to all serotonin-specific reuptake inhibitors (SSRIs), tricyclic antidepressants (TCAs), and continued suicidal ideation
(C) known history of psychotic symptoms in the context of her depressive symptoms
(D) known history of bipolar illness
(E) poor compliance with medications

259. Lifetime prevalence rates for major depression in the general population are approximately

(A) 1%
(B) 5%
(C) 15%

(D) 25%

(E) 35%

260. The most important diagnosis to rule out in this patient before administering an antidepressant medication would be

(A) panic disorder

(B) bipolar disorder

(C) obsessive–compulsive disorder (OCD)

(D) drug-induced depressive disorder

(E) malingering

261. If the patient were prescribed the following medications, which would you suggest discontinuing based on her diagnosis of depression?

(A) atenolol

(B) cimetidine

(C) warfarin

(D) phenytoin

(E) erythromycin

262. Which of the following substances would you expect to contribute to this patient's current symptoms?

(A) LSD

(B) caffeine

(C) peyote

(D) tobacco

(E) cocaine

263. Which of the following conditions, if present, can help in differentiating between major depression and atypical depression?

(A) hypersomnia

(B) anxiety

(C) onset after age 50

(D) no identifiable stressor

(E) increased energy

264. Which of the following factors increases this patient's risk for major depression?

(A) her race

(B) her marital status

(C) her socioeconomic class

(D) her religion

(E) a family history of panic disorder

265. Prior to developing depression, this woman's lifetime risk of being afflicted with depression, compared to a male, is

(A) half

(B) double

(C) the same

(D) triple

(E) one third

Questions 266 through 270

A 34-year-old white man complains of "feeling blue" at his first visit to you. MSE reveals disheveled appearance, a depressed mood, psychomotor retardation, and suicidal thoughts. Thought processes are significant for thought blocking and some slowing. Deficits with remote and short-term memory are noted. Judgment and insight are also impaired. Your diagnosis is a major depressive episode.

266. The type of sleep disturbance you would most expect to see in this patient is

(A) sleeping too deeply (difficulty being awakened)

(B) early morning awakening

(C) increased REM (rapid-eye movement sleep) stage latency

(D) decreased response to sedative drugs

(E) sleeping too lightly (awakened too easily)

267. This patient's memory problems would most likely be attributed to which of the following?

(A) dementia

(B) pseudodementia

(C) concurrent substance abuse

(D) associated neuroendocrine abnormalities

(E) learned helplessness

268. This patient's affect, if consistent with a diagnosis of major depressive episode, would most likely be expected to be

   (A) blunted
   (B) labile
   (C) anxious
   (D) guarded
   (E) bizarre

269. You would expect the biochemical/hormonal profile of this patient to be significant for

   (A) increased catecholamine activity
   (B) increased cortisol secretion
   (C) increased sex hormones
   (D) increased immune functions
   (E) decreased monoamine oxidase (MAO) activity

270. The cognitive model of depression, based on Aaron Beck's triad, is characterized by which of the following?

   (A) negative self-view, negative cognition, negative input from society
   (B) negative self-view, negative interpretation of experience, negative superego
   (C) negative id, negative interpretation of experience, negative view of the future
   (D) negative self-view, negative interpretation of experience, negative view of the future
   (E) negative id, ego, and superego

271. A patient diagnosed with major depression has a lifetime suicide risk of

   (A) 1%
   (B) 5%
   (C) 35%
   (D) 25%
   (E) 15%

272. A patient with dysthymia differs from a patient with major depression in which of the following ways?

   (A) lack of depressed mood
   (B) lack of anhedonia

   (C) presence of concurrent thyroid illness
   (D) meeting fewer major depression criteria
   (E) having atypical depression features

273. Major depression may present in a similar manner to

   (A) antisocial personality disorder
   (B) bereavement
   (C) dysphoria
   (D) psychogenic fugue
   (E) hypnagogic phenomena

274. The term *double depression* refers to which of the following?

   (A) two back-to-back depressive episodes with less than a week in between
   (B) two depressive episodes with no intervening manic illness
   (C) extremely severe depression
   (D) shared depressive disorder
   (E) a major depressive episode following or superimposed on a dysthymia

275. *Kindling* refers to

   (A) the relevance of childhood experience to that of the adult
   (B) the interplay between id and superego
   (C) the process by which a psychotic decompensation begins
   (D) the theory that one decompensation increases the risk for another, worse decompensation
   (E) a theory of Jung's about the importance of young childhood schooling

276. Which of the following choices is true about postpartum depression?

   (A) is more likely to occur in later pregnancies
   (B) can have psychotic features
   (C) occurs at equal rates in women with previous psychiatric/mood illness
   (D) is not dangerous to the child
   (E) is rarely as severe as major depression

Questions 277 through 282

A 52-year-old man with a history of major depression is treated with paroxetine (Paxil). He has been your patient for 2 years and has recently missed his last two appointments, reporting to you that "I've been spectacular!" You have documented two calls from his wife since his last visit. She initially reported that her husband has been "very different." You learn that he has spent more money on frivilous items than he ever has. In addition, when she went to the bank to withdraw money for groceries she was told that the account was overdrawn. Recently, his wife called again to make an appointment for her husband. She reports that one moment her husband is giddy and without notice he quickly becomes agitated and angry.

During the interview the patient questions your credentials and accuses you of being more loyal to his wife than to him. Most of the interview is spent interrupting the patient as you try to decipher his rapid speech.

277. This patient's affect would best be described as

(A) expansive and irritable
(B) guarded and suspicious
(C) labile and dysphoric
(D) euphoric and bizarre
(E) euthymic

278. His speech would best be described as

(A) uninterruptible
(B) pressured
(C) hypermotoric
(D) agitated
(E) tangential

279. Which of the following statements is true?

(A) Patients with bipolar disorder usually have a more favorable course than depressive patients.
(B) A lower percentage of patients with bipolar disorder eventually get treatment as compared to patients with unipolar depression.
(C) Bipolar disorder has a stronger genetic link than patients with depression.

(D) More women are diagnosed with bipolar disorder than with major depression.
(E) Bipolar disorder is more common than major depression in the Northern Hemisphere.

280. Features in this patient most suggestive of mania are

(A) lack of need for sleep, grandiosity, irritability
(B) sexual indiscretions, prominent mood swings, substance abuse
(C) substance abuse, lack of need for sleep, grandiosity
(D) prominent mood swing, lack of need for sleep, irritability
(E) irritability, excessive spending, substance abuse

The patient returns for a follow-up visit 4 weeks after you initiate treatment with valproic acid. He presents looking irritable and demonstrates pressured speech and grandiose delusions. He reports that he is the lost son of a famed millionaire. He exhibits symptoms of depression characterized by decreased sleep, poor appetite and concentration, and thoughts of suicide. He admits to drinking alcohol every day since his last visit. His wife reports that his moods seem to change with the seasons.

281. In addition to starting valproic acid, the other pharmacologic management change indicated at the prior visit would have been to

(A) check the patient's serum paroxetine level
(B) select a more effective antidepressant
(C) stop the antidepressant
(D) select a medication as needed for insomnia
(E) start lithium

282. The most likely diagnosis at this time for this patient is

(A) hypomania
(B) seasonal affective disorder (SAD)
(C) mixed episode
(D) rapid cycling
(E) bipolar II disorder

283. Features of hypomania that differentiate it from mania are

(A) concurrent depressive symptoms and/or need for hospitalization for safety
(B) lack of psychotic features and/or lack of impairment in social functioning
(C) need for hospitalization for safety and/or less sleep impairment
(D) lack of psychotic features and/or lack of hypersexuality
(E) concurrent depressive symptoms and/or impairment in social functioning

Questions 284 through 286

284. A patient places a call after hours to the practice you are covering. You do not have access to the patient's chart but learn that the history suggests the patient experiences dysthymia followed by episodes of hypomania. In making a decision about the patient's medication you quickly recognize the diagnosis. Which of the following choices best categorizes the patient's diagnosis?

(A) bipolar II disorder
(B) bipolar I disorder
(C) cyclothymia
(D) bipolar III disorder
(E) double depression

285. The prevalence of bipolar illness in the general population is approximately

(A) 1%
(B) 5%
(C) 25%
(D) 35%
(E) 15%

286. On a subsequent visit, the patient brings his brother to your office. His brother asks what his risk of developing bipolar illness is. You answer

(A) the same as anyone in the general population
(B) 25%
(C) 10%
(D) 1%
(E) the answer is unknown

Questions 287 through 292

A 26-year-old white woman presents to a psychiatric emergency department in an acutely distressed, nervous state. Emergency department staff are unable to calm her down or gain an adequate history from the patient. She complains of "terrible anxiety." She is slightly diaphoretic, tachycardic, and pupils are mildly dilated. She is on no medications.

287. The cause of anxiety important to rule out in this patient is

(A) cocaine-induced
(B) hypochondriasis
(C) serotonin syndrome
(D) specific phobia
(E) LSD-induced

288. Abdominal pain in this patient might cause you to investigate

(A) blood alcohol level
(B) acetaminophen level
(C) urinary porphobilinogen
(D) urine toxicology screen
(E) serum catecholamine metabolites

289. If the patient suffered from panic disorder, she would likely describe symptoms of

(A) fear that someone is stalking her
(B) fear of a specific situation or object
(C) fear that she was having a heart attack
(D) exaggerated startle response
(E) fears about infection or uncleanliness

290. If the patient suffered from posttraumatic stress disorder (PTSD), her presentation would likely include

(A) fear that someone is stalking her
(B) fear of a specific situation or object
(C) fear that she was having a heart attack
(D) exaggerated startle response
(E) fears about infection or uncleanliness

291. If the patient suffered from OCD, her presentation would likely include

(A) fear that someone is stalking her
(B) fear of a specific situation or object
(C) fear that she was having a heart attack
(D) exaggerated startle response
(E) fears about infection or uncleanliness

292. Given her present state, one would expect which area of this patient's brain to be hyperactive at this time?

(A) locus ceruleus
(B) hippocampus
(C) thalamus
(D) amygdala
(E) basal ganglia

Questions 293 through 302

A 46-year-old man is admitted to the emergency department acutely diaphoretic, tachycardic, hypertensive, tremulous, and agitated. He refuses to give a urine sample for toxicology studies. He is apparently hallucinating, judging from his insistence that he be allowed to "squash those bugs on the wall," of which there are none.

293. One would expect to most likely see this patient's type of hallucinations in the context of

(A) delirium
(B) delusional disorders
(C) schizophrenia
(D) conversion disorder
(E) brief psychotic disorder

294. You are most worried about withdrawal from which of the following drugs of abuse in this patient?

(A) heroin
(B) alcohol
(C) LSD
(D) cocaine
(E) crack

295. You get a report from a family member of the patient that he "has been living off booze and drugs and nothing else for weeks." The emergency department nurse is about to go in to draw blood from the patient and offer him food. The most important thing to do next for this patient is

(A) be sure liver function tests are included in the blood draw
(B) listen for a murmur
(C) administer lorazepam (Ativan) prophylactically for probable agitation
(D) administer thiamine
(E) get a vitamin B_{12} level

296. In general, more severe drug withdrawal syndromes are seen with

(A) drugs with short half-lives
(B) drugs with long half-lives
(C) drugs that are more lipophilic
(D) drugs that are less lipophilic
(E) intravenous drugs

297. In general, drugs of abuse are more popular if they

(A) cross the blood–brain barrier
(B) have antidepressant effects
(C) have a shorter onset of action
(D) have a longer onset of action
(E) can be smoked

298. Alcohol withdrawal is usually treated in the medical setting with

(A) benzodiazepines
(B) barbiturates
(C) clonidine
(D) phenytoin
(E) disulfiram

299. In sudden alcohol intake reduction or abstinence, which of the following is usually seen last chronologically?

(A) withdrawal tremulousness
(B) seizures
(C) confabulation
(D) delirium tremens
(E) disinhibition

300. In a patient with alcoholism in whom you suspect impaired liver function, the most appropriate drug to treat withdrawal symptoms is

(A) phenobarbital (Luminal)
(B) chlordiazepoxide (Librium)
(C) lorazepam (Ativan)
(D) alprazolam (Xanax)
(E) clonidine (Catapres)

301. On neurologic exam, the above patient is found to have nystagmus, confusion, and ataxia. The most likely diagnosis is

(A) Wernicke's encephalopathy
(B) alcoholic cerebellar degeneration
(C) subacute combined degeneration
(D) alcoholic peripheral neuropathy
(E) Ménière's disease

302. In Korsakoff's dementia (alcohol-induced persisting amnestic disorder)

(A) the treatment is vitamin B_{12}
(B) one often sees focal neurologic signs
(C) lesions are seen in the mammillary bodies and thalamus
(D) confabulation is a rare finding
(E) Lewy bodies are often found

Questions 303 and 304

A 62-year-old woman presents to the nursing home where you work as a consulting psychiatrist. She has had a history of bilateral temporal lobectomy for an intractable seizure disorder. After a few weeks at the new facility, the staff report the following observations about the patient in addition to her short-term memory difficulties: She is extremely docile and displays very little emotion. She has a large appetite and compulsively puts both food and nonfood items in her mouth. She also displays sexual disinhibition, often walking out of her room without her pants on.

303. This patient's clinical condition is most consistent with

(A) Pick's disease
(B) Klüver–Bucy syndrome
(C) Arnold–Chiari syndrome
(D) punch-drunk syndrome
(E) Möbius syndrome

304. The loss of what temporal lobe structure is most closely associated with this condition?

(A) hippocampus
(B) insula
(C) superior temporal gyri
(D) amygdala
(E) inferior horn of the lateral ventricle

Questions 305 and 306

A 22-year-old woman is referred by her gynecologist for treatment of a possible eating disorder. The gynecologist informs you that the patient presented to him with a chief complaint of amenorrhea that had been present for 4 months. In addition, the patient is at 83% of her expected body weight. Upon evaluation, the patient describes a repeated pattern of bingeing on large meals, followed by forced vomiting. She also uses laxatives every night before she goes to bed "to prevent constipation." The patient reports that she had been running 3 miles every day, but in the last few weeks she has become too tired to run.

305. The most accurate diagnosis for this patient is

    (A) exercise-induced amenorrhea
    (B) OCD
    (C) psychogenic gastritis
    (D) anorexia nervosa
    (E) bulimia nervosa

306. Laboratory findings associated with severe cases of this disorder include

    (A) decreased serum cortisol levels
    (B) blunted thyroid-stimulating hormone (TSH) response to thyrotropin-releasing hormone (TRH)
    (C) polycythemia
    (D) low serum growth hormone
    (E) high serum blood urea nitrogen (BUN)

307. A 23-year-old college student has experienced frequent episodes of feeling utter doom for the past 3 months. During these episodes he also experiences tremulousness, sweating, dizziness, and tingling in his extremities. He reports experiencing these episodes at least once a week and is now becoming fearful of attending classes, lest he have an episode. The medication of choice for this condition is

    (A) alprazolam (Xanax)
    (B) fluoxetine (Prozac)
    (C) chlordiazepoxide (Librium)
    (D) phenelzine (Nardil)
    (E) valproic acid (Depakote)

Questions 308 and 309

A 34-year-old woman complains of a 3-month history of "feeling down" that has steadily worsened. After losing her job as a sales representative 1 month ago, she has been living with her parents and has not looked for work. The patient reports that she is unmotivated to do anything, even the things she used to enjoy. She says that "nothing really matters . . . I don't matter." She has been sleeping 10 to 14 hours a night and has no appetite. More than once she has pondered suicide as a possible escape route.

308. Given this patient's diagnosis, what is the likelihood that she would fail to suppress her cortisol levels in a dexamethasone suppression test?

    (A) 10%
    (B) 30%
    (C) 50%
    (D) 70%
    (E) 90%

309. What is the likelihood that she would have a blunted response of TSH to an administration of TRH?

    (A) 10%
    (B) 30%
    (C) 50%
    (D) 70%
    (E) 90%

310. A 37-year-old woman who works the night shift at a local grocery store taking inventory reports that her childhood and college years were uneventful, but happy. She spends most of her time alone when she is not at work. She does not venture out of her house, and her social contacts are limited to work-related interactions with coworkers. She is an avid plant lover, and she spends most of her free time taking care of her indoor plants. She reports that she is quite content with her life. The most accurate diagnosis for this patient is

    (A) agoraphobia
    (B) avoidant personality disorder
    (C) schizoid personality disorder
    (D) schizotypal personality disorder
    (E) autistic disorder

Questions 311 through 313

An 18-year-old pregnant HIV-positive white woman presents for treatment of heroin addiction. She reports using heroin for the last 8 months, with substantial efforts to quit for the last 4 months. She is now homeless and has recently been arrested for shoplifting.

311. Detoxification would be preferred in this case over long-term methadone treatment because of

    (A) the age of the patient
    (B) the patient's criminal record
    (C) the patient's HIV-positive status
    (D) the fact that patient has less than 1 year of heroin addiction
    (E) the patient's pregnancy

312. When considering methadone maintenance, it is important to discuss with the patient that

    (A) methadone may cause bone decay
    (B) methadone substantially reduces libido
    (C) methadone worsens dependence on heroin
    (D) effective treatment is likely to require more than 60 mg/day of methadone
    (E) methadone may cause Cushing syndrome

313. Methadone maintenance treatment outcomes generally do not include

    (A) reduction in criminal behavior
    (B) increases in employment
    (C) increases in school attendance
    (D) reduced risk of contracting HIV
    (E) increased risk of depression

314. A 42-year-old business executive presents for his first contact with a mental health provider. He reports that for the last 4 months he has been feeling depressed. His low energy level and poor motivation are affecting his job performance, and the CEO of his company advised him to "take a couple of weeks off." The patient reports that he started feeling down when his wife discovered that he was involved in his third extramarital affair. Since then, he has moved into a small apartment by himself. He is sleeping almost 12 hours every night, has a poor appetite, and is experiencing financial difficulty due to indiscriminate purchases. He laments the loss of his former self. He reports that he used to need only 4 to 5 hours of sleep and once was able to "party all night and work all day."

This case best illustrates an Axis I diagnosis of

    (A) bipolar I disorder
    (B) bipolar II disorder
    (C) major depressive disorder (MDD)
    (D) narcissistic personality disorder
    (E) impulse control disorder not otherwise specified

315. A 52-year-old woman who has been treated with medication for 3 years for a chronic mood disorder reports that although she feels well, she wonders if her medication is causing side effects. She complains of dry mouth, trouble urinating, and occasional dizziness when she gets out of bed. Which of the following medications is she most likely being prescribed?

    (A) fluoxetine (Prozac)
    (B) imipramine (Tofranil)
    (C) phenelzine (Nardil)
    (D) lithium
    (E) valproic acid (Depakote)

Questions 316 and 317

A 72-year-old man is brought in by his wife to your geriatric psychiatry clinic. The patient's wife is concerned about his progressive confusion over the last year. She is particularly distressed that he repeatedly asks the same questions throughout the day. She also notes that her husband has become increasingly unsteady on his feet and needs to use a walker when they go out. She wonders if these symptoms may be related to the meningitis he suffered from 3 years ago.

316. In order for you to make a diagnosis of normal pressure hydrocephalus (NPH), further investigation in this case would have to reveal

    (A) elevated opening pressure upon lumbar puncture
    (B) a history of incontinence
    (C) oculomotor difficulties
    (D) frontal release signs
    (E) perseveration

317. Neuroimaging with noncontrast computed tomography (CT) in this case of NPH is most likely to reveal

(A) dilated lateral ventricles

(B) normal ventricles

(C) frontal sulcal widening

(D) focal subcortical hypointensities

(E) cerebellar atrophy

Questions 318 through 321

A 48-year-old man has been drinking up to six beers per night during the week and up to 12 beers a night on the weekend. A year ago he had his driver's license suspended for drunk driving. His marriage is failing. Last month, he was diagnosed with a gastric ulcer as a result of alcohol consumption. He admits to an alcohol problem, and has tried to stop on numerous occasions. He finds that he experiences insomnia if he doesn't drink for more than 2 days.

318. The feature of this case that suggests alcohol dependence rather than alcohol abuse is

(A) the patient's inability to stop drinking despite knowledge of its harmful effects and his desire to quit

(B) the high quantity of alcohol consumed on a regular basis

(C) the patient's history of drunk driving

(D) the fact that the patient can't sleep if he doesn't drink

(E) a medical complication due to drinking

319. On laboratory examination, this patient is likely to have

(A) increased alanine aminotransferase (ALT) and aspartate aminotransferase (AST), with increased ALT/AST ratio

(B) decreased uric acid

(C) increased gamma-glutamyl transpeptidase (GGT)

(D) microcytic anemia

(E) decreased serum triglycerides

320. The comorbid condition least likely to be found in this patient is

(A) nicotine dependence

(B) generalized anxiety disorder

(C) MDD

(D) antisocial personality disorder

(E) OCD

321. A diagnosis of Wernicke's encephalopathy would be considered in this case if the patient demonstrated

(A) hyperreflexia, visual hallucinations, seizures

(B) headaches, expressive aphasia, hypersomnolence

(C) oculomotor disturbance, ataxia, confusion

(D) urinary incontinence, ataxia, dementia

(E) myoclonus, tactile hallucinations, aggression

322. A 26-year-old computer programmer without a past psychiatric history has been married for 4 years. His wife is expecting their first child. She reports that 3 months ago the patient became preoccupied with the idea that she became pregnant by another man. During this time, he began missing work and isolated himself in his bedroom. His affect has progressively become more blunted. Recently, he believes that his wife is carrying a child conceived by "extraterrestrial forces." He urged her to have an abortion and she refuses. The patient denies any history of substance abuse, and his recent medical evaluation was within normal limits. Which of the following is the most appropriate diagnosis?

(A) brief psychotic disorder

(B) delusional disorder

(C) psychosis not otherwise specified

(D) schizophreniform disorder

(E) schizophrenia

323. A 27-year-old woman was involved in a major automobile accident in which a friend, sitting next to her in the passenger seat, was killed. Since the accident, she has experienced recurrent thoughts of the accident and has recurrent nightmares each night. Lately, she is reluctant to drive and has chosen to ride a bus to work. When she does ride in the car as a passenger, she feels nervous and is overly concerned about the safety of her companion's driving. The most appropriate diagnosis for this patient is

(A) acute stress disorder

(B) adjustment disorder

(C) PTSD

(D) generalized anxiety disorder

(E) MDD

Questions 324 and 325

An 18-year-old woman diagnosed with schizophrenia presents to the psychiatric emergency department after a suicide attempt by carbon monoxide poisoning. Medical evaluation was noncontributory and a urine toxicology screen was negative. The patient reports that she sat in her mother's car with a glove stuck into the exhaust pipe, and eventually fell asleep awaiting death. She relates that she believes that she was personally responsible for the Holocaust and that she should therefore die in a similar way. The patient's mother reports that she has been refusing to take haloperidol for the past 3 weeks.

324. An aspect of this case that is most typical of the epidemiology of suicide and suicide attempts is that

(A) carbon monoxide poisoning is the most common form of suicide attempt

(B) the patient's age is the time of highest risk of death by suicide

(C) as in most cases of suicide, patients are most often psychotic or otherwise without capacity for decision making

(D) the patient survived the attempt

(E) the suicide attempt was completely unexpected

325. The lifetime risk of death by suicide in patients with schizophrenia is closest to

(A) 1%

(B) 5%

(C) 10%

(D) 30%

(E) 50%

326. A 27-year-old internal medicine resident is working in an outpatient clinic. He prefers the inpatient service and is unhappy most of the time he is there. Today, however, he is looking forward to his clinical work because one of his appointments is a follow-up visit for a single, attractive 31-year-old woman who is finishing her antibiotic regimen for treatment of pneumonia. The psychodynamic term for this doctor's response to his patient is best termed

(A) countertransference

(B) empathy

(C) identification

(D) projection

(E) transference

Questions 327 through 329

A 31-year-old woman was admitted to a psychiatric hospital after a failed suicide attempt by medication ingestion. Recently, she broke up with her boyfriend, whom she met in a bar 4 months ago. She is noted for episodes of mood lability, marked by feelings of depression, and anger directed toward the psychiatric resident who completed the rotation 5 days after her admission. When the resident left, she reported that she was having urges to cut her wrists. As the patient was nearing her discharge date, she reported that "all the staff hates me except for Dr. Johnson." Dr. Johnson, a medical student, had a recent difference of opinion with the nursing staff regarding the patient's discharge.

327. The single most appropriate diagnosis for this patient is

(A) psychotic disorder not otherwise specified

(B) major depressive disorder

(C) histrionic personality disorder

(D) cyclothymic disorder

(E) borderline personality disorder

328. The psychodynamic term best used to describe the patient's conflict is

(A) acting out

(B) externalization

(C) regression

(D) splitting

(E) sublimation

329. The outpatient treatment of choice for patients with the diagnosis illustrated in this case is

(A) antidepressant medications

(B) benzodiazepine medications

(C) mood stabilizer medications

(D) neuroleptics

(E) psychotherapy

Questions 330 and 331

A 34-year-old woman presents for treatment of her severe, medication-refractory, major depression. She is referred to you by her outpatient psychiatrist because of your expertise in ECT. After reviewing her past psychiatric history and interviewing the patient, you conclude that she should indeed have ECT.

330. In discussing the effects of ECT with the patient, you should relate that the most likely side effect may be

(A) amnesia

(B) anesthesia-related respiratory complications

(C) fractures from convulsions

(D) abnormal cardiac arrhythmias

(E) psychosis

331. You tell the patient to expect the best possible outcome, she is likely to require

(A) 2 treatments

(B) 4 treatments

(C) 10 treatments

(D) 20 treatments

(E) 40 treatments

Questions 332 and 333

A 38-year-old woman presents to your clinic telling you that she has had disturbing, recurrent thoughts about harming her 7-month-old infant. She imagines using a knife to stab her child. Since having these distressing thoughts, she has removed all sharp objects from her kitchen. Because of this, she has not been able to prepare meals at home and has chosen to buy fast food or take-out food for the family meals. She has not shared these thoughts with her husband.

332. The most accurate diagnosis for this condition is

(A) impulse control disorder not otherwise specified

(B) OCD

(C) obsessive–compulsive personality disorder

(D) psychosis not otherwise specified

(E) schizotypal personality disorder

333. The first-line pharmacotherapy for this condition is

(A) lorazepam (Ativan)

(B) benztropine (Cogentin)

(C) nortriptyline (Pamelor)

(D) haloperidol (Haldol)

(E) fluvoxamine (Luvox)

334. A 72-year-old woman presents to the emergency department from a nursing home. On physical exam she appears malnourished and dehydrated. The medical service initiates intravenous fluid replacement. On MSE, she is alert and oriented to person only. She reports that the president is "Lyndon B. Johnson." During the interview, the patient is easily distracted. She often forgets things shortly after she learns them. One hour later her MSE has improved, reporting the correct day, time, and place. However, she cannot remember why she is there. When asked about the current president she cannot remember his name but describes his appearance. She is able to perform serial sevens slowly but accurately without distraction. Based on the information in this case, the most appropriate diagnosis for this patient's presenting symptoms is

(A) amnestic disorder not otherwise specified

(B) cognitive disorder not otherwise specified

(C) delirium

(D) dementia not otherwise specified

(E) major depression

Questions 335 and 336

You are a research psychiatrist conducting a double-blind, placebo-controlled trial of a new antidepressant. You have enrolled 200 patients into the study, all of whom meet criteria for uncomplicated major depression. You plan to randomize 100 patients to a placebo medication, and the other 100 patients will be randomized to the experimental antidepressant.

335. Of the 100 patients taking the placebo, approximately how many patients would be expected to improve after 4 to 6 weeks?

(A) 5

(B) 10

(C) 30

(D) 50

(E) 70

336. Of the 100 patients taking the experimental antidepressant (assuming this drug is as efficacious as standard antidepressants), approximately how many patients would be expected to improve after 4 to 6 weeks?

(A) 10

(B) 30

(C) 50

(D) 70

(E) 90

Questions 337 and 338

A 24-year-old man is brought to the psychiatric emergency department by his parents. They report that he has been living with them since he dropped out of college a year ago. In the last few months, he has spent an increasing amount of time by himself in his room. Rather than look for employment, he is absorbed in doing crossword puzzles. The parents also report that in the last 2 months, their son's behavior has become increasingly bizarre. His sleep schedule has become disorganized, and he has started wearing his clothes inside out. They note that he makes strange gestures while at the dinner table. In addition, he has begun smiling for very long periods of time, although there is nothing to laugh at. At times, the patient does not respond to questions asked of him, and at other times, he simply repeats the questions.

337. The type of schizophrenia that best describes the presentation is

(A) catatonic type

(B) disorganized type

(C) paranoid type

(D) residual type

(E) undifferentiated

338. Recent epidemiologic trends concerning this type of schizophrenia are notable for

(A) increased prevalence compared to 35 years ago

(B) about the same prevalence compared to 35 years ago

(C) its being the most common subtype of schizophrenia

(D) decreased prevalence compared to 35 years ago

(E) its having an association with history of LSD use

339. A 32-year-old, single, successful Wall Street executive tells you that on the weekends he likes to visit a dominatrix. His regular, paid appointment with this person is described as humiliating and somewhat painful, but also very sexually arousing. He describes his life as otherwise normal. The best way to describe this case by *Diagnostic and Statistical Manual of Mental Disorders*, 4th edition, Text Revision (DSM-IV-TR) diagnostic criteria is

(A) fetishism

(B) frotteurism

(C) no diagnosis

(D) sexual masochism

(E) sexual sadism

340. Which of the following is the most common mental disorder in the United States?

(A) MDD

(B) dementia, Alzheimer's type

(C) generalized anxiety disorder

(D) schizophrenia

(E) phobias

Questions 341 through 343

A 28-year-old woman presents complaining of falling asleep during the day. She says this problem has been ongoing for 3 months. It has been interfering with her work as a telephone operator because she falls asleep two or three times a day while speaking with customers. At times, she finds herself falling asleep at her desk and she is awakened when her head hits the computer console in front of her. Oddly enough, she reports, this can happen when she becomes particularly stressed out as she is managing many calls. The patient also reports that this disturbance has not improved even though she is sure she sleeps 8 hours each night.

341. The most appropriate diagnosis for this case is

(A) circadian rhythm sleep disorder

(B) dyssomnia not otherwise specified

(C) narcolepsy

(D) nightmare disorder

(E) primary hypersomnia

342. The term used to describe the phenomenon of sudden loss of muscle tone associated with stressful situations is

(A) cataplexy

(B) catalepsy

(C) catatonia

(D) sleep jerks

(E) primary atonia

343. The most useful pharmacotherapy for this condition is

(A) lorazepam (Ativan) at bedtime

(B) bupropion (Wellbutrin)

(C) phenelzine (Nardil)

(D) methylphenidate (Ritalin)

(E) fluoxetine (Prozac)

Questions 344 through 346

A 27-year-old woman is brought into the psychiatric emergency department by her distraught husband because she has been acting strangely. She reports that for about 1 year the neighborhood children have been watching and following her, sometimes even breaking into her home. She adds that for the last 6 months she has been hearing a conversation between two voices, typically when she is alone. Her husband says that she has been increasingly withdrawn and rarely talks anymore with her family and friends. She now spends most of the day in their bedroom. He reports that he often hears her talk to herself and has seen her checking the telephone for "bugs."

344. The most likely diagnosis is

(A) delusional disorder

(B) schizophreniform disorder

(C) schizoaffective disorder

(D) schizophrenia

(E) major depression with psychotic features

345. As you begin to discuss the possible diagnosis and treatment options with the patient, she tells you that she is 6 months pregnant. Which of the following psychiatric medications is proven safe in pregnancy?

(A) lithium

(B) valproic acid

(C) haloperidol

(D) chlorpromazine

(E) none of the above

346. The patient's husband tells you that he does not believe the patient needs medication. He is a spiritual man and wants to take her to a healer from his community. What can you tell him about prognosis of this disorder?

(A) The majority of people spontaneously recover.

(B) If she does not take medication, the patient will suffer a chronic deteriorating course.

(C) Prognostic factors may be taken into account, but the actual course of the illness for this patient cannot be predicted.

(D) If the patient does not take medication, she will require permanent commitment in a psychiatric facility.

(E) none of the above

Questions 347 through 349

A 28-year-old woman presents for her annual gynecology appointment. She complains that in the week before her period, she often experiences marked anger and irritability and argues more with her boyfriend. She also reports diminished energy and concentration and sleeping more than is usual for her. These symptoms, in addition to breast tenderness and headaches, always remit in the week after her menses is finished.

347. The most likely diagnosis is

(A) MDD

(B) normal female behavior

(C) premenstrual dysphoric disorder (PMDD)

(D) generalized anxiety disorder

(E) dysthymic disorder

348. Treatment of the above condition may include which of the following?

(A) oral contraceptives

(B) paroxetine

(C) spironolactone

(D) alprazolam

(E) all of the above

349. What is the prevalence of this disorder among women in the United States?

(A) 42 to 50%

(B) 32 to 40%

(C) 22 to 30%

(D) 12 to 20%

(E) 2 to 10%

Questions 350 through 353

A 36-year-old man is brought to the emergency department in respiratory arrest. On exam he is unresponsive, and the medical student rotating through the emergency department observes pinpoint pupils and antecubital "track marks" on her examination. There is suspicion that the patient's condition may be the result of a drug overdose.

350. The patient most likely has overdosed on which of the following drugs?

(A) cocaine

(B) phencyclidine (PCP)

(C) heroin

(D) alcohol

(E) inhalants

351. Which of the following is the best test to document use of the suspected drug?

(A) blood test

(B) urine test

(C) Breathalyzer

(D) skin sample from the site of injection

(E) there is no definitive test

352. For how many days after last use would the suspected drug be noticeable in the above test?

   (A) 6 to 12 hours
   (B) 12 to 24 hours
   (C) 36 to 72 hours
   (D) 7 days
   (E) 14 days

353. The antidote of the suspected drug is

   (A) acetylcysteine
   (B) naloxone
   (C) deferoxamine
   (D) methylene blue
   (E) none of the above

Questions 354 through 356

A 70-year-old white woman with no prior psychiatric history comes into her primary care physician's office and says she has felt very sad since the death of her husband 8 months earlier. During this time, she reports low energy, difficulty falling asleep at night, and problems with her memory. She says that she used to cook for her extended family, but now does not enjoy cooking or even eating; she has lost 10 pounds in the last few months. She has been so disappointed with her inability to cope with the loss of her husband that she has been thinking about "finding a way to get up to heaven with him."

354. The most likely diagnosis is

   (A) bipolar disorder
   (B) normal grieving
   (C) MDD
   (D) dysthymic disorder
   (E) sleep disturbance

355. Which of the following should be considered in the differential diagnosis of any patient with the above disorder?

   (A) hypothyroidism
   (B) viral hepatitis
   (C) systemic lupus erythematosus (SLE)

   (D) Parkinson's disease
   (E) all of the above

356. Which of the following should be avoided when treating a patient with a monoamine oxidase inhibitor (MAOI)?

   (A) aged cheese
   (B) alcohol
   (C) sauerkraut
   (D) salami
   (E) all of the above

357. You are treating a 48-year-old housewife on an inpatient medical unit for an exacerbation of her asthma. On the day that you inform her of her pending discharge, she complains of feeling feverish and achy and has a non-productive cough. The nursing staff reports that she has a sudden fever of 103°F. You treat the fever with acetaminophen and perform a physical exam, order chest x-rays, draw blood, and order a urinalysis. While you are awaiting these results, the nurse informs you that she witnessed the patient dipping her thermometer into a hot cup of tea before another nurse went back into the patient's room to read the thermometer. The most likely diagnosis to account for this woman's behavior is

   (A) conversion disorder
   (B) factitious disorder
   (C) hypochondriasis
   (D) malingering
   (E) somatoform disorder

358. The psychiatric diagnosis that has the highest comorbidity with nicotine dependence is

   (A) alcohol dependence
   (B) bipolar disorder
   (C) generalized anxiety disorder
   (D) MDD
   (E) schizophrenia

Questions 359 through 361

A 32-year-old man is brought to the psychiatric emergency department by police after having been arrested for public nudity. Laboratory tests show a negative drug screen and alcohol levels. On MSE, you find that the patient cannot sit down and is only partly cooperative. He interrupts the interview several times, demanding to be allowed to contact his lawyer "because my rights given to me by God and ordained by the Jeffersonians and Washingtonians and Lincolnians have been infringed . . . and you, sir, are committing illegalities of the highest order." His speech is pressured. He describes his mood as "great," and his affect is variably irritable and euphoric. He can only vaguely describe his rationale for walking naked in the middle of a basketball court during a local high school basketball game: "It is not for you to understand. I am but one in a long line of those who have been known as Jesus, Gandhi, Martin Luther King, John Lennon, and others . . . I'm in training for the drinking of the difficult but luxurious cup . . . It begins with my pronouncements uncovered by the shackles that society has placed on all of this."

Examination of the patient's psychiatric records indicate that he has a history of a major depressive episode treated successfully with an SSRI for 1 year when he was age 23. The patient's parents arrive in the emergency department and tell you that the patient is a college graduate and a computer programmer. Lately, his job has been rather stressful as he has been overlooked for promotion, and his girlfriend left him 1 month ago. He is also in a great deal of credit card debt.

359. The most likely diagnosis for this patient is

    (A) adjustment disorder

    (B) bipolar disorder

    (C) MDD

    (D) PTSD

    (E) schizophrenia

360. The mean age of onset for this disorder is closest to age

    (A) 10

    (B) 20

    (C) 30

    (D) 40

    (E) 50

361. The prevalence of this disorder in the general population is closest to

    (A) 1%

    (B) 3%

    (C) 5%

    (D) 7%

    (E) 9%

362. A 68-year-old man has a history of a left middle cerebral artery stroke. Which of the following psychiatric disturbances is most common following such a neurologic event?

    (A) anxiety

    (B) OCD

    (C) depression

    (D) mania

    (E) panic symptoms

363. A 32-year-old woman presents in the psychiatric emergency department with symptoms of a severe psychosis. You have no psychiatric records available on this patient and, due to her symptoms, she is unable to supply the name of anyone who could supply collateral information. Based on this limited information, this patient is least likely to have a diagnosis of

    (A) bipolar disorder

    (B) major depression

    (C) paranoid personality disorder

    (D) schizophrenia

    (E) substance-induced psychotic disorder

364. A 48-year-old man presents with a chief complaint of impotence that has troubled him for the last year. Based on epidemiology of known causes of this disorder in this patient's age group, the chance that his problem is due to a "psychological" cause rather than a "medical" cause is closest to

    (A) 10%

    (B) 30%

    (C) 50%

(D) 70%

(E) 90%

365. Post-mortem studies and cerebrospinal fluid (CSF) sampling from living patients have revealed a correlation between aggression, impulsivity, and suicide and a decrease in the metabolites of which of the following neurotransmitters compared to control subjects?

(A) dopamine

(B) gamma-aminobutyric acid (GABA)

(C) glutamate

(D) norepinephrine

(E) serotonin

366. A 38-year-old woman diagnosed with multiple sclerosis of moderate severity has had symptoms of depression and memory loss increasing over the last year. On MSE, you notice blunted affect and decreased speed of mental processing. An MRI examination is likely to reveal

(A) normal brain

(B) global cerebral atrophy

(C) ventricular enlargement

(D) multiple plaques of frontal white matter

(E) rare periventricular plaques

367. Which of the following statements best characterizes the set of disorders categorized as paraphilias?

(A) Half of all paraphilias have onset after age 30.

(B) Persons with paraphilic disorders often have three or more types of paraphilias throughout their psychiatric history.

(C) The prevalence of paraphilias is distributed between the genders in near equal ratios.

(D) Voyeurism is the most common form of paraphilia.

(E) Five percent of women are victims of paraphilic acts.

Questions 368 and 369

A 45-year-old married woman, formerly employed as an accountant, had onset of severe anhedonia, amotivation, anergia, and flattened affect when she was 40 years old. Initially, her psychiatrist thought she might be suffering from major depression because of her prominent family history of depression on her father's side. At age 41, she had the sudden onset of auditory hallucinations and a fixed false belief that the government was harassing her. Her psychiatrist then diagnosed her with schizophrenia and placed her on neuroleptics. After starting these medications, her auditory hallucinations disappeared, and she no longer believed in her delusions. However, she continued to have amotivation, anhedonia, and flattened affect, and she was unable to return to her employment as an accountant.

368. Which of the following groups of medications is least likely to effectively treat this patient's negative symptoms?

(A) atypical antipsychotics

(B) SSRIs

(C) high-potency neuroleptics

(D) TCAs

(E) neuroleptics with high 5-hydroxytryptamine-2 (5-HT$_2$) blocking activity

369. Which prognostic indicator suggests a poorer prognosis in this case?

(A) the onset of symptoms relatively late in the patient's life

(B) the fact that the patient is married

(C) a positive family history of depression

(D) the sudden onset of psychotic symptoms

(E) the predominance of negative symptoms

Questions 370 and 371

A 34-year-old woman with schizophrenia has been stable on her psychiatric medications for 3 years and has become pregnant for the first time. Her family psychiatric history is not known because she was adopted. The father of the unborn child does not have schizophrenia.

370. Which percentage most closely approximates the likelihood that this patient's child will have schizophrenia?

(A) 1%

(B) 5%

(C) 10%

(D) 20%

(E) 30%

371. Suppose adoption records indicate that the patient has an identical twin that was adopted into another family. Which percentage most closely represents the likelihood that her twin sister has schizophrenia?

(A) 10%

(B) 30%

(C) 50%

(D) 70%

(E) 90%

372. You are a research psychiatrist who is studying signs and symptoms associated with certain psychiatric disorders that are not mentioned in the DSM-IV-TR for those disorders. Your spreadsheet contains a category of patients who have sensory gating deficits, short-term memory difficulties, and abnormalities in smooth pursuit eye movements. The most frequent DSM-IV-TR diagnosis you are likely to find in this category is

(A) attention deficit–hyperactivity disorder (ADHD)

(B) major depression

(C) OCD

(D) PTSD

(E) schizophrenia

Questions 373 through 376

A 23-year-old single white medical student comes to your office complaining of difficulty sleeping. During the past year he has been worrying excessively about a number of things, including his studies, his relationship with his parents, and that his girlfriend of 2 years is going to break up with him, despite being happy with their relationship. He admits that he has difficulty controlling the time he spends worrying. He notes feeling irritable at times and has been experiencing muscle tension. Due to his symptoms, he has trouble with schoolwork, and his grades have suffered. He does not endorse a depressed mood and asks, "Can you help me with my problems?"

373. The most likely diagnosis for this patient is

(A) social phobia

(B) generalized anxiety disorder

(C) major depression

(D) substance abuse

(E) panic disorder

374. Treatment for this patient's symptoms may include

(A) psychotherapy

(B) benzodiazepines

(C) antidepressants

(D) beta blockers

(E) all of the above may be indicated

375. Three months later, the patient comes back to your office reporting that his mood has been "down in the dumps," and he feels like he may never feel better. Recently, he has been thinking that life wasn't worth living anymore and has passive thoughts of suicide. When asked about specific suicidal plans he reports recent thoughts of taking an overdose of pills. The most appropriate next step would be to

(A) tell the patient he is going to get better and schedule weekly outpatient visits

(B) prescribe lorazepam for his excessive worries

(C) refer the patient to the psychiatric emergency department

(D) prescribe an antidepressant and instruct him to follow up with you in 1 month

(E) call his parents to pick him up and arrange for a family meeting

376. This patient is experiencing symptoms consistent with

(A) panic disorder

(B) major depression

(C) social phobia

(D) substance-induced mood disorder

(E) B and D

Questions 377 and 378

A 29-year-old married white woman is brought into the psychiatric emergency department by her husband who reports that despite feeling depressed 1 month ago, she now has been acting bizarre for the past week. On initial interview, the patient states, "I feel superbly supreme, and you have no idea what an amazing person I am! I am a direct descendant of Queen Elizabeth!" The patient is talking so fast you cannot interrupt her. Her husband reports that the patient has not slept in over a week and that she has recently been adjusting her own medication(s) since her last appointment over a month ago. In addition, her husband reports that this past week alone she has bought a new car, a diamond tennis bracelet, and her third designer handbag.

377. The most likely diagnosis is

(A) a mood disorder

(B) a psychotic disorder

(C) a personality disorder

(D) an anxiety disorder

378. Which of the following medications did the patient most likely inappropriately adjust?

(A) buspirone

(B) ranitidine (Zantac)

(C) valproic acid (Depakote)

(D) propranolol

DIRECTIONS (Questions 379 through 393): Each group of items in this section consists of lettered headings followed by a set of numbered words or phrases. For each numbered word or phrase, select the ONE lettered heading that is most closely associated with it. Each lettered heading may be selected once, more than once, or not at all.

Questions 379 through 386

(A) heroin

(B) Rorschach

(C) alprazolam (Xanax)

(D) Alzheimer's disease

(E) Hamilton

(F) schizophrenia

(G) glucocorticoids

(H) shared psychosis

(I) PCP

(J) Korsakoff syndrome

379. Most common diagnosis among psychiatric hospitalized patients in the United States

380. Folie à deux

381. Often causes psychotic and/or depressive symptoms

382. Amyloid plaques

383. Most dangerous withdrawal syndrome

384. Depression rating scale

385. "Dementia praecox"

386. Confabulation

Questions 387 through 393

Choose the diagnosis that best fits the scenario given.

(A) borderline personality disorder

(B) somatization disorder

(C) conversion disorder

(D) antisocial personality disorder

(E) schizoid personality disorder

(F) schizotypal personality disorder

(G) factitious disorder (Munchausen syndrome)

(H) hypochondriasis

(I) agoraphobia

387. A 46-year-old married white woman is referred to you by a neurologist. She has had an extensive neurologic workup, which was entirely negative, for the sudden onset of right arm paralysis 1 month ago. She says her husband was initially worried she'd had a stroke. When describing the onset of the paralysis, she relates that she was just about to punish her 15-year-old daughter, who has been involved in heavy drug use and increasingly difficult to discipline lately.

388. A 33-year-old divorced white woman is admitted to an inpatient psychiatric ward for apparently attempting suicide by cutting her wrists. When asked why she did it, she describes that "the physical pain makes my emotional pain go away, for a little while, anyway." She vacillates about whether this was a suicide attempt. She relates multiple complaints about various levels of strife with roommates and family members. She is known from previous admissions to the ward for labeling certain staff as her favorites and others as people "I hate." On MSE you note significant emotional lability. Her father committed suicide when she was 9 years old.

389. A 35-year-old man who has spent much of the past decade in jail or on parole for various misdemeanors and felonies initially presents to your substance abuse unit under a false name. He gives you his history in extensive detail, but it nonetheless seems implausible. You talk to his sister, who tells you, "He's the biggest con artist there is—don't believe a thing he says!" She then relates that the patient stole his mother's car last weekend. She believes he sold it for drugs, which he's done in the past, she says.

390. A 36-year-old woman is referred to you by her gynecologist, who reports a long history of sexual and other nonspecific complaints that have apparently shown no evidence of verifiable disease. The gynecologist further relates that she believes this patient has a long history of "doctor shopping." On interview, the patient demands your attention to multiple physical complaints: her back, belly, and chest pain; her dyspareunia and excessive menstrual bleeding; and her constipation and "lactose intolerance." She points out additionally that "nobody's been able to figure out why I can't feel anything on the back side of my arm." She has had multiple surgeries for abdominal complaints in the past, all with no significant findings or findings inconsistent with her complaints. She relates that "I've always been sickly, most of my life."

391. A 41-year-old woman claims she is "certain I have breast cancer." Workup by her internist, including physical exam and mammogram, is negative.

392. A 26-year-old woman is admitted for sepsis. Her roommate reports that a few days before admission she found the patient with a needle and syringe full of what the patient admitted was toilet water. The patient's physical exam reveals intravenous needle marks not made by any hospital staff. Records reveal she was admitted a year ago for gastrointestinal distress and later admitted drinking drain cleaner.

393. A 44-year-old stockbroker has discovered over the last few months that he experiences intense anxiety while taking the subway to work. He relates that "I can't go to the supermarket or any large store anymore, especially when they're crowded. I'm afraid my heart's going to jump out of my chest!"

Answers and Explanations

235. **(C)** The patient's 3- to 4-year history of bizarre behavior, delusions, and decline in social functioning strongly suggest that his illness is schizophrenia. Its prevalence is 1%.

236. **(C)** In twin studies, schizophrenia's monozygotic concordance is 50%, suggesting that there is a strong genetic component to the illness.

237. **(C)** As many as 75% of patients with schizophrenia use tobacco, for multiple reasons. Studies suggest that it increases the metabolism of antipsychotic drugs, thus potentially decreasing their side effects. Research also suggests that it aids in processing of certain auditory information, difficulty with which is one of the many identified "soft" neurologic problems in schizophrenia. About 30 to 50% abuse alcohol, about 15 to 25% use marijuana, and about 5 to 10% use cocaine. Substance abuse often correlates with a poor prognosis.

238. **(A)** More than half a dozen well-controlled studies of schizophrenics have shown decreases in the size of the hippocampus, parahippocampal gyrus, and amygdala. The other regions mentioned in the question have not been conclusively shown to be altered in schizophrenia by MRI or computerized tomography (CT) scans.

239. **(D)** Nihilistic delusion content is classic for Cotard syndrome, a psychotic/delusional theme seen potentially in multiple psychotic illnesses. The belief that people have been replaced by imposters is the hallmark of Cap-

gras syndrome. Folie à deux is a shared delusion aroused in one person by the influence of another. Although nihilism and negativism can be observed in patients with major depressive disorder (MDD), the predominance of psychosis in this patient makes that diagnosis unlikely. Similarly, this patient does not meet criteria for delusional disorder, which is characterized by nonbizarre delusions.

240. **(B)** The belief that people have been replaced by imposters is the hallmark of Capgras syndrome. Simple schizophrenia is a disorder consisting entirely of negative symptoms, with no positive symptoms. See the answer to question 239 for definitions of the other choices.

241. **(C)** Antisocial personality disorder is the only one of the choices that is not characterized by delusional or bizarre, near-psychotic thought content. Schizotypal personality disorder is marked by a pattern of difficulty with close relationships as well as cognitive and perceptual disturbances. Schizoid personality disorder differs from schizotypal personal disorder by the absence of cognitive and perceptual disturbances. The hallmarks of borderline personality disorder are unstable interpersonal relationships and marked impulse dyscontrol. Patients with paranoid personality disorder are mistrusting and suspicious, but do not maintain delusions.

242. **(A)** Schizophreniform disorder is the diagnosis given when symptom criteria of schizophrenia are met, but the duration of symptoms is less than 6 months and longer than 1 month. For a duration of symptoms less than 1 month, brief psychotic disorder is the proper term, while for over 6 months it is schizophrenia. Psychosis not otherwise specified is generally reserved for single episodes that do not fit into other categories. The patient's marked bizarre behavior makes delusional disorder unlikely.

243. **(C)** Onset of schizophrenia has been linked to the use of certain drugs of abuse, most classically LSD and marijuana, but others as well. Patients with mood disorders are generally higher functioning than are those with schizophrenia. Frequently, the onset of schizophrenia is indeed in the setting of some stressor or social change. Negative symptoms are usually the prominent, early, prodromal symptoms. Only about 30% of patients with schizophrenia are able to lead productive lives.

244. **(C)** Progressive social withdrawal is commonly seen as part of the prodrome. All other choices—low intelligence, head trauma, a neglectful mother, and abuse—have not been proven in any conclusive way to be significantly linked to the disease, although early theories held that a history of one or more was a predisposing factor.

245. **(E)** Poor orientation, while possible, is seldom seen in schizophrenics and would rather suggest delirium, dementia, or some other process at work. Each of the other choices are very commonly associated with first-break schizophrenia.

246. **(C)** Ideas of reference is the delusion that others are focusing on you in some positive or negative way, commonly seen in paranoid schizophrenia. For example, a patient might believe that the television is speaking directly to him. Formication is the sensation that bugs are crawling on one's skin. Trichotillomania is compulsive hair pulling accompanied by significant hair loss. Reaction formation, a defense mechanism, involves an unacceptable impulse being expressed as its opposite. Hallucinations are sensory phenomena that should not be confused with delusions.

247. **(D)** Flattened affect is one of the negative symptoms of schizophrenia and is much more likely to be seen than hyperactivity or elective mutism, neither of which is necessarily a schizophrenic manifestation. Tactile hallucinations are much more commonly linked to delirium. Catatonia (resistance to, absence of, or even stereotypes of movement) is not seen in this patient, although it is linked to a now rarer type of schizophrenia (catatonic type).

248. **(E)** Acetylcholine is not thought to be nearly as significant in the pathophysiology of schizophrenia as are serotonin and dopamine. Abnormalities in each of the latter two neurotransmitter systems have been clearly shown to cause schizophrenic symptoms. The mesolimbic tract is a dopaminergic tract specifically implicated in schizophrenia, and the amygdala is thought to be involved in the emotional components of schizophrenia, along with the rest of the limbic system.

249. **(C)** Parkinsonism, a side effect of neuroleptics, is frequently mistaken for flattened affect. Auditory hallucinations are more predominant in schizophrenia than are other hallucinations. There is an increased incidence of schizotypal personality disorder in family members of those affected by schizophrenia. Siblings also have a higher risk of developing schizophrenia than does the general population. Kraepelin developed the concept of dementia praecox (a cognitive deterioration occurring at an early age) and emphasized its progressively declining course.

250. **(E)** Loss of ego boundaries is commonly manifested as inappropriate conversational distance. Formication is the sensation that bugs are crawling on one's skin. Flight of ideas is flow of nonconnected speech/thoughts; circumstantiality is speech/thoughts with identifiable connections between thoughts, but which drift off the point and ramble, eventually coming back to the point. Ideas of reference is the delusion that others are focusing on you in some positive or negative way.

251. **(B)** The downward drift hypothesis points out chronic mental illness's tendency to cause its sufferers to move downward through the social strata. This downward movement has to do with the effects of the illness itself, not the side effects of medications or the stress-diathesis model, which addresses the entirely different issue of susceptibility to illness. The socioeconomic cost of schizophrenia is the *result* of above drift, not its cause. Bleuler is known for his four "A's"—association, affect, autism, and ambivalence—used to describe schizophrenia.

252. **(D)** Clearly, on previous occasions, this patient's presentation has strongly suggested schizophrenia, and now he is presenting with classic catatonic features: negativism, hypomotorism, and echolalia with echopraxia. The diagnosis of schizophrenia makes elective mutism very unlikely. There is no evidence of secondary gain, making a diagnosis of malingering similarly unlikely. Drug-induced psychosis is unlikely to result in the classical symptoms of catatonic schizophrenia.

253. **(A)** This woman's high social and occupational functioning rules out any of the psychotic/schizophrenia-spectrum diagnoses as possibilities, and she is not paranoid. Her illness clearly is well circumscribed and is of delusional intensity only (i.e., it does not significantly impair social or occupational functioning).

254. **(B)** Patients with schizophrenia have significantly increased suicidal risk compared with the general population. Studies suggest that they have no increased homicide or unreliability risk, but do have an increased substance abuse and mood disorder risk.

255. **(B)** Prodromal schizophrenia is normally composed of increasing negative symptoms in the absence of positive symptoms. Negative symptoms do not include affective lability or become milder over time, nor are they easy to tell apart from depressive symptoms. They include autistic features.

256. **(B)** Positive symptoms frequently respond to antipsychotics. Negative symptoms are less likely to do so, although clozapine is thought to decrease negative symptoms. Positive symptoms do not include apathy or social withdrawal or remain static over the course of the illness; most studies suggest that they decrease with time. They are difficult to distinguish from delirium, and they include hallucinations.

257. **(C)** Loss of interest in formerly enjoyed activities, also known as anhedonia, is one of the two criteria that must be one of the observed symptoms in order to make the diagnosis of major depression (the other is depressed mood). All other choices are symptoms of depression but are not essential to the diagnosis.

258. **(A)** Depression severity, history of poor response to many medications (many clinicians believe that all medication options should be exhausted), and need for quick antidepressant action are really the only universally agreed-upon criteria that encourage the clinician to use ECT in major depression. Poor compliance would push a clinician toward ECT only if all other methods of encouraging compliance had failed. The other options all describe diagnoses that would likely respond to ECT, but would not necessarily move the clinician to ECT over medications.

259. **(C)** MDD has a prevalence of 15% (approximately 20% for women and 10% for men).

260. **(B)** It is always essential to rule out bipolar disorder before administering antidepressants, because all antidepressants can induce mania in susceptible patients. However, antidepressants are sometimes carefully administered to bipolar patients who are predominantly depressed. All the other diagnoses mentioned would likely respond favorably to antidepressants, with the exception of drug-induced depression, for which the treatment is removal of the inciting agent.

261. **(A)** All beta blockers have been implicated in depression, not just those that are thought to be more lipophilic and therefore cross the blood–brain barrier more easily. There is recent evidence that they may not be as culpable as once thought, but they are still known as the prototypical "depression-causing drugs," and are more likely than any of the other choices to cause depression, although cimetidine and phenytoin have been implicated.

262. **(E)** Although cocaine can cause euphoria in the short term, it quickly leaves the patient with a "crash" afterward, during which a profound depression can often set in. None of the other substances have such strong potential to cause depression, although each has been implicated in depression, many in withdrawal states.

263. **(A)** Atypical depression is defined as hypersomnic, hyperphagic depression. Otherwise, symptoms are identical to normal major depression. Some also believe that there is an increased sensitivity to rejection in patients with the syndrome, and that certain medications (SSRIs and MAOIs) may be more effective than others.

264. **(B)** Being single (or divorced or separated) has been shown to be a risk factor for the development of major depression. None of the other choices has been clearly shown to increase risk of depression.

265. **(B)** Women have twice the lifetime risk of major depression as that of males.

266. **(B)** Although many sleep disturbances have been described in depression (e.g., the other choices, among others), early morning awakening has been most consistently linked with major depression.

267. **(B)** Pseudodementia is a syndrome of dementia-like features (memory, cognitive deficits) that seems to result from major depression, the diagnosis for this patient. At this patient's age, dementia from other common causes would be unlikely. Although the other choices represent possible causes of his

cognitive deficits, pseudodementia is far more likely.

268. **(A)** Blunted, or constricted, affect, or in more severe cases, flattened affect, is often seen in those patients suffering from major depression. Anxiety commonly afflicts depressed patients, but this is less commonly a prominent part of their presentation as blunted affect. The other choices would suggest other diagnoses; lability suggests bipolar disorder or an organic disorder, while guarded or bizarre affect suggests a psychotic disorder such as paranoid schizophrenia.

269. **(B)** Increased cortisol in depression is one of the earliest observations in biological psychiatry, and is well borne out in subsequent studies. Catecholamines are decreased in depression, as are sex hormones and immune function. Levels of MAOs are unknown.

270. **(D)** Aaron Beck proposed a triad of beliefs or cognitive styles that he felt predisposed patients to depression, which are sometimes otherwise stated as: "I'm bad, things have always been bad, things will continue to be bad." Id, ego, and superego refer to Freud's model of the mind.

271. **(E)** A patient with major depression has a lifetime suicide risk of 15%. (*Memory aid:* Note the similarity to the prevalence of MDD.)

272. **(D)** The criteria for dysthymia are the same criteria as those of MDD but patients must have only two symptoms, whereas MDD requires five. These symptoms may or may not indicate an atypical depressive syndrome.

273. **(B)** Bereavement can (and often does) present with identical symptoms to MDD; one must look for a precipitating death or loss of some sort to clarify the diagnosis. Antisocial personality disorder describes individuals with long histories of disregard for the rights of others and often dishonesty used in attempts to gain something for themselves. Dysphoria describes the mood of depression

and is not a diagnosis. Psychogenic fugue is a type of dissociative disorder that can involve sudden, unexplained travel away from one's home. Hypnagogic phenomena are vivid hallucinations that occur just as someone is falling asleep.

274. **(E)** Double depression occurs when a major depressive episode is superimposed on dysthymic disorder. It is thought to affect as many as 40% of patients with MDD and to carry a poorer prognosis.

275. **(D)** Kindling, based on a model of neural activity in which repeated subthreshold stimulation of a given neuron results in discharge of an action potential, is a theory that suggests that one decompensation can lead to a second episode. The theory does not involve Jung, childhood development, or the id and superego.

276. **(B)** Postpartum depression can, and often does, present with psychosis. Later pregnancies are at no higher risks than earlier pregnancies. It is more prevalent in women with previous mood/psychotic illness and is potentially dangerous to the child. For example, women sometimes have impulses to harm their own children. Finally, it is commonly indistinguishable from major depression in the severity of symptoms.

277. **(A)** This is a typical presentation for mania, an episode that seems to have been at least partially induced by treatment with an antidepressant (all antidepressants can induce/exacerbate mania). This patient's affect, like that of many patients with mania, is expansive and irritable. He is to a lesser extent guarded and suspicious, but this does not capture the full picture of his mania. He is labile but hardly dysphoric, and he is euphoric but not bizarre. He is not euthymic.

278. **(B)** Although all of the other choices might explain part of his speech characterization, pressured is used to describe speech that is difficult to interrupt and at a fast rate.

279. **(C)** Bipolar I disorder clearly has a stronger genetic link than major depression and probably has the strongest genetic link of all the major psychiatric illnesses. Bipolar II disorder has a strong genetic link, but not as strong as bipolar I disorder. Bipolar illness usually carries a poorer prognosis than unipolar depression. A higher percentage of patients with bipolar disease are eventually treated compared with patients with unipolar depression. Bipolar disorder has no sexual predilection and has not been shown to be any more common in broad geographic areas.

280. **(A)** Each of these three features is a criterion for manic episode. In each of the other answers, at least one answer is not a criterion. Prominent mood swings, substance abuse, and excessive spending are not criteria for the diagnosis, although all are common during manic episodes.

281. **(C)** Antidepressants can precipitate or exacerbate mania in patients with bipolar disorder, who are not infrequently first diagnosed as suffering from unipolar depression. SSRI levels have not been shown to correlate with efficacy. Because the paroxetine appears to have precipitated a mania, the drug should have been stopped. Insomnia would have likely resolved itself with the discontinuation of the SSRI and resolution of the manic episode. Starting two mood stabilizers at once is not supported by clinical trial evidence.

282. **(C)** Diagnosis of a mixed episode requires that criteria of both a manic and major depressive episode are met simultaneously. The patient's manic symptoms exceed those of hypomania, which excludes bipolar II disorder. Despite his comments, there are no data particularly supporting a diagnosis of SAD. The rapidity of his cycling is unclear.

283. **(B)** Features of mania not shared by hypomania include impairment in social functioning, lack of psychotic symptoms, and lack of

need for hospitalization. Other choices include symptoms other than these.

284. **(C)** Cyclothymia is defined as cycling between hypomania and dysthymia. Treatment is the same as in bipolar disorder. Bipolar III disorder does not exist. Double depression occurs when a major depressive episode is superimposed on dysthymic disorder.

285. **(A)** The prevalence of bipolar disorder is 1%.

286. **(B)** First-degree relatives of patients with bipolar disorder have a 25% risk of the illness.

287. **(A)** Dangerous drug abuse should be ruled out first in this patient; cocaine is more acutely dangerous than LSD. She is on no medications, so she would have no reason to develop serotonin syndrome, a rare, severe adverse reaction to serotonergic drugs. Carcinoid tumor, another cause of serotonin syndrome, is equally unlikely. Hypochondriasis and specific phobia are seldom acutely life threatening.

288. **(C)** Porphyria is manifested not uncommonly by psychiatric (manic or psychotic-appearing) symptoms. It rarely occurs without abdominal pain. Each of the other choices would have psychiatric symptoms less directly connected to the abdominal pain.

289. **(C)** Fear that one is having a heart attack or that "I am going crazy" are classic features and criteria of panic disorder. The fear that someone is stalking her is more likely to suggest a paranoid disorder. Fear of a specific situation or object suggests a specific phobia, while an exaggerated startle response is classic for PTSD. Fears about infection or uncleanliness are common in patients with OCD.

290. **(D)** As described in answer 289, an exaggerated startle reflex is classic for PTSD.

291. **(E)** As described in answer 289, excessive fears about infection or uncleanliness are suggestive of OCD.

292. **(A)** The locus ceruleus is the "alarm" center of the brain and is hyperactive in anxiety states. It is the center of most of the norepinephrine-containing neurons in the brain. The hippocampus, part of the limbic system, and the amygdala are involved in memory formation. The thalamus is the brain's relay center. The basal ganglia coordinate motor activity.

293. **(A)** Any type of hallucinations can be seen in delirium. In schizophrenia-spectrum illness, including brief psychotic disorder, one rarely sees hallucinations other than auditory. Nonauditory hallucinations, then, as a general rule, suggest delirium of some cause. Delusions are thoughts (fixed false beliefs) and do not include sensory phenomena like hallucinations. Conversion disorder does not usually show hallucinations of any sort.

294. **(B)** Alcohol (and benzodiazepines, because they also act on GABA receptors) is generally associated with the most dangerous withdrawal syndrome of all the drugs of abuse. Despite the profound discomfort of withdrawal from heroin and other opiates, opiate withdrawal is not life-threatening. Similarly, withdrawal from crack and cocaine is uncomfortable but not life-threatening. Withdrawal from LSD is not well-characterized.

295. **(D)** Serious, chronic alcoholics often take in calories from little else besides alcohol and are thus at risk for thiamine deficiency. If a thiamine-deficient patient is given food, he or she can develop Wernicke's encephalopathy from the body's attempts to metabolize glucose in the absence of thiamine pyrophosphate. While the other choices are important concerns, none are of the acute significance of thiamine deficiency.

296. **(A)** This is a general rule that almost always applies, at least in the cases in which a drug has a withdrawal syndrome. Lipophilia gen-

erally is related to half-life in the sense that body stores of the drug are available for a "self-taper," but is not directly related to severity of withdrawal. Route can have some effect on withdrawal severity, as intravenous drugs can be shorter acting, but is not necessarily directly related, as some intravenous drugs can still have long half-lives.

297. **(C)** The shorter the onset of action, the quicker the "high" and the quicker the addiction potential; hence, users simply like, and get addicted to, such drugs more easily.

298. **(A)** Benzodiazepines and alcohol have near-identical modes of action in their modulation of GABA receptors in the brain. This similarity makes benzodiazepines a sensible and popular choice for treatment of alcohol withdrawal. Much less commonly (although more common in the distant past), barbiturates (which also act on GABA) and clonidine (which modulates autonomic instability) are used. Phenytoin is not used, and disulfiram is used to encourage alcohol abstinence by its inhibition of aldehyde dehydrogenase.

299. **(D)** Delirium tremens is commonly seen as a late manifestation of alcohol withdrawal, the order usually being: withdrawal tremulousness (within 12 to 24 hours), seizures (within about 2 days), and delirium tremens (at about the 2- to 8-day mark).

300. **(C)** In cases of suspected liver impairment, it is advisable to use a benzodiazepine minimally metabolized by the liver, of which there are two: lorazepam (Ativan) and oxazepam (Serax). Other benzodiazepines, such as those listed, are mostly metabolized by the liver and could thus quickly build to toxic levels. Phenobarbital and clonidine are no longer used to treat alcohol withdrawal.

301. **(A)** This is a classic presentation of Wernicke's encephalitis: ataxia, confusion, and eye movement findings (mnemonic: ACE). The other responses describe similar, but distinct, syndromes. Alcoholic cerebellar degeneration is a disorder of the cerebellar vermis

in which patients have difficulty with gait and stance but characteristically do not have arm ataxia nor nystagmus. Subacute combined degeneration results from B_{12} deficiency, which leads to demyelination and axonal degeneration of the peripheral nerves, posterior and lateral columns of the spinal cord, and the cerebrum. Patients have cognitive impairment, diminished position and vibration sensation, and abnormal gait. Alcoholic peripheral neuropathy is a sensory peripheral neuropathy in which alcohol may directly cause axonal damage, although malnutrition may also play a role. Ménière's disease is a vestibular disorder in which distention of the endolymphatic sac causes intermittent vertigo, tinnitus, and hearing loss.

302. **(C)** Pathologic lesions in Korsakoff's are found in the mammillary bodies and thalamus. Confabulation is a common finding. Treatment is with thiamine, not vitamin B_{12}. The neurological findings are ataxia and nystagmus. Lewy body disease, which presents as a dementia similar to Alzheimer's disease, involves deposition of inclusion bodies in the cerebral cortex.

303. **(B)** Klüver-Bucy syndrome presents with docility, lack of fear response, anterograde amnesia, hyperphagia, and hypersexuality. Pick's disease is a form of dementia, often indistinguishable from Alzheimer's disease, in which the frontal and temporal lobes are atrophied. Arnold–Chiari syndrome describes a condition with hydrocephalus and cerebellar anatomic and functional abnormalities. Punch-drunk syndrome describes an acquired movement disorder associated with traumatic damage to the substantia nigra. Möbius syndrome is congenital absence of the facial nerves and nuclei with resulting bilateral facial paralysis.

304. **(D)** Klüver-Bucy syndrome is most closely associated with severe damage to, or disconnectivity of, the amygdala bilaterally. The hippocampus, although important to short-term memory, is not directly involved with regulating aggression drives, sexual behaviors, and fear responses. The insula, found deep within the central sulcus, is medial to the temporal lobe and generally not considered a part of it. Superior temporal gyri are more generally involved with processing complex auditory information such as the understanding of language. The lateral ventricle is a cerebrospinal fluid–containing space that has no direct neuropsychiatric functional role.

305. **(D)** This patient would meet criteria for bulimia except that she missed three consecutive periods, which automatically places her in the category of anorexia. Her anorexia appears similar to bulimia, however, and she would likely be further qualified as having the binge eating–purging type of anorexia. Exercise can induce amenorrhea, but other clues in this case indicate a more complex etiology of the loss of menses. OCD is often found comorbid with eating disorders in women, and indeed many of the food-associated behaviors in anorexia may seem similar to OCD-related rituals. In this case, all of the patient's symptoms are explained in the context of an eating disorder. Psychogenic gastritis is not a DSM-IV-TR diagnosis.

306. **(E)** As with many forms of starvation, a predominance of catabolic over anabolic processes tends to elevate BUN. Cortisol levels tend to be elevated in anorexia, reflecting the stress state of the body. In anorexia, TSH responsiveness to TRH remains normal. Persons with anorexia also tend to be anemic. Serum growth hormone is often elevated in anorexia.

307. **(B)** Fluoxetine (Prozac), an SSRI, is the treatment of choice for panic disorder, with or without agoraphobia. Alprazolam (Xanax), although commonly used for panic disorder, is a benzodiazepine that is effective in the short term but has considerable dependence liability. In addition, its short half-life may actually cause withdrawal states that mimic panic. Chlordiazepoxide (Librium) is a long-acting benzodiazepine that is also effective in

panic disorder but also carries some dependence liability. SSRIs have been shown in trials to be as effective as benzodiazepines but without the abuse potential. Phenelzine (Nardil), an MAOI, has been shown to be effective in some studies in anxiety disorders, but its side effect profile is regarded as problematic. Valproic acid (Depakote), has not been demonstrated to be effective for panic.

308. **(C)** This is one of the most important biological findings in affective disorder research. Studies show that in major depression, about half of all patients do not have blunted cortisol levels to an administration of dexamethasone the night before. This is thought to be indicative of abnormal feedback control in the hypothalamic–pituitary–adrenal axis in major depression. Patients with psychotic depression are even more likely to have poor dexamethasone suppression.

309. **(B)** About one third of all patients with major depression do not show an increase of TSH with administration of TRH.

310. **(C)** Persons with schizoid personality are reclusive and do not mind the lack of social interaction. Agoraphobia is tied to fear of panic symptoms in public. Such symptoms are not mentioned in this case. Persons with avoidant personality are shy and fearful of social rejection. However, their lack of socialization is distressing to them. Schizotypal persons can have schizoid features, but they also have bizarre thinking. Patients with autism have pronounced deficits in language, communication, and socialization, which are not prominently reflected in this case of a woman who had uneventful but happy formative years.

311. **(D)** Federal standards require a minimum of 1 year of addiction to opiates, with exceptions made for recent discharge from penal institutions or long-term treatment centers. Federal standards require that the minimum age for treatment is 18. The patient's tendency toward criminal activity is likely related to her need to buy heroin and would

likely diminish with methadone treatment. HIV status has no bearing on methadone treatment. Pregnancy outcomes have been shown to improve with methadone treatment.

312. **(D)** Studies show that most addicts do not experience a sufficient decrease of their cravings at less than 60 mg/day during initial treatment. The fear of bone decay and loss of libido are popular misconceptions about the effects of methadone. Although an opiate, methadone has a longer half-life than heroin (and thus a milder withdrawal syndrome) and is given in a treatment setting in which complete opiate detoxification is more likely to succeed if the patient desires this route. There is no association of methadone treatment with Cushing syndrome.

313. **(E)** Studies have shown that methadone maintenance treatment helps eliminate unstable lifestyles that hinder employment, further education, and criminal activity. Furthermore, HIV risk is reduced. These factors, along with engagement in a supportive psychiatric treatment center, may lessen risk of psychiatric morbidity while in treatment. There is thus no increased risk of depression with methadone treatment.

314. **(B)** This patient's history is most consistent with a mood pattern defined by prolonged periods of hypomania (symptoms of mania not severe enough to cause occupational dysfunction or psychiatric treatment) and now a major depressive episode. Hypomania with major depression defines bipolar II disorder. In bipolar I disorder, the mania is more severe, causing notable occupational dysfunction and usually contact with psychiatrists. This patient is in the midst of a major depressive episode, but his history of mania indicates a bipolar diagnosis. This is an important distinction to make in diagnosis, because improper treatment with antidepressants can precipitate a manic episode. Narcissistic personality disorder is an Axis II diagnosis. This patient does display impulsivity, but impulse control disorder not otherwise specified can

be diagnosed only after the exclusion of major mental illness such as bipolar disorder, which may have impulsive features.

315. **(B)** Dry mouth, dizziness (associated with hypotension), and urinary hesitancy are due to anticholinergic and adrenergic blocking effects of TCAs such as imipramine. Fluoxetine, an SSRI, is most often associated with gastrointestinal upset, sexual dysfunction, and agitation. Phenelzine, an MAOI, can be associated with hypotension but is less likely to have anticholinergic effects. Lithium is most often associated with polyuria, polydipsia, tremor, and mental confusion at higher doses. Valproic acid may cause gastrointestinal upset, but is otherwise commonly associated with sedation and tremor at higher doses.

316. **(B)** The classic triad of NPH is confusion, gait ataxia, and incontinence. Elevated opening pressure is not found in NPH (thus the "normal pressure" part of the diagnosis). Oculomotor difficulties are a part of the Wernicke–Korsakoff syndrome. Frontal release signs and perseveration are nonspecific findings common in demented patients.

317. **(A)** CT scan commonly reveals dilated ventricles, thought to be the result of increased pressure waves impinging within the ventricular system. Normal ventricles would not be expected in NPH patients. Frontal sulcal widening is found in dementias that have underlying cerebral atrophy. Hypointensities found in subcortical areas are often indicative of lacunar strokes. Cerebellar atrophy is seen most often in congenital disorders and alcoholism.

318. **(A)** The patient's inability to quit drinking regardless of a desire to quit or knowledge of its negative aspects best differentiates dependence from abuse. Neither dependence nor abuse is determined based on quantity of alcohol consumed. The patient's history of drunk driving and gastric ulcer are both consequences of the abuse construct of DSM-IV-TR. The patient's statement that he can't

sleep when he tries to quit drinking does imply physiologic dependence, but the alcohol dependence criteria can be met with a "without physiologic dependence" qualifier.

319. **(C)** Patients with alcoholism often are found to have elevated GGT on routine laboratory screening. They also may have an increased ALT and AST, but with an increased AST/ALT ratio, not increased ALT/AST. Patients with alcoholism also commonly have increased uric acid levels, macrocytic anemia, and increased serum triglycerides.

320. **(E)** There is no particularly increased rate of OCD in alcoholism. On the other hand, many patients with alcoholism have underlying or associated smoking habits, depression, and anxiety disorders (as high as 50% in some studies). There is also an increased rate of antisocial personality disorder in alcoholism.

321. **(C)** Oculomotor difficulty, ataxia, and confusion or dementia is the classic triad of Wernicke's encephalopathy. While hyperreflexia, tactile hallucinations, and seizures are symptoms of alcohol withdrawal, they are not part of the Wernicke's triad. Ataxia and aggression can be symptoms of alcohol intoxication.

322. **(D)** This patient would meet criteria for schizophrenia except the duration of his illness has been less than 6 months. Brief psychotic disorder may present with psychosis, but the duration of the disturbance must be 1 month or less in duration. This patient's delusions are too bizarre to meet criteria for delusional disorder. Psychosis not otherwise specified is reserved for cases of psychosis in which the etiology may be related to substance abuse, a medical condition, or an endogenous psychotic illness of unknown duration.

323. **(A)** This patient has symptoms consistent with PTSD or acute stress disorder (i.e., traumatic event, intrusive memories of trauma, avoidance of reminders, hypervigilance), but the fact that the trauma was only 3 weeks prior means that she would be diagnosed with acute distress disorder. If her symptoms persist after 4 weeks, then she would be diagnosed with PTSD. Adjustment disorder most often represents a change in mood, anxiety, or conduct that happens after a nontraumatic event. In generalized anxiety disorder, there is no associated trauma. The patient has no evidence of MDD.

324. **(D)** Female patients typically attempt suicide without succeeding. The attempt-to-success ratio has been reported to be as high as 20:1 for women. Overdose with pills is by far the most common modality of suicide attempt. Suicide becomes increasingly common with advancing age, although there has been a recent increase in rates of teenage suicide. Most patients attempting and completing suicide are not psychotic or otherwise incompetent. Patients allude to four fifths of suicide attempts to others before the attempts are made. Unexpected suicidal gestures are atypical.

325. **(C)** The lifetime incidence of suicide in patients with schizophrenia is about 10%, compared with less than 1% in the general population.

326. **(A)** Feelings and attitudes originating from the treater, evoked by the patient, are called countertransference. Transference denotes feelings and attitudes about the treater coming from the patient. Empathy is the ability of the treater to psychologically "put himself in his patient's shoes" and thereby understand his patient's thinking, feelings, or behavior. Identification is a rather unconscious incorporation of someone else's traits into one's own manner; for example, adolescents have hairstyles similar to admired rock stars. Projection occurs when one assigns emotions to another person in an attempt to psychologically cover up the presence of those emotions within himself. For example, the doctor in the case may tell his fellow resident that he believes that his female patient is attracted to him, when in actuality he is attracted to her.

327. (E) This patient displays symptoms of fear of loss and abandonment, intense interpersonal relationships, recurrent suicidal behavior or threats, affective instability, and difficulty controlling intense anger. Patients with borderline personality disorder have depressive symptoms that may become "full-blown" as a result of their social isolation, but this scenario does not mention full criteria for major depression. Patients with histrionic personality disorder, like those with borderline personality disorder, may display excessive emotionality and attention seeking, but their core symptoms center around superficial seductiveness and theatricality. Patients with cyclothymia often present as a diagnostic question with regard to the possibility of a borderline personality diagnosis. This is due to their prominent mood instability and impulsivity, which happens in both disorders. In this case, the other criteria for a borderline diagnosis resolves this dilemma. Psychotic disorder not otherwise specified is reserved for more frank delusional symptoms of unclear etiology than are evident with this patient who is paranoid that "all the staff hates me."

328. (D) Borderline patients classically split groups that comprise their social milieu. This is achieved in part by their own views that people around them are either all good or all bad, and partly by members of the group, who may act to collude in this view and come in conflict with one another. Acting out generally represents the enactment of a behavior of coming from an impulse that had presented conflict in order to relieve the sense that the conflict exists at all. Externalization, a generalized form of projection, represents the tendency to believe in the existence of patterns of behavior in others that is really true about oneself. Regression is a return to patterns of relating, thinking, or feeling that had come before one's current developmental stage. For example, many medical students who return home act as if they are teenagers with regard to their parents or other hometown friends. Sublimation is the channeling of drives or conflicts into goals that eventually become gratifying. For example, some people remember being afraid of blood and hospitals, and worked out these fears upon medical school training.

329. (E) Psychotherapy and steady social support represent the best long-term method for the management of borderline personality disorder. Dialectic behavioral therapy has gained recent popularity as a form of psychotherapeutic intervention for these patients. Neuroleptics, mood stabilizers, and antidepressants have all been shown to have some efficacy in treating target symptoms in some borderline patients. Benzodiazepines may treat anxiety in these patients, but they have particular abuse liability in these impulsive patients.

330. (A) Amnesia is a common side effect, presenting in the form of short-term memory deficits. Anesthesia-induced respiratory dysfunction, fractures, and arrhythmias are rare side effects. Psychosis can be improved rather than worsened; indeed, ECT is regarded as most indicated in psychotic depressions.

331. (C) For catatonic conditions, 2 or 4 ECT treatments may be effective. In major depression, 6 to 12 sessions are generally optimal for a good risk–benefit ratio of positive treatment effects versus memory impairment (which is more likely with 20 or 40 treatments). When ECT is given for psychosis or mania, 20 or more treatments may be necessary for a positive response.

332. (B) This patient has recurrent thoughts that are distressing. They are conceived as a product of her mind and not as "implanted messages" as may happen in schizophrenia. She attempts to ignore or suppress her symptoms by not explaining to her husband how she feels or by getting rid of all the knives in her kitchen. Impulse control disorder not otherwise specified is reserved for the inaction of impulses that are not as directly ego-dystonic (disturbing) as in this case, and that do not have an obsessional nonenacted (thinking) component. Obsessive–compulsive personality disorder is a pervasive character style marked by a "pattern of preoccupation with orderliness, perfectionism, and mental and interpersonal control." These persons are often described as "control freaks" by laypersons and are noted to be particularly inflexible. Psychosis not otherwise specified is inappropriate because this patient has fair insight regarding her obsessional thinking. She does act on her thoughts, and they are disturbing to her. She is thus not psychotic. This patient does not display a thinking style that is marked by magical thinking. There is no mention of a history of strangeness prior to the birth of her child. Therefore, schizotypal personality disorder is not appropriate.

333. **(E)** Fluvoxamine (Luvox) and other SSRIs (paroxetine, fluoxetine, sertraline) are known for their antiobsessional effects as well as their antidepressant and antianxiety effects. Lorazepam (Ativan), a benzodiazepine, may decrease anxiety but has no direct antiobsessional effects. Benztropine (Cogentin) is an anticholinergic typically used to counter neuroleptic-induced extrapyramidal symptoms. Nortriptyline (Pamelor) and other TCAs have not proven efficacious for OCD. Haloperidol (Haldol) is a typical high-potency neuroleptic that may be useful in forms of OCD in which there is a psychotic component. However, it does not ameliorate purely obsessional thinking.

334. **(C)** This patient's MSE is most consistent with delirium in that it is remarkable for relatively *rapidly fluctuating* memory, orientation, and attention. Also, her apparent dehydration and malnourishment provides evidence for an underlying medical cause of her mental status change. Amnestic disorder is not likely given this patient's shifts in attention and memory fluctuations. Cognitive disorder not otherwise specified is reserved for cases exclusive of dementia and delirium such as cases of traumatic brain injury. Although this patient would seem a likely person to have dementia because she came from a nursing home, her fluctuating mental status is indica-

tive of a delirium. Dementias should be diagnosed in the context of a relatively stable set of deficits on an MSE, and the underlying causes are rarely associated with acute medical insults. Importantly, however, the presence of dementia does predispose to delirium. Major depression can cause cognitive deficits on MSEs that are reversible with antidepressant treatment. These *pseudodementias*, like dementia, most often present as a more stable exam than is illustrated in this case.

335. **(C)** About one third of all patients with depression will respond to the surprisingly powerful placebo effect. However, this response is not as well sustained as in patients placed on antidepressant medications.

336. **(D)** Standard antidepressant therapies, including SSRIs and tricyclic antidepressants, will effect a positive response in 65 to 75% of patients.

337. **(A)** Schizophrenia, catatonic subtype, is defined by a predominance of symptoms that involve motor behaviors and nonverbal forms of communication such as facial expression. This category includes famous cases of "waxy flexibility," echolalia (repeating another's words inappropriately), and echopraxia (repeating another's gestures inappropriately). Disorganized schizophrenia, traditionally known as *hebephrenia*, is notable for pronounced and severe thought disorder that can be relatively refractory to neuroleptic treatment. Such patients may present with a chief complaint such as "I came to restore my tranquility so that I can get what's coming to me upside down." Patients with paranoid schizophrenia may be relatively high functioning between episodes of psychosis. They may have relatively little thought disorder and may not have other bizarre manners. The diagnosis of residual schizophrenia is reserved for patients who have not had prominent positive symptoms (primarily thought disorder and psychosis) for some time and present with primarily chronic negative symptoms (anergia, anhedonia, and flattened affect). A diagnosis of undifferentiated schiz-

ophrenia is reserved for cases in which the clinician cannot distinguish a subtype. Often, these cases can present with mild components of all the types.

338.   **(D)** Catatonic schizophrenia has always been the least prevalent subtype of schizophrenia according to most studies, but has also become increasingly rare in recent decades. It has been suggested that changes in diagnostic criteria over these years may account for this finding. Additionally, some forms of mental illness that were diagnosed as catatonic schizophrenia may have been cases of neurosyphilis, which with antibiotics has become increasingly rare. It is possible also that the advent of neuroleptic and other modern medications may have extinguished catatonic symptoms in schizophrenic populations.

339.   **(C)** There is no evidence of occupational or social dysfunction or marked distress caused by this patient's activities. Virtually all DSM-IV-TR diagnoses are qualified by these criteria. If the patient did describe such concerns, the diagnosis would most likely be sexual masochism, in which patients are aroused by psychologically or physically punishing acts by another person (or fantasies of punishment). In sexual sadism, the patient is aroused by giving such punishment (or fantasies of giving it) to others. Fetishism involves sexual arousal connected to nonliving objects. In frotteurism, the patient is sexually aroused by touching or rubbing up against a nonconsenting person.

340.   **(E)** Phobic disorders, including social phobia and the simple phobias (fear of animals, heights, closed spaces, blood, injections), have a prevalence of about 15%. MDD is present in between 5 and 10% of the population. Alzheimer's disease affects about 5% of the population older than 65, rising to 15 to 25% of patients aged 85 and older. Although not the most prevalent mental disorder, it is becoming increasingly common as the elderly population continues to increase. Generalized anxiety disorder has been estimated to have a 1-year prevalence rate of about 3 to

8%. Schizophrenia is found in about 1% of the worldwide population.

341.   **(C)** Narcolepsy is a disorder often affecting persons in their teens or 20s. It is a disorder of REM sleep mechanisms that also affects dogs. Circadian rhythm sleep disorder is a sleep disorder caused most often by sleep scheduling changes such as jet lag or night-shift work. Dyssomnia not otherwise specified is reserved for sleep disturbances of unknown cause or causes associated with environmental disturbances such as those that produce prolonged sleep deprivation. Restless legs syndrome falls under this category. Nightmare disorder is diagnosed in the absence of other predisposing mental illness (e.g., PTSD) in which the patient has repeated nightmares, causing significant distress. Primary hypersomnia is excessive daytime drowsiness or hours spent sleeping at night that is not better accounted for by an identifiable environmental or medical cause, substance abuse, or mental disorder (e.g., major depression). Additionally, it is not associated with specific stigmata of narcolepsy such as cataplexy or sleep paralysis.

342.   **(A)** Sudden loss of muscle tone associated with stressful situations is a special stigmata of narcolepsy and points to the connection of this disorder with REM sleep mechanisms (which inhibit movement and muscle tone during REM sleep). Catalepsy and catatonia are used to describe bizarre movement and posture behaviors found in catatonic schizophrenia and some psychotic depressions. "Sleep jerks" and "primary atonia" are meaningless terms.

343.   **(D)** Methylphenidate (Ritalin) has been shown to be useful in inhibiting onset of narcoleptic episodes, likely owing to the capacity for the drug to enhance central nervous system arousal mechanisms that inhibit REM-related mechanisms. Nighttime benzodiazepine regimens are not particularly effective for narcolepsy. Antidepressant treatment with TCAs has been found to be useful in combination with methylphenidate in some

patients with narcolepsy. However, the efficacy of bupropion, MAOIs such as phenelzine, and SSRIs such as fluoxetine has not been well studied.

344. **(D)** This woman's symptoms fit the DSM-IV-TR criteria for schizophrenia. She has had auditory hallucinations and persecutory delusions for at least a 1-month period, with evidence of the disturbance for at least 6 months as suggested in the history, leading to declining social function and problems with interpersonal relations. Delusional disorder can be excluded because the patient has other prominent symptoms (auditory hallucinations, social decline) in addition to prominent delusions. Schizophreniform disorder describes symptoms of duration more than 1 month but less than 6 months. Neither schizoaffective disorder nor MDD fit the symptoms, as the patient has not described any prominent mood symptoms.

345. **(E)** None of the listed medications are proven safe in pregnancy. Haloperidol and chlorpromazine are Class C drugs by Food and Drug Administration (FDA) rating, signifying that adverse fetal effects have been seen in animals, but there are no human data available. Lithium is a Class D drug, meaning that there is known human fetal risk, but the drug may be used in a life-threatening situation or when clinical circumstances justify its use. Valproic acid is Category X, indicating that there is proven fetal risk in humans such that the risk outweighs the benefit.

346. **(C)** Positive prognostic factors include late onset of illness, obvious precipitating stressors, acute onset, good premorbid social and work function, marriage, family history of mood symptoms, and positive symptoms (hallucinations). Negative prognostic factors include early onset of illness, lack of precipitating stressors, insidious onset, poor premorbid social and work function, withdrawn/autistic behavior, positive family history of schizophrenia, poor social supports, negative symptoms (disorganized behavior, amotivation), neurologic symptoms,

and history of perinatal trauma. Choice A is not true; while some patients may recover (often with the proper treatment), the majority do not spontaneously recover. Choices B and D may be possible scenarios but cannot be conclusively stated about the prognosis of this patient.

347. **(C)** This patient's symptoms fit DSM-IV-TR criteria for premenstrual dysphoric disorder (PMDD). Her symptoms are not severe enough nor of sufficient duration (2 or more weeks) to diagnose MDD. The remittance of symptoms in the week after menses is typical of PMDD. In adults, dysthymic disorder is characterized by subthreshold depressive symptoms, for more days than not, over a 2-year period. The patient does not describe prominent anxiety symptoms, making generalized anxiety disorder unlikely. This is not just "normal female behavior."

348. **(E)** All of the choices have been shown to treat at least some of the symptoms of PMDD in clinical trials.

349. **(E)** A number of studies place the prevalence of PMDD at 2 to 10%.

350. **(C)** Heroin overdose is most likely to have caused the clinical situation described. Cocaine use causes pupillary dilatation, not constriction. PCP and alcohol intoxication may cause coma, but both are associated with nystagmus rather than pupillary size changes. Inhalants are also known to cause coma but are not classically associated with pupillary constriction.

351–352. **(351-B, 352-C)** The only test available to document heroin/opiate use is a urine toxicology screen. Heroin may be detected in the urine for 36 to 72 hours after last use.

353. **(B)** Naloxone is used to reverse the acute effects of opiate overdose by blocking CNS opioid receptors. Acetylcysteine is administered in acetaminophen overdose, while deferoxamine is used in iron overdose. Methylene blue is used to treat methemoglobinemia.

354. **(C)** This woman's symptoms, including depressed mood, decreased appetite, diminished energy, insomnia, lack of interest in previously pleasurable activities, and recurrent thoughts of suicide fit criteria for MDD. A diagnosis of bipolar disorder requires a history of at least one previous manic episode; while this diagnosis cannot be ruled out based on the information provided in the question, the lack of a prior psychiatric history makes bipolar disorder less likely than major depression. Normal grieving may involve mild depressive symptoms such as low mood, sleep problems, and difficulty concentrating; however, if symptoms persist beyond 2 months, involve suicidal behavior, or lead to marked functional disturbance, major depression should be diagnosed. Criteria for dysthymic disorder requires exclusion of a major depressive episode and that subthreshold symptoms of depression be present for at least 2 years in adults (one year in children). This patient does have a sleep disturbance, but this does not best account for her entire clinical picture.

355. **(E)** All of the listed medical conditions can be associated with depressive symptoms and should be considered in the differential diagnosis.

356. **(E)** All of the listed foods have high tyramine content and when consumed while taking an MAOI may cause a potentially lethal hypertensive crisis.

357. **(B)** This case best depicts a case of a patient who is feigning or producing symptoms of an illness in order to gain gratification from assuming the sick role. There is little reason to believe this act could help her achieve financial or other material gain as in malingering. In conversion disorder, patients are primarily preoccupied with the idea that they have an illness that presents with a constellation of neurologic symptoms that are usually not physiologic. In hypochondriasis, a patient believes that he or she has some particular medical diagnosis. It is the worry about this illness that causes much of the distress.

Patients with somatoform disorder tend to have clusters of subjective symptoms over time affecting multiple possible organ symptoms or anatomic parts that do not usually correlate to any specific medical diagnosis.

358. **(E)** Studies show that 70 to 90% of patients with schizophrenia smoke. Other studies have shown that 30 to 70% of patients with alcoholism smoke. Up to 70% of patients with bipolar disorder smoke. Patients with anxiety and major depression have a 40 to 60% incidence of smoking.

359. **(B)** This patient meets criteria for a current manic episode with symptoms of psychomotor agitation, pressured speech, grandiose thinking, flight of ideas, and history of excessive spending as evidenced by his credit card debt. His history of good premorbid functioning and a remitted major depression are also consistent with a diagnosis of bipolar disorder rather than schizophrenia. Adjustment disorders present with an identifiable stressor creating a milder mood, anxiety, or behavioral disturbance than is present in this case. The patient's presentation of mania rules out major depression. In fact, although he may have future major depressive episodes, he should never be diagnosed with MDD due to the current episode of mania. This patient's history does not reveal an exposure to an acute severe psychological stressor, and he does not present with symptoms of reliving past traumas, hypervigilance, and avoidance as in PTSD.

360. **(C)** Bipolar disorder usually presents in a range of ages from childhood to age 50, with a mean age of onset of 30.

361. **(A)** Bipolar disorder, like schizophrenia, has a substantial genetic component and affects about 1% of the general population.

362. **(C)** Classically, infarcts of the left frontal hemispheres (part of left middle cerebral artery distribution) present with depression, while those of the right frontal hemisphere present with euphoria, inappropriate indifference, or mania. Obsessive–compulsive behaviors present occasionally after diffuse bilateral frontal injury. Panic and anxiety symptoms have not been described as having any particular association with left middle cerebral artery strokes, although such comorbid cases probably exist.

363. **(C)** Patients with paranoid personality disorder rarely present to psychiatrists. If they presented with a severe psychosis, as in this case, they would probably be given a schizophrenia spectrum disorder diagnosis. Patients using a variety of recreational substances represent a major fraction of patients presenting to emergency departments with psychotic symptoms. Patients with severe affective disorders may commonly present with mood-congruent psychoses (e.g., grandiose delusions in mania, delusions of guilt in major depression).

364. **(E)** About 90% of cases of impotence in the age group 30 to 50 have a psychological etiology. After 50, the etiology becomes increasingly medically related to causes such as medications, diabetes, hypertension, and alcoholism.

365. **(E)** The serotonin metabolite designated 5-HIAA measured in the CSF has been shown to be lower than control groups in postmortem analysis of victims of suicide and patients with impulsivity and violence or aggression. No such associations have been established with the other neurotransmitters listed.

366. **(D)** Depression is the most common presenting psychiatric symptom in patients with multiple sclerosis. It may present during the course of mild progressive cognitive decline that is consistent with a subcortical dementia (slowing of mental processing, motor difficulties, blunted or inappropriate affect, relative preservation of language-dependent skills). Neuroimaging of these patients usually shows diffuse white-matter plaques affecting the frontal lobes. Ventricular enlargement and cerebral atrophy are associated with the most common form of cortical dementia, Alzheimer's disease.

367. **(B)** It is very common for persons with paraphilia to have more than one form of paraphilia. For example, a person may be both voyeuristic and exhibitionistic as well as stimulated by acts of frotteurism. Half of all paraphilias have onset before age 18 years, not 30. There is a clear predominance of male patients with paraphilias, rather than a balance between the genders. Pedophilia, rather than voyeurism, is the most common paraphilia. Ten to 20% of women have been victims of childhood molestation of some form. While adults, up to 20% of women may experience being the object of exhibitionism or voyeurism.

368. **(C)** High-potency and other typical neuroleptics are known to have a lack of efficacy for the negative symptoms of schizophrenia. Atypical antipsychotics, including clozapine, risperidone, and olanzapine, all have relatively high $5-HT_2$-blocking activity compared to typical neuroleptics. These medications have in some studies been shown to reduce the negative symptoms of schizophrenia, although controversy still remains whether this effect represents the lack of extrapyramidal symptoms with the atypicals that would often come along with typical neuroleptic treatment. This controversy hinges on the issue of the large overlap of symptoms between the negative symptom syndrome and motor and behavioral side effects of typical neuroleptics. SSRIs and TCAs have not been particularly effective for negative symptoms of schizophrenia, although they may treat a comorbid depression that may be complicating the negative symptoms.

369. **(E)** Generally speaking, patients with pronounced negative syndromes have greater social and occupational difficulty, refractoriness to medications, and more chronicity of illness compared to patients whose diseases are more episodic with acute psychotic exacerbations. Onset of symptoms late in life is a good prognostic indicator for patients with

schizophrenia, as is good premorbid functioning. Patients who are married also do better than those who are single, possibly reflecting the advantages of social support in the marriage. Marriage is more likely be an option for those patients who are less socially impaired on account of having milder negative symptoms. Patients with a positive family history of affective disorders, rather than schizophrenia, have a better prognosis in schizophrenia. Generally speaking, the more schizophrenia-like the clinical picture and the family history, the worse the prognosis, while the more affective-like, the better the prognosis. The sudden-onset symptoms in schizophrenia, as opposed to insidious onset, is a good prognostic indicator, possibly because it reflects less chronicity of symptoms and a greater chance of medical or psychoactive agent–related psychosis.

370. **(C)** About 12% of children who have one parent with schizophrenia suffer from schizophrenia, while the risk climbs to 40% if both parents have schizophrenia.

371. **(C)** About half of all identical twin siblings with schizophrenia also have schizophrenia. These data have served as important evidence that schizophrenia represents the result of a combination of environmental stressors and genetic vulnerability. About 12% of dizygotic twins of schizophrenic patients also have schizophrenia. A nontwin sibling of a person with schizophrenia has about an 8% risk of having schizophrenia.

372. **(E)** There are a number of stigmata associated with schizophrenia that are not included in the diagnostic criteria. These include "soft" neurologic signs such as short-term memory deficits, unstable smooth pursuit eye movements, and decreased ability to habituate to repeated sensory stimuli (sensory gating abnormalities). In addition, patients with schizophrenia have difficulty in conceptualizing complex visual compositions. Patients with major depression, PTSD, OCD, and ADHD also have been shown to have

short-term memory difficulties, but not the other stigmata mentioned.

373. **(B)** The most likely diagnosis is generalized anxiety disorder (GAD). This patient meets criteria for GAD, including excessive uncontrollable worry about numerous events for at least 6 months, a sleep disturbance, muscle tension, and an irritable mood. Social phobia is incorrect as there is no evidence that he fears social or performance situations. Major depression is unlikely because he denies a depressed mood and does not report neurovegetative symptoms (appetite and energy changes) of depression other than a sleep deficit. There is no report of substance abuse or panic attacks in the vignette, thus making the last two diagnoses unlikely.

374. **(E)** Psychotherapy, benzodiazepines, antidepressants, and beta blockers can all be used in the treatment of GAD. Dynamic, supportive, and cognitive behavioral therapy are also used to treat GAD.

375. **(C)** The most appropriate next step is to send the patient to the psychiatric emergency department. This patient is experiencing an acute episode of major depression, and because of his suicidal ideation with thoughts of overdosing he should be referred to the emergency department for further assessment while assuring his safety. Telling the patient he will be fine, prescribing medication, or contacting his parents about transportation and a family meeting does not adequately address his immediate safety.

376. **(E)** The most likely additional diagnosis is major depression, but a mood disorder secondary to substance use cannot be ruled out at this time. A complete history and physical exam, including obtaining a urine sample to test for drugs of abuse, will help clarify the diagnosis. Social phobia and panic disorder are not diagnostic possibilities at this time.

377. **(A)** The most likely diagnosis is bipolar disorder, classified in the DSM-IV-TR as a mood

disorder in which the individual will experience symptoms of a depressive disorder and symptoms of mania, independently, during the course of the illness. The current episode exemplifies a manic episode with symptoms that include inflated self-esteem and grandiosity, pressured speech, a decreased need for sleep, and an impulsive shopping excursion without considering possible consequences. A psychotic disorder like schizophrenia cannot be diagnosed, as there is no indication of prominent psychotic symptoms (hallucinations, disorganized thought processes and speech) present for at least 6 months. Personality and anxiety disorder do not present with the classic signs of mania.

378. **(C)** From the choices given, the patient was most likely taking either lithium or valproic acid (Depakote), which are both mood stabilizers and both indicated for the treatment of bipolar disorder. Buspirone, an anxiolytic, and propranolol, a beta blocker used occasionally for GAD and panic disorder, are not likely to have been prescribed for this patient's bipolar disorder. Ranitidine (Zantac), while sometimes confused by patients for the benzodiazepine alprazolam (Xanax), is an antacid.

379. **(F)** Schizophrenia is the most common illness in hospitalized psychiatric patients in the United States.

380. **(H)** Folie à deux is a shared delusion aroused in one person by the influence of another.

381. **(G)** Glucocorticoids (e.g., prednisone) are a common iatrogenic cause of reversible psychiatric symptoms such as depression and psychosis.

382. **(D)** Beta-amyloid plaque buildup is seen in Alzheimer's dementia.

383. **(C)** Like alcohol, benzodiazepines have potentially extremely dangerous withdrawal syndromes, which have essentially identical clinical features (due to their near-identical actions on GABA modulation in the brain). The danger of withdrawal is even greater with the short-acting benzodiazepines (short-acting drugs in general cause more acute withdrawal), and alprazolam (Xanax) is one of the very shortest. Despite the profound discomfort of withdrawal from heroin and other opiates, opiate withdrawal is not life threatening. Withdrawal from PCP is not well characterized.

384. **(E)** The Hamilton Depression Scale is a commonly used measure of depressive symptoms. The Rorschach Test is a projective test, using inkblots, which measures perceptual accuracy, reality testing, and integration of affective and intellectual functioning.

385. **(F)** Dementia praecox was an early term for schizophrenia, coined by Kraepelin.

386. **(J)** Korsakoff's dementia (alcohol-induced persisting amnestic disorder) commonly evinces confabulation.

387. **(C)** Conversion disorder is described as the often sudden onset of a singular neurologic deficit, often in the setting of stress. As in this case, there can be (often subconscious) guilt linkage to the development of the symptom.

388. **(A)** Characteristic features of borderline personality disorder, as demonstrated in this patient, include self-mutilative behavior (which can temporarily bring relief of emotional angst), emotional volatility, and instability of relationships with others, including tendencies to view others as either "all good" or "all bad" (also referred to as "splitting"). Borderline personality disorder often arises in patients who have histories of abandonment and/or abuse at a young age.

389. **(D)** Antisocial personality disorder describes individuals with long histories of disregard to the rights of others and dishonesty used in attempts to gain something for themselves. Often comorbid with substance abuse, this disorder is extremely common in prison inmates (30 to 50%). Schizotypal personality disorder is marked by a pattern of difficulty with close relationships as well as cognitive and perceptual disturbances. Schizoid per-

sonality disorder differs from schizotypal personal disorder by the absence of cognitive and perceptual disturbances.

390. **(B)** Somatization disorder describes the condition suffered by individuals who have a long history of multiple somatic complaints (gastrointestinal, sexual, and neurologic) that, despite exhaustive medical workups, have either no identifiable cause or are out of proportion to the medical findings. These patients often describe themselves as having been sickly all their lives and, presumably in their frustration with doctors' inability to find reasons for their problems, chronically "doctor shop."

391. **(H)** The hallmark of hypochondriasis is the belief by a patient that he or she has a specific medical illness. Patients with the disorder often interpret somatic complaints as signifying definite serious illness.

392. **(G)** Factitious disorder, Munchausen's type, describes the condition suffered by patients who intentionally produce signs and/or symptoms of medical illness. Commonly, patients will be former health care workers or have such workers in their families.

393. **(I)** Agoraphobia describes the condition suffered by individuals who fear open, crowded spaces, particularly ones from which "escape" may be difficult. It is often comorbid with panic disorder, as suggested by this patient's symptom of palpitations.

CHAPTER 5

Somatic Treatment and Psychopharmacology

Frank G. Fortunati, MD, JD, and Raziya Sunderji, MD

Questions

DIRECTIONS (Questions 394 through 491): Each of the numbered items or incomplete statements in this section is followed by answers or by completions of the statement. Select the ONE lettered answer or completion that is BEST in each case.

Questions 394 through 396

A 32-year-old man is admitted to a general hospital after ingesting an unknown quantity of phenelzine (Nardil) in a suicide attempt. After gastric lavage and administration of a charcoal slurry, he is transferred to the medical intensive care unit for monitoring. Twenty-four hours later, he begins to see horses running in the halls and pulls out his intravenous (IV) lines.

394. The most important treatment at this time should include

   (A) chlorpromazine (Thorazine)
   (B) bretylium (Bretylol)
   (C) lorazepam (Ativan)
   (D) phenytoin (Dilantin)
   (E) meperidine (Demerol)

395. Twelve days after his suicide attempt, he receives venlafaxine (Effexor) to treat his depression. One hour after ingestion of the venlafaxine, he becomes tachycardic and diaphoretic and develops myoclonic jerks. This condition is known as

   (A) neuroleptic malignant syndrome
   (B) akathisia
   (C) serotonin syndrome

   (D) rapid-cycling bipolar disorder
   (E) opisthotonos

396. In the central nervous system (CNS), the neurotransmitter associated with the above reaction is mostly synthesized in the

   (A) nucleus accumbens
   (B) locus ceruleus
   (C) raphe nucleus
   (D) caudate nucleus
   (E) substantia nigra

Questions 397 through 399

A 24-year-old woman presents to her primary care physician for a regular checkup. During the exam, her doctor notes a 15-pound weight gain. She complains that she always feels tired during the day despite sleeping from 8 P.M. to 9 A.M. daily. On further questioning, the physician learns that the patient feels sad and empty, often thinks about death, cannot concentrate at work, and lacks the energy to care for her two children. However, her mood picks up when her physician questions her about her children.

397. The most effective agent would be

   (A) fluoxetine (Prozac)
   (B) nortriptyline (Pamelor)
   (C) phenelzine (Nardil)
   (D) sertraline (Zoloft)
   (E) trazodone (Desyrel)

398. Her physician initiates treatment with citalopram (Celexa). Which of the following is considered an adequate trial of this agent?

(A) 2 weeks

(B) 6 weeks

(C) 3 months

(D) 6 months

(E) 8 months

399. What symptoms can her physician expect to improve last?

(A) depressed mood

(B) hyperphagia

(C) hypersomnia

(D) daytime fatigue

(E) poor concentration

Questions 400 through 404

While on call in a general hospital, you are called at 4:30 A.M. to evaluate a patient who wants to be discharged. Upon arriving on the floor, the nurse tells you he just pulled out his third IV of the day and started to swing the IV pole in the air while yelling profanities. He tells a nurse's aide he must capture the tiger that is loose in the parking lot. You quickly look at his chart and see that he is a 55-year-old man admitted 36 hours earlier for abdominal pain, nausea, and vomiting. His transaminases were elevated on admission, but his hepatitis profile is still pending. His orders are for Tylenol and Maalox as needed, normal saline at 125 cc/hr, and NPO for upper endoscopy in the morning.

400. The most appropriate initial medication at this time is

(A) oxazepam (Serax)

(B) chlordiazepoxide (Librium)

(C) haloperidol (Haldol)

(D) chlorpromazine (Thorazine)

(E) disulfiram (Antabuse)

401. The receptor most closely associated with these symptoms is

(A) dopamine-2 (D_2)

(B) dopamine-4 (D_4)

(C) gamma-aminobutyric acid (GABA)-A

(D) GABA-B

(E) 5-hydroxytryptamine-2 (5-HT$_2$)

402. You speak briefly with this patient and are able to settle him down. His temperature is 102.1°F, pulse is 130, and blood pressure is 220/120. The most appropriate medication and route should be

(A) labetalol (Normodyne) IV

(B) haloperidol (Haldol) IM

(C) haloperidol IV

(D) lorazepam (Ativan) IM

(E) lorazepam IV

403. This syndrome usually occurs

(A) within the first 12 hours after admission

(B) within the first 2 days after admission

(C) within the first 5 days after admission

(D) within the first 10 days after admission

(E) anytime during this admission

404. Another medication that this patient should receive promptly is

(A) thiamine (vitamin B$_1$)

(B) pyridoxine (vitamin B$_6$)

(C) phenytoin (Dilantin)

(D) valproic acid (Depakote)

(E) disulfiram (Antabuse)

Questions 405 through 410

A 32-year-old single woman presents to the emergency department escorted by her family after she revealed to them a plan to take a full bottle of Tylenol and drink a bottle of wine in a suicide attempt. She claims that she cannot handle work any longer because her boss is trying to have her fired and her coworkers are helping him find fault in her work. She states they have even tapped her phone and are having her followed. Your detailed history reveals the following: She has never attempted suicide before and has never seen a psychiatrist; she was engaged to be married 2 years ago, but her fiance was killed in an auto accident; she has difficulty falling asleep at night and wakes up often during the night; she can no longer concentrate on her work; and she does not enjoy painting as she once did. She has lost 10 pounds over the past 2 months without dieting. She denies hallucinations of any type. There is no significant family history of psychiatric illness.

405. Which of the following medications would be the most appropriate first-line therapy?

(A) phenelzine (Nardil)

(B) trazodone (Desyrel)

(C) sertraline (Zoloft)

(D) amoxapine (Asendin)

(E) amitriptyline (Elavil)

406. One theory regarding the mechanism of action for antidepressants, taking into account the delayed therapeutic response, involves

(A) downregulation of postsynaptic 5-HT$_2$ binding sites

(B) upregulation of postsynaptic 5-HT$_2$ binding sites

(C) increased serotonin in the synaptic cleft

(D) increased mitochondrial serotonin

(E) downregulation of dopamine receptors

407. In addition to the above medication, her physician should strongly consider the addition of

(A) benztropine (Cogentin)

(B) thyroxine (Synthroid)

(C) propranolol

(D) lithium

(E) olanzapine (Zyprexa)

408. After 5 weeks of the treatment you prescribed above, the patient no longer has suicidal thoughts and is able to function well at work. She has begun to date again and is considering resuming a sexual relationship with an old boyfriend. The most common side effect of sexual function of the medications you prescribed for her is

(A) anorgasmia

(B) dyspareunia

(C) decreased desire

(D) vaginismus

(E) female analog of premature ejaculation

409. Two months after starting treatment with you, the patient reports that she feels "back to normal" and asks when she can stop the medication you initially prescribed. You tell her that she can safely stop the medication

(A) now

(B) in 2 months

(C) in 4 months

(D) after 10 months

(E) after 5 years

410. She returns 3 months after starting treatment and reports a poor sexual relationship with her boyfriend. Which of the following antidepressants could be considered in place of your original therapy if the sexual dysfunction becomes intolerable?

(A) bupropion (Wellbutrin)

(B) fluvoxamine (Luvox)

(C) fluoxetine (Prozac)

(D) clomipramine (Anafranil)

(E) citalopram (Celexa)

Questions 411 through 416

A 25-year-old man presents to the emergency department accompanied by his family, who report that the patient has not left his bedroom in 3 weeks. They report that he spends his day reading science fiction novels that they provide for him. He was once prescribed perphenazine (Trilafon), which they tell you seemed to help him, but he refuses to take it. On exam, you find him to be malodorous and disheveled. He is guarded when you speak with him. He does not make eye contact, and he avoids looking at the television in the waiting room because, he says, he wants to prevent intruders from controlling his thoughts. After completing the exam, you admit him to the inpatient psychiatric unit.

411. Because the patient did not take the perphenazine, you decide to try fluphenazine (Prolixin). After 5 days, he is no longer afraid to look at the television but he spends much of the day pacing the floor. He claims he paces the floor because he does not like sitting in his room. His family informs you that he often walked the streets of his neighborhood when he was taking perphenazine. After reducing the fluphenazine to the lowest dose you feel he needs, he still paces the halls. Next, you

    (A) discontinue fluphenazine (Prolixin) and try another agent
    (B) add propranolol
    (C) add lorazepam (Ativan)
    (D) add benztropine (Cogentin)
    (E) add diphenhydramine (Benadryl)

412. One week later, he leaves the hospital and returns home. He continues the medications you prescribed and on a follow-up visit you notice he moves slowly and has a festinating gait. Which of the following antipsychotic agents is least likely to cause this effect?

    (A) risperidone (Risperdal)
    (B) haloperidol (Haldol)
    (C) olanzapine (Zyprexa)
    (D) thiordiazine (Mellaril)
    (E) chlorpromazine (Thorazine)

413. The receptor most likely to account for the above side effect is

    (A) nigrostriatal D_2 receptors
    (B) mesolimbic D_2 receptors
    (C) basal ganglia acetylcholine receptors
    (D) D_4 receptors
    (E) 5-HT$_2$

414. His parents ask you about clozapine, which has been recommended by previous psychiatrists. Clozapine's side effect that causes the greatest alarm is

    (A) thrombocytopenia
    (B) sustained sinus tachycardia

    (C) sialorrhea
    (D) agranulocytosis
    (E) orthostatic hypotension

415. Despite your treatment, the patient still has psychotic symptoms. He and his parents agree to try clozapine. You have initiated treatment slowly and he has shown some improvement; however, he has been producing a large amount of saliva and drool, soaking his shirts. You should

    (A) stop treatment with clozapine
    (B) initiate propranolol
    (C) initiate propylthiouracil
    (D) increase the dose of clozapine
    (E) initiate amantadine

416. In addition to the above side effect, he has developed an increase in his resting heart rate. An electrocardiogram (ECG) revealed a sinus tachycardia without other changes from his baseline. This has been repeated several times over the past month, and the heart rate remains elevated. You should consider

    (A) stopping treatment with clozapine
    (B) initiating benztropine
    (C) checking creatinine phosphokinase levels
    (D) initiating treatment with propranolol
    (E) initiating treatment with labetalol

Questions 417 through 420

A 33-year-old mentally retarded male resident of a group home presents to the emergency department escorted by staff members who believe he has become confused and disoriented over the past few days. He has been a resident there for several years without incident, but last week his thioridazine was changed to haloperidol because of concerns about the long-term use of high doses of thioridazine. On exam, you find him to be disoriented to place and time; he is diaphoretic with a temperature of 105.8° F, a heart rate of 130 beats/min, and a respiratory rate of 20/min. His extremities are stiff. Routine labs reveal a white blood count (WBC) of

15,000; blood urea nitrogen (BUN) 75 mg%, creatinine 1.2 mg%, and creatinine phosphokinase 2,300 mg%.

417. The most likely diagnosis is

   (A) acute dystonia
   (B) neuroleptic malignant syndrome (NMS)
   (C) serotonin syndrome
   (D) sepsis
   (E) renal failure

418. The most common serious complication this patient may experience is

   (A) respiratory failure
   (B) pulmonary embolism
   (C) rhabdomyolysis
   (D) myocardial infarction
   (E) diffuse intravascular coagulation

419. The most appropriate treatment for this patient is

   (A) dialysis
   (B) urine acidification
   (C) urine alkalinization
   (D) dantrolene
   (E) benztropine

420. The long-term consequence of high-dose thioridazine use that probably caused his physician to switch to haloperidol is

   (A) tardive dyskinesia
   (B) priapism
   (C) retinal pigmentation
   (D) hyperprolactinemia
   (E) agranulocytosis

Questions 421 through 424

A 45-year-old unemployed investment banker presents to your office accompanied by his wife. He has been out of work for 1 month because he is afraid to take the train into work. He never had difficulty traveling until 2 months ago, when on a train during a family vacation, he suffered chest pain, shortness of breath, nausea, and a fear of dying. These symptoms lasted about 15 minutes. A workup by a cardiologist was negative. However, these symptoms, also accompanied by intense fear and a feeling of being detached from himself, have continued. He has had about two attacks a week and also has fear just thinking about returning to work because he fears he will die on the train. He tells you that he could not have come to see you without his wife's help.

421. A reasonable first choice of pharmacotherapy for this patient would be

   (A) bupropion (Wellbutrin)
   (B) trazodone (Desyrel)
   (C) propranolol
   (D) buspirone (BuSpar)
   (E) fluoxetine (Prozac)

422. A frequent side effect when starting the above medication in patients such as this is

   (A) sedation
   (B) anxiety
   (C) constipation
   (D) mania
   (E) paranoia

423. The most frequently used benzodiazepine to help reduce symptoms acutely is

   (A) oxazepam (Serax)
   (B) chlordiazepoxide (Librium)
   (C) diazepam (Valium)
   (D) alprazolam (Xanax)
   (E) temazepam (Restoril)

424. The most potent antianxiety agent is

   (A) alprazolam (Xanax)
   (B) buspirone (BuSpar)
   (C) clonazepam (Klonopin)
   (D) chlordiazepoxide (Librium)
   (E) diazepam (Valium)

Questions 425 through 429

A 22-year-old single male college music student reluctantly presents to your office on the request of his parents. His parents are worried because he has not been eating, talks constantly, and never seems to sleep. He says he has never felt better, he's writing several songs a day, and needs only a few hours of sleep. He believes he will be the next John Lennon and wants to get back to writing, but he can't even stay focused long enough to answer any of your questions. He does not have any psychiatric history and denies using any substances.

425. The most appropriate agent for initial and maintenance treatment of this patient is

   (A) clonazepam (Klonopin)
   (B) lithium
   (C) topiramate (Topamax)
   (D) haloperidol (Haldol)
   (E) gabapentin (Neurontin)

426. The minimum initial laboratory data that should be obtained before starting treatment is

   (A) serum creatinine, BUN and electrolytes, thyroid studies, urinalysis
   (B) liver function tests, serum creatinine, BUN and electrolytes
   (C) complete blood count (CBC) with differential
   (D) prothrombin and partial thromboplastin times
   (E) serum ammonia

427. A common initial side effect of the above treatment is

   (A) priapism
   (B) delayed ejaculation
   (C) psoriasis
   (D) increased appetite
   (E) polydipsia

428. The most common neuropsychiatric side effect of the above treatment is

   (A) amnesia
   (B) paresthesias
   (C) cogwheel rigidity
   (D) seizures
   (E) hand tremor

429. After starting appropriate treatment, he sprains his ankle while exercising. His primary care doctor told him to take over-the-counter ibuprofen, which he started 2 days ago. His ankle still hurts, and he plans to continue taking the medication. You advise him to

   (A) increase the dose of ibuprofen
   (B) decrease the dose of ibuprofen
   (C) continue ibuprofen at the prescribed dose
   (D) switch to aspirin
   (E) stop the medication you prescribed

Questions 430 through 432

A 9-year-old boy is brought to the physician because his parents have received a note from his second-grade teacher complaining that he is disruptive in class. His teacher believes he could achieve better grades if he could sit still and pay attention. His parents report he has always been an active child but does have difficulty getting along with other children in the neighborhood. In the exam room, he can't sit still and has difficulty completing a task you have assigned.

430. The most appropriate medication for initial management of this condition is

   (A) lorazepam (Ativan)
   (B) lithium
   (C) fluoxetine (Prozac)
   (D) desipramine (Norpramin)
   (E) methylphenidate (Ritalin)

431. The most common side effect of this treatment is

(A) difficulty falling asleep

(B) daytime drowsiness

(C) slowed growth

(D) increase in appetite

(E) decrease in systolic blood pressure

432. Treatment with the above medication has been reported to exacerbate

(A) bedwetting

(B) tics

(C) poor impulse control

(D) reading difficulties

(E) myopia

Questions 433 and 434

A 9-year-old boy is brought to your office by his mother because of his "compulsions," which have worsened over the past year. She first noticed them last year when several times a day he would repeatedly blink his eyes and frown while clearing his throat. He continues to do this despite trying not to, and in addition, he often sticks out his tongue and smells his shirt while speaking with classmates. These "compulsions" have caused him to lose friends at school.

433. Pharmacologic blockade of which of the following receptors provides the greatest relief of these symptoms?

(A) norepinephrine

(B) serotonin

(C) dopamine

(D) alpha-2

(E) GABA

434. Which of the following agents is most effective to treat this disorder?

(A) amitriptyline (Elavil)

(B) haloperidol (Haldol)

(C) clonidine (Catapres)

(D) alprazolam (Xanax)

(E) paroxetine (Paxil)

Questions 435 through 438

You have been treating a 55-year-old man with schizophrenia for 20 years with haloperidol (Haldol) and benztropine (Cogentin). Generally, he has done well and has not required major medication changes or hospitalizations. About 2 years ago, you noticed some lip smacking and tongue protrusions that did not bother him; however, now he also has odd, irregular movements of his arms that make it difficult for him to eat.

435. The syndrome that best describes these symptoms is

(A) Meige syndrome

(B) anticholinergic toxicity

(C) tardive dyskinesia

(D) Huntington's disease

(E) Sydenham's chorea

436. The most appropriate next step is to

(A) order a magnetic resonance imaging (MRI) scan of the brain

(B) decrease the dose of haloperidol

(C) increase the dose of haloperidol

(D) decrease the dose of benztropine

(E) increase the dose of benztropine

437. The only medication that may improve these symptoms is

(A) benztropine (Cogentin)

(B) trihexyphenidyl (Artane)

(C) olanzapine (Zyprexa)

(D) levodopa (Dopar)

(E) clozapine (Clozaril)

438. Which of the following is a definite risk factor for developing these symptoms?

(A) age over 50 years

(B) male gender

(C) presence of an affective disorder

(D) family history of Parkinson's disease

(E) use of low-potency antipsychotics

439. A 24-year-old married secretary has complained of dizziness, palpitations, and sweaty palms for the past 10 months. Sometimes, she also has extreme muscle tension in her neck that occurs both at work and at home. She has difficulty falling asleep and feels "edgy" most of the day. She also has difficulty concentrating at work. She has gone to a local emergency department three times because of the palpitations, but nothing was found. Her family practitioner placed her on a hypoglycemic diet and referred her to a neurologist, who found no abnormalities. She tells you she has many worries about her family but does not feel particularly depressed. Which of the following will provide the most immediate relief of her symptoms?

(A) alprazolam (Xanax)
(B) fluoxetine (Prozac)
(C) bupropion (Wellbutrin)
(D) buspirone (BuSpar)
(E) imipramine (Tofranil)

440. A 22-year-old woman is admitted to a psychiatric unit after a serious suicide attempt. She has had many suicide attempts in the past with varying severity. Her arms are scarred by prior attempts at hurting herself. She had been a good student until high school, when she took up with a "fast" crowd and began abusing alcohol and marijuana and ran away from home several times. She has had several intense, stormy relationships with men. Outpatient treatment has mostly consisted of her complaints to her therapist about her family. She usually calls her therapist daily about different crises; however, her therapist was on vacation during her most recent crisis. Which of the following classes of agents have been shown to be helpful for this patient?

(A) tricyclic antidepressants (TCAs) and antipsychotics
(B) selective serotonin reuptake inhibitors (SSRIs) and antipsychotics
(C) antipsychotics and benzodiazepines
(D) anticonvulsants and stimulants
(E) stimulants and SSRIs

441. A 36-year-old man is referred to you by his internist for evaluation of his eating disorder. He stands 6 feet 2 inches tall and had weighed 270 pounds until he lost 90 pounds last year because his wife thought he was "fat." Since losing the weight, he is obsessed with becoming fat. He hates feeling full after a meal. Sometimes, he binges on junk food but always induces vomiting afterwards. Now, he can no longer enjoy food and cannot stop dieting. Which of the following medications has shown success in treating such patients?

(A) fluoxetine (Prozac)
(B) mirtazapine (Remeron)
(C) phenytoin (Dilantin)
(D) protriptyline (Vivactil)
(E) quetiapine (Seroquel)

442. A 19-year-old woman is admitted to an inpatient psychiatric facility for her eating disorder. She weighs 82 pounds and stands 5 feet 6 inches tall. She began dieting in high school to lose an unwanted 5 pounds. Encouraged by compliments on her figure, she continued to lose another 10 pounds. Her eating habits are ritualized: She cuts her food into small pieces and moves it around on her plate. She has an intense fear of being overweight. Which of the following statements most accurately reflects pharmacotherapy for this type of patient?

(A) Successful pharmacotherapy should include appetite stimulants such as cyproheptadine (Periactin).
(B) Pharmacotherapy generally has a limited role in the treatment of these patients.
(C) High-dose chlorpromazine (Thorazine) is useful in treating these patients.
(D) Amitriptyline (Elavil) is useful in treating these patients.
(E) Promotility agents such as cisapride (Propulsid) are useful in treating patients who purge.

443. A 36-year-old man whom you have treated for 8 months with paroxetine (Paxil) for his first episode of major depression has done very well. Because of the sexual function side effects, he decided to stop taking it 3 days ago without first informing you. Two days after he stopped it, he became irritable and even had a crying spell. He had the flu 2 weeks ago, but body aches, chills, and general lethargy have returned. Which of the following should you consider?

(A) Start bupropion (Wellbutrin) because it lacks sexual side effects.

(B) Treat his flu symptomatically.

(C) Consider a mood stabilizer for his irritability.

(D) Restart the paroxetine (Paxil) and taper it off.

(E) Prescribe phenytoin (Dilantin) for seizure prophylaxis.

444. A 30-year-old man presents to a general hospital after ingesting 20 tablets of his prescribed carbamazepine (Tegretol) in a suicide attempt. He has no prior psychiatric history, but has a history of seizures. Your detailed history reveals several months of depressed mood, weight loss, anhedonia, sleeplessness, and difficulty concentrating. Four days after admission, his carbamazepine level has returned to normal and has been restarted to treat his seizure disorder. Which of the following medications would be most appropriate for this patient?

(A) fluoxetine (Prozac)

(B) nefazodone (Serzone)

(C) paroxetine (Paxil)

(D) clomipramine (Anafranil)

(E) amitriptyline (Elavil)

Questions 445 through 450

A 65-year-old man presents to your psychiatric office on a referral from his primary care physician for evaluation of depression. He feels depressed and hopeless and has lost his appetite. He no longer enjoys seeing his grandchildren. It takes him several hours to fall asleep at night, and he stays asleep only about 3 hours. He occasionally does not buy food because he is concerned about going broke; however, his family informs you that he is financially well off. He stands 6 feet tall and weighs 155 pounds, much less than his usual 175 pounds. Additionally, he feels guilty about becoming a burden on his family.

445. The most effective treatment for this patient is

(A) amoxapine (Asendin)

(B) phenelzine (Nardil)

(C) electroconvulsive therapy (ECT)

(D) phenelzine and olanzapine (Zyprexa)

(E) mirtazapine (Remeron)

446. The most common immediate side effect of the above treatment is

(A) drowsiness

(B) increased appetite

(C) cognitive impairment

(D) cardiac arrhythmias

(E) increased risk of suicide

447. A factor that, if present, predicts a poor response to the above treatment is

(A) delusions

(B) family history of depression

(C) psychomotor retardation

(D) unusually prolonged length of illness

(E) inability to react to environmental situations

448. Which of the following, if present, would be the strongest contraindication to the above treatment?

(A) chronic obstructive pulmonary disease (COPD)

(B) first-degree heart block

(C) cerebral arteriovenous malformation

(D) history of serious suicide attempts by overdose

(E) treatment with fluoxetine (Prozac) 2 weeks ago

449. An antidepressant medication that might be useful to help him fall asleep at night is

(A) diazepam (Valium)
(B) diphenhydramine (Benadryl)
(C) trazodone (Desyrel)
(D) fluoxetine (Prozac)
(E) bupropion (Wellbutrin)

450. A rare but troubling sexual side effect of the above medication is

(A) priapism
(B) premature ejaculation
(C) anorgasmia
(D) impotence
(E) gynecomastia

Questions 451 through 453

A 57-year-old man whom you have treated for 20 years for bipolar disorder is admitted to the general hospital with chest pain.

451. The hospital physician asks whether the lithium he is receiving can affect his ECG. You inform her that lithium

(A) has no effect on the ECG
(B) can prolong the P-R interval
(C) can invert the T waves
(D) can prolong the QT interval
(E) can shorten the QT interval

452. The most likely abnormality expected on urinalysis of this patient is

(A) low specific gravity
(B) proteinuria
(C) hematuria
(D) hyaline casts
(E) red cell casts

453. The patient was found to have suffered from a myocardial infarction (MI) and underwent angioplasty. He was discharged from the hospital on propranolol, losartan, topical nitroglycerin, hydrochlorothiazide, and one baby aspirin a day, in addition to his lithium. Prior to his MI, his lithium level was always 0.8 mmol/L on 900 mg of lithium carbonate a day. Now it is 1.3 mmol/L on the same dose. The most likely cause for this change is

(A) decreased volume of distribution post-MI
(B) aspirin
(C) hydrochlorothiazide
(D) captopril
(E) propranolol

Questions 454 through 456

A 47-year-old male novelist feared contamination from anything he believed was dirty. In restaurants, he would use his own plastic utensils. Elsewhere, he would wear gloves or use paper towels to avoid touching "dirty objects." Upon returning home, he would wash his hands five times at night before going about his activities. If he accidentally touched anything prior to washing his hands, he would experience a vague uncomfortable feeling and would be unable to perform his usual nightly activities. As a result of these symptoms he was unable to have a meaningful social life.

454. The most effective agent for this syndrome is

(A) clomipramine (Anafranil)
(B) mirtazapine (Remeron)
(C) clonazepam (Klonopin)
(D) phenelzine (Nardil)
(E) olanzapine (Zyprexa)

455. When using an SSRI such as fluoxetine, which of the following statements is often true?

(A) Doses used are higher than those used in depression.
(B) Doses used are lower than those used in depression.
(C) Response occurs more quickly than in depression.
(D) Patients often require divided daily doses.
(E) Psychodynamic psychotherapy is often required.

456. You started treating this patient with fluoxetine at 60 mg daily 4 months ago. He no longer needs to wash his hands quite so often but still has an uncomfortable feeling when he touches "dirty things." Which of the following statements is most accurate regarding treatment at this point?

(A) Buspirone (BuSpar) is not effective as an augmenting agent.

(B) Fenfluramine (Pendormin) has documented efficacy as an augmenting agent.

(C) Lithium has documented efficacy as an augmenting agent.

(D) Cingulotomy should be considered next.

(E) Clozapine (Clozaril) has been effective.

Questions 457 through 460

A 21-year-old college student has been hearing voices telling him to hurt himself for more than a year. Trials with the following agents have reduced the voices: chlorpromazine (Thorazine) 1,800 mg daily for 1 month, then haloperidol (Haldol) 60 mg daily for 6 weeks, then olanzapine (Zyprexa) 20 mg daily for 1 month. Despite a reduction in the voices, he has continued to remain isolated from family and friends.

457. Which of the following agents should be tried next?

(A) fluphenazine (Prolixin)

(B) risperidone (Risperdal)

(C) ziprasidone (Zeldox)

(D) clozapine (Clozaril)

(E) perphenazine (Trilafon)

458. A side effect that limits the use of the above agent is

(A) weight gain

(B) somnolence

(C) agranulocytosis

(D) decreased ejaculatory volume

(E) dystonic reactions

459. One of the leading theories for the efficacy of the above agent involves its action at which of the following receptors?

(A) D_2

(B) D_3

(C) D_4

(D) $5\text{-}HT_1$

(E) $5\text{-}HT_3$

460. The patient has been stable on the above medication for more than a year and wants to try bupropion (Wellbutrin) for smoking cessation. These two agents taken together should be used with caution because

(A) both may cause significant anticholinergic side effects

(B) both may cause orthostatic hypotension

(C) both may lower the seizure threshold

(D) bupropion may interfere with the absorption of clozapine

(E) bupropion may interfere with the metabolism of clozapine

461. A 65-year-old man with major depression and hypertension presents to the emergency department because he fell to the ground after arising from a chair. He has no significant cardiac history and his ECG, electrolytes, and neurologic exam are unremarkable. His family reports that his physician recently started a new antidepressant, but they do not know its name. Which of the following antidepressants is generally associated with this scenario?

(A) bupropion (Wellbutrin)

(B) mirtazapine (Remeron)

(C) nefazodone (Serzone)

(D) imipramine (Tofranil)

(E) nortriptyline (Pamelor)

462. A 35-year-old man with a history of seizures and hypertension has been treated for major depression with sertraline (Zoloft) at 200 mg daily for 2 months with no improvement in symptoms. He is not acutely suicidal, but he is frustrated by his lack of improvement. His primary care doctor has referred him to you for further evaluation. He has not had a seizure for years and is not taking any anticonvulsant medications. At this time, you should consider

(A) adding lithium to his regimen

(B) adding thyroid hormone

(C) switching to imipramine (Tofranil)

(D) switching to bupropion (Wellbutrin)

(E) switching to venlafaxine (Effexor)

Questions 463 through 467

A 28-year-old woman whom you have treated for bipolar disorder informs you that she is 3 weeks pregnant and is anxious about the baby's health. You are treating her with lithium, and she has not had a manic episode in 3 years.

463. Which of the following statements is correct regarding bipolar disorder and pregnancy?

(A) Lithium is safe after the first trimester and can be safely continued through birth.

(B) Divalproex sodium (Depakote) is a safe alternative to lithium.

(C) Carbamazepine (Tegretol) is a safe alternative to lithium.

(D) Lithium substantially increases the risk of Ebstein's anomaly of the tricuspid valves by 75%.

(E) Clonazepam (Klonopin) does not carry an increased risk of major fetal malformations.

464. Your patient discontinued her lithium and gave birth without complications. You have restarted her on lithium. Therapeutic levels of lithium are

(A) 0.4 to 0.6 mEq/L

(B) 0.8 to 1.2 mEq/L

(C) 5 to 10 mEq/L

(D) 10 to 20 mEq/L

(E) 50 to 100 mEq/L

465. Her lithium level is therapeutic. One year later, however, she enters a deep depression. She is unable to get out of bed, she cannot feed or care for her baby, and she weighs 15 pounds less than her pre-pregnancy weight. Which of the following medications should you consider at this time?

(A) olanzapine (Zyprexa)

(B) valproic acid (Depakote)

(C) bupropion (Wellbutrin)

(D) phenelzine (Nardil)

(E) desipramine (Norpramin)

466. Three years later, she has recovered from her depressive episode but has developed a goiter and clinical hypothyroidism. Her internist suspected the lithium as the culprit and discontinued it. She also placed her on thyroxine. Two months after the lithium is discontinued, she begins to spend more money than she has. She sleeps only a few hours each night. She has grandiose ideas of becoming a famous songwriter and is admitted to an inpatient psychiatric unit after driving recklessly to escape from another famous songwriter who was trying to steal her songs. All her thyroid indices are normal. Which of the following statements is true regarding treatment in this setting?

(A) Neuroleptic medications are contraindicated in the acute phase of treatment.

(B) Lithium is twice as effective as valproic acid in this setting.

(C) Response to treatment with lithium should occur in 2 days.

(D) A loading dose of lithium will not improve the response time.

(E) Valproic acid is as effective as carbamazepine.

467. Treatment with valproic acid is instituted. Which of the following statements regarding valproic acid treatment is correct?

(A) Weight gain may be seen with maintenance therapy.

(B) Serum creatinine needs to be monitored during treatment.

(C) Hirsutism may be seen with maintenance therapy.

(D) Gastrointestinal complaints are rare.

(E) Polycythemia is the most common hematologic side effect.

Questions 468 through 471

A 67-year-old woman presents to your office for evaluation of a 20-pound weight loss over a 4-month period and insomnia for the past 4 weeks. Her daughter informs you that her mother no longer enjoys any of her hobbies and has been speaking lately about dying. They have already consulted an internist, who performed an extensive medical workup, including chemistries, blood count, thyroid studies, gastrointestinal imaging, and endoscopy, all of which were normal.

468. You would like to start an antidepressant medication but would like to minimize adverse side effects while exploiting other side effects. Which of the following agents has a side effect profile that may be beneficial?

(A) nefazodone (Serzone)

(B) fluoxetine (Prozac)

(C) nortriptyline (Pamelor)

(D) mirtazapine (Remeron)

(E) bupropion (Wellbutrin)

469. Upon further history, you learn that antidepressants have failed in several previous trials. You would like to start a TCA. Which of the following would preclude using such an agent?

(A) lacunar infarcts

(B) treatment with the antihypertensive amlodipine

(C) left bundle branch block on ECG

(D) urinary retention

(E) estrogen replacement therapy

470. The pharmacology of TCAs involves

(A) 5-HT$_{2a}$ antagonism

(B) 5-HT$_{2a}$ agonism

(C) dopamine blockade

(D) inhibition of norepinephrine and serotonin reuptake

(E) inhibition of dopamine reuptake

471. Which of the following antidepressants would be least likely to exacerbate her pre-existing urinary retention?

(A) desipramine (Norpramin)

(B) nortriptyline (Pamelor)

(C) clomipramine (Anafranil)

(D) amitriptyline (Elavil)

(E) doxepin (Sinequan)

Questions 472 through 474

A 72-year-old man is admitted to a general hospital's intensive care unit because of altered mental status. His medical workup has revealed pneumonia and congestive heart failure (CHF). On the second hospital day, he is agitated and pulls out his IV access. He also has been noted to speak out loud with no one in the room. His level of consciousness seems to wax and wane. He does not have a psychiatric history and is not allergic to any medications. Besides his CHF and pneumonia, he does not have other comorbid conditions.

472. Which of the following agents would be the most appropriate to administer for his agitation?

(A) thioridazine (Mellaril)

(B) chlorpromazine (Thorazine)

(C) lorazepam (Ativan)

(D) olanzapine (Zyprexa)

(E) haloperidol (Haldol)

473. Which of the following agents would be least likely to cause orthostatic hypotension?

(A) haloperidol (Haldol)

(B) perphenazine (Trilafon)

(C) thioridazine (Mellaril)

(D) risperidone (Risperdal)

(E) quetiapine (Seroquel)

474. Intravenous use of haloperidol has been associated with which of the following adverse effects?

(A) NMS
(B) torsade de pointes arrhythmias
(C) increased anaphylaxis
(D) increased incidence of extrapyramidal side effects
(E) longer half-life

Questions 475 and 476

A 32-year-old man presents to your clinic after losing his job because he was intoxicated while working. He has been drinking daily since he was 16 years old. He was able to complete college and went to work full-time right after graduation, but has lost several jobs since then. After the loss of his last job, his wife threatened to leave him if he does not get help.

475. Which of the following agents can be used to sensitize him to the effects of alcohol?

(A) metronidazole (Flagyl)
(B) fluoxetine (Prozac)
(C) flumazenil (Romazicon)
(D) disulfiram (Antabuse)
(E) naloxone (Narcan)

476. Further history reveals that he does not have a mood disorder. He tells you that often he simply cannot control his craving to have another drink. Which of the following agents has shown some success in decreasing cravings for alcohol?

(A) fluoxetine (Prozac)
(B) disulfiram (Antabuse)
(C) naltrexone (ReVia)
(D) bupropion (Wellbutrin)
(E) diazepam (Valium)

Questions 477 and 478

A 36-year-old woman is referred to you by her primary care physician for management of anxiety and fear that has persisted for several months. She reports that she was raped and held hostage on a boat for several days by two armed men. During this, she experienced intense fear for her life. Since then, she has had intense stress whenever she is near the water and has frequent nightmares. She cannot recall details of the ordeal but tries to avoid driving her car within sight of the ocean, which has been difficult because of the location of her home. She feels detached from her husband and family and has abandoned plans to pursue her career as a painter. She has difficulty falling asleep and is easily startled by phone calls. She no longer goes to public places alone.

477. Which of the following agents is believed to help relieve the numbing symptoms she is experiencing?

(A) alprazolam (Xanax)
(B) fluoxetine (Prozac)
(C) carbamazepine (Tegretol)
(D) thioridazine (Mellaril)
(E) naltrexone (ReVia)

478. Whenever she drives near the water, which is unavoidable, she experiences intense anxiety, fear, and palpitations, and feels that she is re-experiencing her abduction. Which of the following agents may help reduce these symptoms?

(A) olanzapine (Zyprexa)
(B) naltrexone (ReVia)
(C) perphenazine (Trilafon)
(D) divalproex sodium (Depakote)
(E) clonidine (Catapres)

479. You have been asked to evaluate an 80-year-old male nursing home resident because of a change in mental status. The nursing staff reports that he has been a patient there for about a year without any problems until about 1 month ago when he was having difficulty sleeping. The staff physician prescribed lorazepam (Ativan) 2 mg at bedtime; however, he was still unable to sleep. He started wandering during the day and has been restricted to his room. Because he remains agitated during the day, they have been giving him lorazepam 2 mg every 6 hours for agitation. His other medications include hydrochlorothiazide 25 mg daily, digoxin 0.125 mg every other day, diltiazem (Cardizem) 240 mg sustained release daily, and transdermal nitroglycerin 0.4 mg/hr. His electrolytes are normal except for a potassium of 3.4 mmol/L. A recent digoxin level is not available. The first intervention you should consider is

(A) stopping the room seclusion
(B) replacing the potassium
(C) tapering the lorazepam
(D) checking the hydrochlorothiazide level
(E) monitoring orthostatic vitals

Questions 480 and 481

A 64-year-old man presents to your office, accompanied by his wife, complaining of memory loss. He is a retired stockbroker who can no longer recall stock quotes like he did several years ago. His wife has become both concerned and annoyed because he seems to immediately forget whatever she has told him. These memory problems have slowly progressed over several years, and recently he has had difficulty getting dressed. More than once, he has put his underwear on over his pants. His wife has also noted that he speaks much less than he once did over dinner. He does not have any medical illnesses.

480. Which of the following agents may play a role in improving his memory?

(A) fluoxetine (Prozac)
(B) trazodone (Desyrel)
(C) aspirin
(D) donepezil (Aricept)
(E) pemoline (Cylert)

481. On further questioning, his wife reports that he does not sleep well and will infrequently wander around the house. He then sleeps for a large part of the day. Which of the following would be useful to control this behavior?

(A) trazodone (Desyrel)
(B) haloperidol (Haldol)
(C) lorazepam (Ativan)
(D) triazolam (Halcion)
(E) chlorpromazine (Thorazine)

Questions 482 and 483

A 25-year-old man is brought into the emergency department lethargic and stuporous. He responds only to painful stimuli, wakes up briefly and yells, then goes back to sleep. Ambulance personnel report that they found him near a house known for drug trafficking. There is no evidence of physical injury.

482. Medications that he should receive first are

(A) dextrose and flumazenil (Romazicon)
(B) dextrose, flumazenil, and naloxone (Narcan)
(C) dextrose, flumazenil, naloxone, and thiamine
(D) dextrose and naloxone
(E) dextrose, naloxone, and thiamine

483. The patient is treated, and a urine toxicology screen is positive for the presence of opioids. When he is more alert, he informs you that he has been using intravenous heroin daily for several weeks. His last use was about 8 hours ago. His heroin use escalated several weeks ago from snorting to intravenous use when he no longer felt a good "high" from snorting. He has never detoxified before. He has no other comorbid medical conditions, and he does not abuse alcohol. To detoxify him, many clinicians might use

(A) clonidine (Catapres)
(B) propranolol
(C) methadone
(D) naloxone (Narcan)
(E) chlordiazepoxide (Librium)

484. A 45-year-old woman presents to your practice with depression. Her mother recently passed away from lung cancer, and her father died 4 years ago from lung cancer. She has seen therapists to help with her grief, but she continues to have symptoms of major depression 6 months after her mother's death. Despite several attempts to quit smoking, she still smokes two packs of cigarettes a day. Which of the following should be considered as pharmacotherapy for her depression and smoking?

(A) imipramine (Tofranil)

(B) bupropion (Wellbutrin)

(C) buspirone (BuSpar)

(D) trazodone (Desyrel)

(E) phenelzine (Nardil)

485. A 52-year-old man who has poorly controlled diabetes is referred to you for evaluation of medication noncompliance. You learn that he cannot fall asleep at night and has no energy during the day. His appetite is gone, and he does not enjoy activities as he once did. Overall, he feels depressed. Additionally, he has been experiencing chronic pain in his feet, which is not relieved by analgesics. Which of the following may help his mood and his pain?

(A) alprazolam (Xanax)

(B) citalopram (Celexa)

(C) amitriptyline (Elavil)

(D) bupropion (Wellbutrin)

(E) nefazodone (Serzone)

486. A 47-year-old woman presents to your office for psychiatric care because she has just relocated to your town. She has a history of bipolar disorder, but her prior psychiatrist recently stopped her lithium because she developed thyroid autoantibodies. She complains of being irritable and not able to sleep for several weeks. She tells you that her thoughts are racing, and you have a difficult time redirecting her answers. However, she believes her biggest problem is her facial pain, which was diagnosed as trigeminal neuralgia and has not improved with anal-

gesics. A medication that may potentially help both conditions is

(A) lithium

(B) amitriptyline (Elavil)

(C) fluoxetine (Prozac)

(D) gabapentin (Neurontin)

(E) thyroxine

487. A 33-year-old woman with a history of schizophrenia has recently started treatment with olanzapine (Zyprexa). She has tolerated the medication well and is living in a group home, anticipating moving into her own apartment. She no longer hears voices and no longer has a desire to hurt herself. Which of the following side effects of olanzapine is most likely to interfere with her continued use of the drug?

(A) increased prolactin

(B) increased excitability

(C) weight gain

(D) agranulocytosis

(E) development of cataracts

488. A 42-year-old man who is being treated for auditory hallucinations responds very well to haloperidol (Haldol) while in the hospital but typically stops taking the medications soon after leaving the hospital. He is generally agreeable to taking the haloperidol and benztropine (Cogentin), and there is no evidence of any significant adverse effect. However, his outpatient clinicians believe that he simply forgets to take it. This quickly allows his hallucinations to return and the cycle to start again. An alternative for this patient may be

(A) depot haloperidol every 1 weeks

(B) depot haloperidol every 4 weeks

(C) depot fluphenazine every 2 weeks

(D) depot fluphenazine every 4 weeks

(E) depot risperidone every 4 weeks

Questions 489 and 490

A 76-year-old man who has felt depressed for several months presents to your office for evaluation. He has had weight loss, decreased appetite, and no interest in his hobbies, and cannot concentrate on your cognitive exam. He has passing thoughts of dying. He admits that he frequently hears voices telling him that he is going to die soon. You have decided to start an antidepressant and risperidone (Risperdal) at 0.5 mg twice a day.

489. A side effect of risperidone that should be monitored for is

(A) agranulocytosis
(B) leukocytosis
(C) anticholinergic side effects
(D) orthostatic hypotension
(E) weight loss

490. As his dose of risperidone increases, the likelihood of which of the following can also be expected to increase?

(A) extrapyramidal side effects
(B) leukocytosis
(C) anticholinergic effects

(D) agranulocytosis
(E) weight loss

491. A 26-year-old woman who gave birth to her first child 2 months ago presents to your office on a referral for evaluation of depression. She is not breast feeding. She has a history of depression from before her pregnancy, and her depression is usually accompanied by voices that tell her to harm herself. In the past, she has responded well to nortriptyline (Pamelor) and risperidone (Risperdal). A side effect of risperidone that could possibly limit its use is

(A) weight gain
(B) galactorrhea
(C) sedation
(D) akathisia
(E) parkinsonism

Answers and Explanations

394. **(C)** Phenelzine and tranylcypromine are the only nonselective monoamine oxidase inhibitors (MAOIs) currently approved for use in the United States. They are extremely dangerous in overdose and, after a brief asymptomatic period of 12 to 24 hours, may produce hyperpyrexia and autonomic excitability sufficient enough to cause rhabdomyolysis. Supportive care should be instituted. If delirium develops, small doses of intravenous benzodiazepines should be used. Lorazepam is preferred because of its short elimination half-life. Neuroleptics, especially short-acting agents such as chlorpromazine, should be avoided because of their tendency to contribute to hypotension. If ventricular arrhythmias develop, they can be treated with lidocaine. Bretylium may contribute to the adrenergic crisis and should be avoided. Phenytoin may be used if seizures develop. Meperidine should be avoided as it may contribute to the adrenergic crisis. Other medications that are contraindicated with MAOIs include stimulants, decongestants, amine precursors such as L-dopa and L-tryptophan, and the antihypertensives methyldopa, guanethidine, and reserpine.

395. **(C)** Blocking reuptake of catecholamines and indolamines in patients already using an MAOI can result in a potentially life-threatening drug interaction known as a serotonin syndrome. Medications that block such reuptake include the SSRIs, TCAs, buspirone, and other antidepressants, such as venlafaxine. Features of mild serotonin syndrome include tachycardia, flushing, fever, hypertension, ocular oscillations, and myoclonic jerks. Severe serotonin syndrome may result in severe hyperthermia, coma, autonomic instability, convulsions, and death; therefore, wait at least 14 days after discontinuing an MAOI before starting a serotonergic agent. Rapid cycling bipolar disorder is an affective disorder, while neuroleptic malignant syndrome is an idiosyncratic reaction to neuroleptic drugs. Akathisia and opisthotonos are both extrapyramidal side effects of neuroleptics.

396. **(C)** Most serotonin in the CNS is synthesized in the dorsal and median raphe nucleus of the brain stem. The substantia nigra synthesizes dopamine, and the locus ceruleus synthesizes norepinephrine.

397. **(C)** This patient is likely suffering from a major depressive episode. Because of her increase in weight, hypersomnia, and mood reactivity, her depression has atypical features. Although atypical features respond best to MAOIs such as phenelzine, these medications are rarely used because of the potential risk of a fatal hypertensive crisis when eating certain tyramine-containing foods. SSRIs such as fluoxetine and sertraline are also beneficial even though response rates to SSRIs may not match those of the MAOIs. Due to their favorable safety profile, SSRIs have become a first line treatment in major depression. TCAs such as nortriptyline are less effective than MAOIs for atypical depression. Trazodone inhibits serotonin reuptake and may also be serotonomimetic.

398. **(B)** Approximately 50% of patients who meet criteria for major depression will recover after treatment for 6 weeks with an adequately dosed antidepressant. Initially, sleep may improve within the first 2 weeks; however, this response may not be predictive of efficacy. Substantial effects may not be seen for 4 weeks, and maximal effects may require up to 8 weeks of treatment.

399. **(A)** Mood often improves last, while neurovegetative symptoms improve earlier.

400. **(A)** Alcohol withdrawal should be strongly considered in this patient. Benzodiazepines are the drug of choice for control of alcohol withdrawal symptoms and for prophylaxis against withdrawal seizures and the potentially life-threatening delirium tremens. Long-acting benzodiazepines such as chlordiazepoxide and diazepam are appropriate; however, both are extensively metabolized by the liver. Since this patient has elevated transaminases, oxazepam, or lorazepam, which only undergoes glucuronidation prior to elimination, is preferable. A high-potency antipsychotic agent such as haloperidol may be necessary to help control this patient. However, low-potency antipsychotics, such as chlorpromazine, should be avoided because they may lower the seizure threshold. Disulfiram is used to treat alcohol dependence, not acute alcohol withdrawal.

401. **(C)** In the central nervous system, GABA is an inhibitory neurotransmitter. At the postsynaptic GABA-A receptor, GABA facilitates chloride ion influx into a cell via a chloride channel, resulting in inhibition of that neuron. Alcohol and benzodiazepines both allosterically modulate the GABA-A receptor to facilitate GABAergic inhibition. Abrupt removal of alcohol or benzodiazepines after prolonged use results in a relative deficit of GABAergic inhibition, which can lead to anxiety, insomnia, delirium, and seizures. GABA-B is the site of action of the muscle relaxant baclofen. Alcohol does not act at the dopamine or serotonin receptors.

402. **(E)** This patient has delirium tremens, which is a medical emergency. He should be trans-

ferred to an intensive care setting where intravenous benzodiazepines can be administered with greater safety. The intravenous route is preferred in this situation to ensure adequate absorption. Haloperidol can be used for its sedative effect, but it should not take the place of a benzodiazepine. Similarly, IV labetalol may be useful in the intensive care unit, but it should not replace a benzodiazepine.

403. **(C)** Alcohol withdrawal can take the form of minor withdrawal symptoms such as tremulousness, withdrawal seizures, or withdrawal delirium, formerly known as delirium tremens. Minor withdrawal symptoms can last for several days. Withdrawal seizures are rarely focal and usually occur within 48 hours after alcohol consumption ceases. Delirium tremens most often occurs within 96 hours of cessation of drinking; therefore, 5 days is the most correct response.

404. **(A)** Thiamine should be administered urgently to all patients suspected of alcohol withdrawal to help prevent Wernicke–Korsakoff syndrome. Wernike's encephalopathy is characterized by altered mental status, ataxia, and sixth nerve palsy. Korsakoff's psychosis can follow Wernicke's and is characterized by anterograde memory deficits that can lead to confabulation. Pyridoxine may also be administered, but failure to do so is not as dire. Seizure prophylaxis is with benzodiazepines. Anticonvulsants such as phenytoin or valproic acid are not usually used but may be added if there is a previous history of withdrawal seizures. Disulfiram is used as an alcohol aversion agent and absolutely should not be given during withdrawal.

405. **(C)** This patient presents with a major depressive episode with psychotic features. There is little evidence that one antidepressant is more effective than another in this condition, so selection is often based on safety and side effect profile. SSRIs (e.g., fluoxetine, sertraline, paroxetine, and fluvoxamine) are the most widely used agents for an initial depressive episode because of their safety and relative lack of side effects. The most common side effects of sertraline are gastrointestinal distress and sexual dysfunction. TCAs, including amitriptyline, are potentially lethal in overdose and have sedating, anticholinergic, and orthostatic effects that limit their use. The efficacy of trazodone has been questioned by many clinicians, and its sedating and orthostatic side effects limit its use as an antidepressant; however, it is frequently used to treat the insomnia associated with SSRI use. Phenelzine is an MAOI and is not an appropriate first-line therapy due to its side effect profile and extensive drug interactions. Amoxapine is a tetracyclic antidepressant, which, similar to neuroleptic medications, causes dopamine receptor blockade, extrapyramidal side effects, and tardive dyskinesia.

406. (A) The precise mechanism of action of SSRIs in depression is not fully understood. Acutely, they enhance serotonergic neurotransmission by permitting serotonin more time to bind at the postsynaptic terminal. However, since therapeutic effect of SSRIs may take several weeks, this acute effect is likely not responsible for the improvement seen in depression. One leading theory is that they cause downregulation of postsynaptic $5\text{-}HT_2$ receptors. However, not all SSRIs have been shown to do this, so the answer is likely much more complicated. SSRIs can inhibit the dopamine system, accounting for the anecdotal reports of SSRIs causing extrapyramidal side effects. However, this is probably unrelated to their effectiveness in depression.

407. (E) Olanzapine is an atypical antipsychotic that should strongly be considered in this patient. When delusions or other psychotic symptoms are present, the addition of low to moderate doses of antipsychotic medications may potentiate an antidepressant response. Olanzapine is an atypical antipsychotic because it has a lower incidence of extrapyramidal side effects. Both thyroid hormone and lithium have been used in depression to augment a partial response from antidepres-

sants; however, one should first monitor for a response to the first-line antidepressant. Benztropine is an antiparkinsonian agent used with typical neuroleptic medications and would not be appropriate here. Propranolol is a beta-blocking agent not indicated in this patient.

408. (A) Anorgasmia is the most common reported sexual dysfunction side effect in females taking SSRIs such as sertraline.

409. (D) The recommended length of treatment of a first episode of unipolar depression is at least 6 months and usually on the scale of 8 to 12 months, and possibly longer, depending on patient factors such as family history of a mood disorder, severity and duration of the depressive episode, and comorbid psychiatric symptoms such as anxiety and substance abuse. Discontinuation within the first 16 weeks of treatment is associated with a high risk of relapse.

410. (A) Bupropion is the one antidepressant listed that does not cause sexual dysfunction. Fluvoxamine, fluoxetine, and citalopram are all SSRIs that have been reported to cause varying degrees of sexual dysfunction. Clomipramine is a TCA that has a greater incidence of sexual dysfunction than other TCAs, possibly due to its potent serotonin reuptake inhibiting properties.

411. (B) Akathisia, an extrapyramidal side effect of neuroleptics, can be difficult to distinguish from anxiety in a psychotic individual; however, based on observation and history from his parents, akathisia should be strongly considered and empiric treatment attempted. Onset usually begins between 5 and 60 days after initiation of treatment but can occur after just one dose. First, the neuroleptic dose should be reduced as much as possible. In general, anticholinergic agents such as Cogentin are used to treat extrapyramidal symptoms. In the absence of other extrapyramidal side effects, however, many clinicians would start treatment with a beta blocker such as propranolol. Antianxiety agents such as lorazepam are generally not helpful. Diphenhydramine is helpful in acute dystonias but not in akathisia.

412. **(C)** The symptoms described resemble antipsychotic drug-induced parkinsonism. These symptoms include bradykinesia, rigidity, cogwheeling, tremor, masked facies, stooped posture, festinating gait, and drooling. Onset is usually after several weeks of treatment and is more common in high-potency typical neuroleptics, such as fluphenazine and haloperidol. Low-potency medications, such as chlorpromazine and thioridazine, have substantial anticholinergic activity, which reduces, but does not eliminate, this effect. The elderly are particularly vulnerable to drug-induced parkinsonism. Atypical neuroleptics such as risperidone and olanzapine are not free of this side effect; however, they are associated with a lower incidence. Of these, olanzapine has the lowest incidence.

413. **(A)** Nigrostriatal D_2 receptors that are blocked by neuroleptic medications cause an imbalance between dopamine and acetylcholine, which accounts for the parkinsonian symptoms. Mesolimbic D_2 receptor blockade is believed to account for the antipsychotic effect of neuroleptics and does not cause extrapyramidal symptoms. Typical neuroleptics block both nigrostriatal and mesolimbic dopamine, whereas atypical neuroleptics preferentially block mesolimbic dopamine, accounting for decreased extrapyramidal symptom liability.

414. **(D)** Clozapine, the first atypical antipsychotic medication, is now believed to be in a class of its own. It has activity at numerous receptors that account for its many side effects. These receptors include alpha-1; histamine-1; D_1, D_2, and D_4; 5-HT$_2$, 5-HT$_3$, and 5-HT$_{2c}$; and muscarinic receptors. Of all the side effects listed, agranulocytosis causes the most concern and necessitates white blood cell differentials weekly for 6 months, then every 2 weeks for the duration of treatment. The incidence of agranulocytosis is 1% or

less, and the incidence of death among those who suffer agranulocytosis is 2.5/10,000.

415. **(C)** Sialorrhea is a common side effect of treatment with clozapine. It can be extremely bothersome to the patient and others but does not usually require discontinuation of treatment. Often, behavioral measures are sufficient, such as the use of lozenges or placing a towel on the patient's pillow at night. Anticholinergic agents such as propylthiouracil often help reduce the volume of saliva. Propranolol is useful in the treatment of akathisia, while amantadine may be helpful in the treatment of parkinsonian symptoms.

416. **(D)** Patients on clozapine often develop a persistent sinus tachycardia that does not require cessation of treatment. Often, the tachycardia resolves without necessitating further intervention; however, should it persist, it may be treated with the beta antagonist propranolol. Clozapine has significant alpha-receptor blockage, which often causes orthostatic hypotension, requiring a gradual titration of the dose. Because of this, labetalol would not be appropriate as it may exacerbate this side effect. Benztropine is an anticholinergic agent that will not help the tachycardia. There is no reason to check creatinine phosphokinase levels, which might be expected to be high in NMS.

417. **(B)** NMS is a serious idiosyncratic reaction to neuroleptic drugs. Its main features include hyperthermia; severe muscular rigidity; and autonomic instability including tachycardia, tachypnea, hyper- or hypotension, diaphoresis, and delirium. It can occur with all antipsychotics, although it is rarely reported when clozapine is used alone. The risk is greater with high doses of high-potency neuroleptics. Other risk factors include medical illness, dehydration, and poor nutrition. Acute dystonia usually occurs early in the treatment of neuroleptics, but rarely involves fever and delirium. This patient's history is not consistent with serotonin syndrome. His prerenal azotemia was likely a contributing

factor, and renal failure is a possible adverse outcome but not the cause of this syndrome. Sepsis or CNS infection, as well as rhabdomyolysis from other causes, malignant hyperthermia, heat stroke, and allergic drug reactions are part of the differential diagnosis, but the likely diagnosis is NMS.

418. **(C)** Rhabdomyolysis is the most common serious complication of NMS, occurring in up to 25% of patients in one series. Dialysis may be required to protect patients from renal failure. Creatinine phosphokinase is usually elevated in NMS, but there are no specific laboratory findings. All of the other listed complications have been reported, but with less frequency.

419. **(D)** Dantrolene, a direct-acting muscle relaxant, is given most frequently to treat NMS. Other agents that have been used with less frequency are the central dopamine agonists bromocriptine and amantadine. Benztropine is also occasionally used with dantroline. Since most neuroleptics are highly protein bound, dialysis or urine acidification or alkalinization will not remove them; however, dialysis may be necessary to prevent renal failure.

420. **(C)** Retinal pigmentation is known to occur when thioridazine is used in high doses (> 1,000 mg/d). It may not remit when thioridazine is discontinued, and it can lead to blindness. The other choices can occur with all neuroleptics.

421. **(E)** This patient is suffering from panic disorder with agoraphobia. There are many medications that have proven benefit for this condition, including TCAs, SSRIs, MAOIs, and high-potency benzodiazepines. Of the agents listed, only fluoxetine, an SSRI, is one of them. Bupropion, an antidepressant with dopamine activity, is not effective. Trazodone, an antidepressant with mixed serotonergic effects, has shown conflicting results. Buspirone, a partial 5-HT$_{1a}$ antagonist with antianxiety activity, is not effective. Propranolol, a beta-adrenergic blocker, may help

alleviate the physical symptoms such as tachycardia but does not prevent the attack.

422. **(B)** Patients with panic disorder are notoriously sensitive to SSRIs and TCAs when these agents are initiated. They experience increased jitteriness and anxiety; therefore, the starting dose of these medications is often half or one quarter of the starting dose used to treat depression. The dose is then carefully titrated up. Sedation is a frequent side effect of benzodiazepine treatment, not of SSRI treatment. Constipation is a side effect of TCAs, not SSRIs. Mania and paranoia are not frequent side effects of SSRI treatment; however, these may occur, particularly in those with a family history of bipolar I disorder.

423. **(D)** Benzodiazepines can be useful additions to the pharmacologic treatment of panic disorder, particularly if accompanied by agoraphobia. However, their sedating side effect limits the use of most of these agents. The agents used most often are the high-potency alprazolam, or the long-acting clonazepam. The other agents listed cause significant sedation and have not been sufficiently studied in panic disorder.

424. **(C)** Clonazepam is the most potent benzodiazepine listed. Using 1-mg lorazepam (Ativan) for equivalent dose in milligrams, the potency relationship of some common benzodiazepines is as follows: clonazepam (Klonopin) 0.25 mg; triazolam (Halcion) 0.25 mg; alprazolam (Xanax) 0.5 mg; diazepam (Valium) 5.0 mg; clorazepate (Tranxene) 7.5 mg; chlordiazepoxide (Librium) 10.0 mg; temazepam (Restoril); and flurazepam (Dalmane) 30.0 mg. Flumazenil is a benzodiazepine antagonist. Buspirone (BuSpar) is a nonbenzodiazepine anxiolytic that is generally considered to be less potent.

425. **(B)** This patient presents with signs and symptoms suggestive of a first manic episode. Lithium and valproic acid (Depakote) remain the mainstay of initial and maintenance treatment of bipolar I disorder. The use of anticonvulsants such as gabapentin and topira-

mate are being utilized for bipolar disorder, but they are not drugs of first choice. Neuroleptics, such as haloperidol, and benzodiazepines, such as clonazepam, may be used with lithium or valproic acid (Depakote) initially; however, they are not routinely used as maintenance treatment.

426. **(A)** These are the minimum initial laboratory studies required before initiating lithium treatment. Because lithium is a Group IA monovalent ion, the kidney handles it much as it does sodium. Ninety-five percent of lithium is excreted unchanged through the kidneys. Therefore electrolytes, creatinine, BUN, and urinalysis are required to check kidney function. Thyroid studies are required because lithium inhibits the synthesis of thyroid hormone and its release from the thyroid. A CBC is optional. Lithium may cause a benign elevation in the WBC. Liver function tests should be performed prior to initiating treatment with valproic acid. Rare cases of fatal hepatotoxicity have been reported with valproic acid. Valproic acid may also elevate serum ammonia levels, but this is rare.

427. **(E)** Polydipsia is a common initial side effect of lithium treatment, and patients should be warned about it prior to initiating therapy. Priapism is a rare but important side effect of trazodone treatment. Delayed ejaculation occurs with SSRIs. Lithium may cause a rash similar to psoriasis, but this is not common. Lithium-induced weight gain is a problem in a small percentage of patients, but not as frequent as polydipsia.

428. **(E)** Hand tremor is the most common neuropsychiatric side effect of lithium therapy. It occurs in 25 to 50% of patients and decreases with a decrease in dose or treatment with a beta blocker. Mild memory impairment may occur but is less common. Extrapyramidal symptoms are infrequent, and seizures rarely occur. Paresthesias are not known to occur.

429. **(D)** The recommendation should be to switch to aspirin. In some individuals, nonsteroidal anti-inflammatory agents cause an increase in lithium levels. Therefore, these agents should be used with caution in patients taking lithium and avoided if possible. Aspirin and sulindac, however, do not affect lithium levels and are therefore safe for use with lithium.

430. **(E)** This patient has symptoms of attention deficit–hyperactivity disorder (ADHD). Stimulants are the most common pharmacologic agents used, and, among them, methylphenidate has been the most widely used. Others include dextroamphetamine and pemoline. TCAs such as desipramine are considered second-line agents. Lorazepam, lithium, and fluoxetine are not used in ADHD.

431. **(A)** Difficulty falling asleep and decreased appetite are the two most common side effects of methylphenidate. Stimulants have been reported to slow growth; however, it is believed to be less common with methylphenidate, and dose related. When drug holidays are given, a growth rebound is seen. Methylphenidate may cause an increase in systolic blood pressure.

432. **(B)** Stimulants have been frequently reported to exacerbate the tics associated with Tourette's disorder and some studies have warned that they should not be given to children with tics or a family history of Tourette's disorder. However, some recent studies have identified frequent comorbidity of ADHD and Tourette's disorder.

433. **(C)** Dopamine D_2 receptor antagonism provides the greatest relief of symptoms in children suffering from Tourette's disorder. Pharmacologic treatment is strictly symptomatic and is not curative. An alpha-2 agonist, not antagonist, would provide some relief, though it is not as effective as D_2 receptor antagonism.

434. **(B)** Haloperidol is the only medication listed that is a strong antagonist at the D_2 receptor. Another agent that is nearly as effective as haloperidol is pimozide. Clonidine, which is an alpha-2 agonist, is also used in Tourette's

disorder, but it is clearly less effective than haloperidol. However, because clonidine is not a neuroleptic, it lacks extrapyramidal side effects and the associated long-term sequelae. Additionally, it may be useful in patients with ADHD and Tourette's disorder.

435. **(C)** The most likely syndrome is tardive dyskinesia (TD). TD is a movement disorder that may occur after long-term treatment with neuroleptic medication, such as haloperidol. It consists of a number of abnormal and involuntary movements such as lip smacking, facial grimacing, and choreoathetoid-like movements of the limbs and trunk. In Huntington's disease, a dominant genetic disorder, the involuntary movements are accompanied by a progressive dementia. Sydenham's chorea, associated with rheumatic fever, occurs in children. Meige syndrome is an oral facial dystonia involving blinking and chin thrusting, sometimes lip pursing or tongue movements, and occasionally shoulder movement. Anticholinergic toxicity, which usually presents as delirium, is not present.

436. **(B)** The most appropriate next step is to decrease the dose of haloperidol to the lowest possible effective dose. If possible, the haloperidol should be discontinued; however, this is often not possible with patients with chronic schizophrenia. When initially decreasing the dose, the symptoms may at first appear worse; however, they should eventually diminish. Maintaining a patient on the lowest possible dose minimizes the risk of TD. Benztropine is used to prevent extrapyramidal symptoms; however, it has been suggested that its use may actually contribute to TD.

437. **(E)** It was once believed that if patients developed signs of TD, they would progress to severe dyskinesias. Recent evidence, however, indicates that most patients stabilize and may spontaneously improve even if they continue taking the antipsychotic. However, the only medication that may improve these symptoms is clozapine.

438. **(A)** The elderly, especially women, are at increased risk for developing TD. In one study, 30% of elderly patients treated with antipsychotics for one year developed TD. Some studies suggest that the presence of an affective disorder may be a risk factor, but the data are not as strong as for the age of the patient. There is no evidence that a family history of Parkinson's disease is a risk factor. All antipsychotic agents, except clozapine, may cause TD. The use of the newer atypical antipsychotic agents such as risperidone, quetiapine, and olanzapine have substantially less risk for TD than the conventional neuroleptics.

439. **(A)** This patient likely has generalized anxiety disorder (GAD). Benzodiazepines are the most effective medications for quickly reducing symptoms of GAD. All benzodiazepines are effective, and the choice should be based on potency, half-life, and side effects. Alprazolam has an intermediate onset, a half-life of 6 to 20 hours, and does not have active metabolites. Buspirone is effective for reducing symptoms but does not work as quickly as benzodiazepines. The tricyclic agent imipramine and SSRIs such as fluoxetine also have anxiolytic properties but also do not work as quickly as benzodiazepines. Bupropion does not have anxiolytic properties.

440. **(B)** This patient likely has the Axis II diagnosis of borderline personality disorder. This disorder can be extremely difficult to treat. SSRIs, particularly fluoxetine, have been shown to reduce the impulsiveness and affective instability in these patients, while antipsychotics such as haloperidol have been shown to decrease the impulsiveness and psychotic thinking. One recent study used low-dose clozapine in a small sample of severe borderline personality disorder patients and found it to be beneficial. Anticonvulsants such as valproic acid (Depakote) may help modulate intense fluctuations in affect but stimulants have not been shown to be effective in borderline personality disorder. TCAs carry a heightened risk in these patients because of their potential lethality in overdose.

441. **(A)** This patient is suffering from bulimia nervosa, purging type, and several studies have shown that fluoxetine can help these patients. Many believe it is related to the high incidence of comorbid depression in this population; however, TCAs, such as protriptyline, have not been as effective. Because electroencephalographic (EEG) abnormalities have been found in patients with bulimia, phenytoin has been tried, but it does not appear to be effective.

442. **(B)** Unless there is a comorbid psychiatric disorder such as obsessive–compulsive disorder (OCD) or depression, pharmacotherapy generally has a limited role in the treatment of anorexia nervosa. Reports on the usefulness of cyproheptadine to stimulate appetite have been mixed. Generally, these patients already have a good appetite. One study suggested that high-dose chlorpromazine is useful, but the results have not been duplicated. The TCA amitriptyline and the promotility agent cisapride are not useful in anorexia nervosa. In particular, cisapride should be avoided because patients with anorexia nervosa are already at high risk for arrhythmias, which can be worsened by cisapride.

443. **(D)** This patient likely has SSRI discontinuation syndrome, which may occur within 1 to 3 days of abruptly stopping an SSRI. The most common physical symptoms are dizziness, nausea and vomiting, fatigue, lethargy, and flulike symptoms. Psychological symptoms are anxiety, irritability, and crying spells. Paroxetine may cause this because of its short half-life and lack of an active metabolite. Fluoxetine has an active metabolite with a half-life ranging from 4 to 16 days, and therefore does not require tapering. The discontinuation syndrome is not known to be lethal; however, restarting the paroxetine and tapering it is a reasonable choice.

444. **(C)** This patient has major depression requiring antidepressant treatment. SSRIs are a good first choice; however, fluoxetine has been reported to increase carbamazepine levels. Paroxetine has not been reported to increase carbamazepine levels. Nefazodone does increase carbamazepine levels, perhaps through interaction with the cytochrome p450 3A3/4 isoenzyme. Clomipramine and amitriptyline are both TCAs that have substantial anticholinergic side effects.

445. **(C)** ECT is effective in up to 80% of patients with either bipolar or unipolar depression. The overall efficacy of antidepressants in uncomplicated unipolar depression has been reported to be approximately 65%. In particular, it is more effective than pharmacotherapy when there is a delusional component as in this case. Additionally, this patient's substantial weight loss weighs in favor of ECT since improvement may be observed after only 2 days.

446. **(C)** Cognitive impairment, and, in particular, memory difficulty, is the most common side effect of ECT. The degree of amnesia is greater with bilateral ECT than with unilateral ECT. Cardiovascular complications usually take the form of hypotension and/or hypertension, as well as tachycardia. In general, ECT is safe in individuals with cardiovascular disease. Potential complications can be reduced with prophylactic medications to reduce the transient hypertension and tachycardia.

447. **(D)** Predicting clinical response to ECT can be difficult. Several studies have reported that patients with a longer current episode of depression may not respond as well. The other factors listed have been reported, though not consistently, to predict a good response to ECT: a psychotic depression; family history of depression; psychomotor retardation; and lack of reactivity to surroundings.

448. **(C)** There are no absolute contraindications to ECT; however, the strongest relative contraindication to ECT of those listed is cerebral arteriovenous malformation. Other strong relative contraindications include recent myocardial infarction, any illness that increases intracranial pressure, medical conditions that may disrupt the blood–brain barrier (e.g., multiple sclerosis), aneurysm, and bleeding disorders. The incidence of arrhythmias during ECT is low. In one study of patients with cardiac disease, only 4% developed minor ECT-induced cardiac complications.

449. **(C)** Trazodone (Desyrel) is an antidepressant medication, unrelated to other antidepressant drugs (except nefazodone), which affects the serotonin system by weak reuptake inhibition and antagonist activity at 5-HT$_{1a}$, 5-HT$_{1c}$, and 5-HT$_2$ receptors. Some clinicians have questioned its efficacy in severe illness, but its use as an adjunct to help with sleep in depressed patients is growing. Some SSRIs can be activating, such as fluoxetine, and trazodone can help with sleep in these patients. Bupropion does not cause significant drowsiness. Diazepam is a benzodiazepine, and diphenhydramine is an antihistamine, although both have been used to help with sleep. Both should be avoided in the elderly, if possible.

450. **(A)** Priapism, though rare, has been reported with trazodone use. The manufacturer has reported the incidence of any abnormal erectile function to be about 1 in 6,000 men. This side effect usually occurs within the first month of treatment but can occur at any time. Any abnormal erectile function should prompt discontinuation of the medication.

451. **(C)** Lithium often causes T-wave flattening or inversion on ECG, but the changes are usually not clinically significant. Sinus node dysfunction and first-degree atrioventricular (AV) block are rare but are the most commonly reported cardiac side effects of lithium. Lithium toxicity can cause sinoatrial block, AV block, AV dissociation, bradyarrhythmias, ventricular tachycardia, and ventricular fibrillation.

452. **(A)** Lithium is almost entirely renally eliminated from the body, but it is not known to cause progressive renal insufficiency. It may affect concentrating ability due to its inhibitory effect on intracellular cyclic adenosine monophosphate formation in renal

tubules. Some studies indicate that this may be decreased by once-daily dosing. In addition, there appears to be a more progressive effect on urine concentrating ability in those treated for a long time or with a history of lithium toxicity.

453. **(C)** Thiazide diuretics can increase lithium levels due to decreased lithium clearance. Other agents that can increase lithium levels are: the diuretics ethacrynic acid, spironolactone, and triamterene; nonsteroidal anti-inflammatory agents except aspirin and sulindac; the antibiotics metronidazole and tetracycline; and angiotensin-converting enzyme inhibitors.

454. **(A)** Clomipramine, a TCA with potent serotonin reuptake inhibition, is the most widely studied agent with efficacy in OCD. Several SSRIs, including fluoxetine, fluvoxamine, sertraline, and paroxetine, have demonstrated efficacy in OCD. Other tricyclic agents are not as effective as clomipramine, probably because they lack the potent serotonin reuptake inhibition of clomipramine. Clonazepam may be used for anxiety associated with OCD, but it is not effective in treating the underlying disorder. Mirtazapine is an antidepressant that is a central alpha-2 antagonist, leading to increased norepinephrine and serotonin release, and an antagonist of both 5-HT$_2$ and 5-HT$_3$. However, it has not been used in OCD. Phenelzine is an MAOI that is not used in OCD. Olanzapine is an atypical neuroleptic. Neuroleptics generally are not effective in OCD.

455. **(A)** Many patients treated for OCD with SSRIs take doses higher than those used in depression, based on the results of early studies that concluded that higher doses were required for a response. However, it may be that many patients require 10 to 12 weeks to respond and that doses are increased due to lack of an early response. Psychotherapy may be helpful for some patients, but it is not often required. There is no particular need for divided doses.

456. (A) Just like treatment of refractory depression, treatment of refractory OCD is largely based on case reports and clinical preferences. There are very few controlled blinded trials in refractory OCD. Several open-label studies reported buspirone was effective as an augmentation to SSRIs or clomipramine; however, a double-blind controlled study found no benefit to the addition of buspirone. There are case reports of fenfluramine and lithium as effective augmenting agents, but these findings require validation. Some studies found that clozapine in patients with schizophrenia worsened OCD symptoms. Cingulotomy, a surgical procedure, should be reserved for severe refractory cases.

457. (D) This patient is suffering from command auditory hallucinations, which have not sufficiently responded to adequate trials of two typical neuroleptic agents, chlorpromazine and haloperidol, and one atypical neuroleptic agent, olanzapine. Therefore, a trial of clozapine is warranted. Clozapine was the first atypical neuroleptic and has been found to be superior to typical neuroleptics in reducing both positive and negative symptoms. It may also improve cognitive deficits in patients with schizophrenia. Fluphenazine and perphenazine are both typical neuroleptics like haloperidol and chlorpromazine. Risperidone is considered an atypical neuroleptic but the rate of response in refractory patients is less than that with clozapine. Ziprasidone is awaiting Food and Drug Administration (FDA) approval, but like olanzapine, it has 5-HT_{2a} and D_2 receptor antagonist properties.

458. (C) Agranulocytosis was once believed to occur in about 3% of patients taking clozapine, a statistic that greatly limited its use in the United States. However, weekly surveillance of WBC and absolute neutrophil count initiated by the manufacturer have resulted in actual rates of agranulocytosis of 1% or less. The fatality rate among those patients with agranulocytosis is 2.5/10,000. Although it can occur anytime, agranulocytosis peaks between 2 and 6 months of therapy; after 6

months, monitoring may be decreased to every 2 weeks. Weight gain is a significant side effect of neuroleptics, and olanzapine in particular. Similarly, somnolence is reported with use of all neuroleptics. Olanzapine has been reported to decrease ejaculatory volume. Dystonia is an extrapyramidal side effect of typical neuroleptics and, to a lesser extent, atypical neuroleptics, with the exception of clozapine.

459. (C) Clozapine acts at many receptors, including D_1, D_2, and D_4; histamine-1; muscarinic; alpha-1 adrenergic; and serotonin types 5-HT_2, 5-HT_{2c}, and 5-HT_3. Efforts to identify the exact mechanism of antipsychotic action of clozapine have revealed at least two possibilities. Unlike "typical" neuroleptics, it has much more potent antagonism at the D_4 receptor compared to the D_2 receptor, especially in the limbic system. This has led to speculation that the D_4 receptor may mediate psychotic symptoms. It also has activity at the 5-HT_2 receptor, activity that typical neuroleptics lack.

460. (C) Both clozapine and bupropion may independently lower the seizure threshold and should be used together with caution. One study speculated that clozapine may not be effective until it induces EEG changes. Unlike clozapine, bupropion does not have anticholinergic side effects or cause orthostatic hypotension.

461. (D) TCAs, including imipramine and nortriptyline, block various receptors, including muscarinic, alpha-1 and -2 adrenergic, dopaminergic, and histaminergic, to varying degrees. As a class, their blockade of alpha-1 receptors is generally believed to be responsible for any orthostatic hypotension that may occur, especially in the elderly. Nortriptyline has relatively less alpha-1 blocking potency, and some clinicians prefer it over other tricyclics in the elderly. Bupropion and mirtazapine are not associated with orthostatic hypotension. Trazodone can cause orthostatic hypotension from alpha-1 blockade; however, nefazodone has a lower affinity and is expected to have a lower incidence of orthostatic hypotension.

462. **(E)** Treatment of refractory depression remains controversial. Unlike evidence for initial selection of antidepressant therapy, there is little well-controlled evidence regarding treatment of refractory depression. Selection is based largely on clinical practice and side effect profile. This patient has had an adequate trial of an SSRI without response. Lithium and thyroid augmentation of antidepressants have been well worked out; however, this patient has not even had a partial response to augment. Additionally, these options are generally reserved for patients who have failed multiple trials of other medications. Imipramine is a tricylic and has the accompanying anticholinergic side effects typical of this class, which make it a less desirable choice. Bupropion is an effective agent; however, the risk of seizures in patients without a seizure history is 0.6 to 0.9% at doses greater than 200 mg/d. At low doses, venlafaxine inhibits only serotonin reuptake, but at doses greater than 225 mg/d it also inhibits norepinephrine reuptake, distinguishing it from the SSRIs. In 3 to 13% of patients, venlafaxine has caused a sustained increase in supine diastolic blood pressure.

463. **(E)** All of the commonly used mood-stabilizing medications, except clonazepam (a benzodiazepine), appear to carry an increased risk of fetal malformations or a potential deleterious effect on later cognitive development. Use of lithium during the first trimester increases the risk of cardiac malformations, including Ebstein's anomaly, to 7.7%. A fetal echocardiogram should be done between weeks 16 and 18 of pregnancy. Lithium may be used in the second and third trimesters, but it should be stopped peripartum because of the rapid fluid shifts and changes in glomerular filtration. Carbamazepine increases the risk of neural tube defects, and valproic acid (or divalproex sodium) increases the risk of intrauterine growth retardation and neural tube defects.

464. **(B)** The most widely cited therapeutic lithium concentration is 0.8 to 1.2 mEq/L. This level should be taken approximately 12 hours after the prior dose. Generally, the level is checked in the morning before the morning dose. Lithium has a narrow therapeutic window. Tremor can be seen at levels below 1.2 mEq/L, and above that level, nausea and vomiting can be seen. Levels above 3.0 mEq/L require emergency medical treatment, and dialysis may be necessary.

465. **(C)** Treatment of the depressed phase of bipolar illness remains controversial. Lithium is not as effective in protecting against acute depressive episodes as it is against mania. Patients with bipolar disorder are more likely than unipolar patients to have an antidepressant response to lithium, but further intervention is often required. Evidence suggests that treating bipolar depression with any antidepressant can induce a manic episode in bipolar patients. Additionally, evidence suggests that TCAs can trigger rapid-cycling bipolar disorder. There is some evidence, however, that bupropion and paroxetine may have a reduced incidence of triggering a manic event. One report suggests that it may help rapid-cycling bipolar II disorder.

466. **(D)** Neuroleptic medications may play an important role in the initial management of acutely manic patients by controlling agitation and assisting with sedation. Valproic acid and lithium are equally effective in the control of an acute manic episode. Initial response to lithium may take 7 to 14 days. Generally, the acute improvement that may be observed on inpatient units is due to the sedative effects of neuroleptics and benzodiazepines. Loading doses of lithium do not decrease the time needed to respond.

467. **(A)** Weight gain is a common complaint of patients on maintenance valproic acid treatment. Hair loss, not hirsutism, is another common complaint. Valproic acid frequently causes gastrointestinal distress. An enteric-coated form known as divalproex, which contains valproic acid and sodium valproate,

is generally better tolerated. Valproic acid is extensively metabolized by the liver, so liver function tests should be performed before and during treatment. It generally does not affect kidney function. Common hematologic side effects include leukopenia and thrombocytopenia.

468. **(D)** Mirtazapine is an antidepressant whose pharmacologic profile is different from other available agents. It is a central alpha-2-adrenergic antagonist and an antagonist of 5-HT$_2$ and 5-HT$_3$ receptors, as well as H$_1$ receptors. Because it blocks alpha-2 receptors, it leads to enhanced serotonin release, but blockade of 5-HT$_2$ and 5-HT$_3$ leads to relative enhancement of 5-HT$_1$ activity, giving it a different side effect profile than SSRIs. For example, it tends to increase appetite and cause weight gain compared to placebo. Also, its H$_1$ antagonism causes sedation. However, at higher doses, alpha-2-adrenergic blockade also leads to increased norepinephrine release, which may counteract the H$_1$-mediated sedation. In this patient, use of mirtazapine to exploit its potential increased appetite and sedation side effects should be considered.

469. **(C)** TCAs produce several cardiovascular side effects, the most significant being a quinidine-like effect slowing cardiac conduction. Some clinicians will avoid tricyclics if there are any ECG changes. Certainly, if there are changes in conduction, such as a prolonged QT interval, widening of the QRS complex, or AV conduction abnormalities, TCAs should be avoided. In overdose, they can produce heart block, widen the QRS complex, cause a bundle branch block, and cause tachyarrhythmias; however, even in therapeutic concentrations, they may have adverse effects on cardiac conduction. TCAs may be used in patients with prior cerebral infarctions. Amlodipine and estrogen replacement are not contraindications. TCAs may exacerbate urinary retention from anticholinergic effects, but it is not a contraindication.

470. **(D)** TCAs inhibit reuptake of norepinephrine and serotonin to varying degrees. Struc-

turally, they can be divided into tertiary amines (amitriptyline, clomipramine, doxepin, imipramine, and trimipramine) and secondary amines (desipramine, nortriptyline, and protriptyline). Tertiary amines tend to inhibit reuptake of serotonin to a greater degree than norepinephrine, while secondary amines primarily inhibit reuptake of norepinephrine. Bupropion is an antidepressant that inhibits both norepinephrine and dopamine reuptake.

471. **(A)** Desipramine is the least anticholinergic of all the TCAs, followed closely by nortriptyline. Both of these are secondary amines that primarily inhibit norepinephrine reuptake. The tertiary amines—doxepin, clomipramine, and amitriptyline—have greater anticholinergic activity. Amitriptyline is the most anticholinergic. This can be particularly bothersome in older men with prostatic hypertrophy. Another TCA, amoxapine, has almost no anticholinergic effects; however, it also has dopamine antagonist activity, which introduces some side effects associated with neuroleptics.

472. **(E)** This patient is likely delirious, and prompt identification and treatment of the underlying cause is indicated. To help control the agitation that may accompany delirium, low-dose haloperidol is frequently used. Haloperidol does not treat the delirium, however. It is used most frequently because it is the most potent of the typical antipsychotics, therefore requiring lower doses with fewer anticholinergic or orthostatic side effects. Additionally, low-potency agents such as chlorpromazine or thioridazine are not only associated with orthostatic hypotension and anticholinergic side effects, but also with prolongation of the QT interval. Olanzapine is not used in the intensive care setting partly because it is not available in a parenteral form. Lorazepam may help sedate the patient, but it will not help his psychosis.

473. **(A)** Of the typical neuroleptics listed (haloperidol, perphenazine, and thioridazine), haloperidol is the most potent and has the

least activity at alpha-1 receptors. Therefore, it is the least likely to cause orthostatic hypotension. The atypical agents listed (risperidone and quetiapine) have activity at alpha-1 receptors and are both associated with orthostatic hypotension.

474. **(B)** Haloperidol is available in a parenteral form. It is FDA approved only for intramuscular injection; however, it is routinely used by clinicians intravenously in the intensive care unit. Intravenously, it is associated with a shorter half-life and a lower incidence of extrapyramidal symptoms. However, several clinicians have reported an association between intravenous haloperidol and torsade de pointes ventricular arrhythmias.

475. **(D)** The metabolism of ethyl alcohol involves a two-step enzymatic process. The first enzyme, alcohol dehydrogenase, metabolizes ethanol to acetaldehyde, which is quickly metabolized by aldehyde dehydrogenase. Disulfiram (Antabuse) inhibits aldehyde dehydrogenase, resulting in an accumulation of acetaldehyde. Acetaldehyde causes facial flushing, tachycardia, hypotension, nausea and vomiting, and physical discomfort. Therefore, a patient on disulfiram has an incentive to remain abstinent. Obviously, disulfiram works only if patients continue to take it. Metronidazole is an antibiotic that has a disulfiram-like reaction but is not used for this purpose. Flumazenil is a benzodiazepine antagonist. Fluoxetine does not sensitize against alcohol use. Naloxone is an opioid antagonist.

476. **(C)** Multiple neurotransmitter systems have been investigated in attempts to control alcohol cravings. One system that may play a role is the opioid system. Naltrexone is an opioid antagonist that has been shown to decrease the number of days a person with alcohol dependence drinks and to increase the time before relapse of heavy drinking. Treatment of depression with an agent such as fluoxetine or bupropion may help control drinking if a comorbid depression exists, but use of antidepressants in the absence of a mood disor-

der has not been effective. Disulfiram is an alcohol-sensitizing agent. Diazepam is a benzodiazepine that may treat withdrawal symptoms but has not been shown to decrease cravings.

477. **(B)** This patient is likely suffering from posttraumatic stress disorder (PTSD). Several studies have found that SSRIs were useful in reducing the numbing symptoms of PTSD. In one trial of rape victims, fluoxetine reduced symptoms of reexperiencing, avoidance or numbing, and hyperarousal. Further double-blind controlled trials are needed to confirm these findings. Benzodiazepines have not been useful for these symptoms. Antipsychotics such as thioridazine have generally not been useful, although some clinicians are beginning to try the atypical neuroleptics. Anticonvulsants are not routinely used, but some studies found that carbamazepine reduced the reexperiencing and arousal symptoms. Naltrexone, an opioid antagonist, has not been extensively studied in PTSD.

478. **(E)** Open-label trials of the antiadrenergic agent clonidine (an alpha-2-adrenergic agonist) have demonstrated decreases in symptoms of reexperiencing and hyperarousal. Double-blind controlled trials are needed to confirm these findings.

479. **(C)** Elderly patients can be sensitive to the adverse effects of benzodiazepines. This patient is taking 8 mg/d of lorazepam, which is a large dose. Slowly tapering the lorazepam while investigating other causes of delirium is a reasonable first step. A digoxin level might be useful as high levels of digoxin can affect mental status, but hydrochlorothiazide levels are not measured.

480. **(D)** This patient may be suffering from Alzheimer's dementia. He has clear cognitive decline and, although reversible causes of cognitive impairment should be investigated, there is no indication that any reversible cause is present. Two cholinesterase inhibitors have been approved for use in Alzheimer's dementia: donepezil (Aricept)

and tacrine (Cognex). There does not appear to be an indication for fluoxetine in this patient. Aspirin or trazodone will not improve cognitive ability. Pemoline is a stimulant that does not appear to be indicated in this case.

481. **(A)** Trazodone (Desyrel) is a serotonergic agent frequently used in the elderly to help with sleep and in turn may help this patient's occasional wandering behavior. It can cause orthostatic hypotension and should therefore be used with caution in those with risk factors for bleeding. Benzodiazepines should generally be used with caution in the elderly. They may actually make behavior worse and may contribute to delirium. If necessary, starting doses should be much lower than recommended. Chlorpromazine and haloperidol are neuroleptics that should also be used carefully in the elderly. Chlorpromazine, a low-potency neuroleptic, has substantial side effects including extrapyramidal symptoms and anticholinergic properties that may exacerbate other problems such as urinary retention and confusion. Haloperidol is a high-potency neuroleptic that may cause substantial extrapyramidal symptoms. Additionally, elderly patients may develop TD much more rapidly than younger patients might.

482. **(E)** Patients who present with altered levels of consciousness need to be medically managed, evaluated, and treated for several reversible causes. These include hypoglycemia, opioid overdose, and alcohol intoxication. Airway protection and monitoring of air exchange and cardiovascular status are required. Several treatments that should be immediately considered include IV dextrose, usually D50, to treat hypoglycemia; thiamine to guard against the development of Wernicke–Korsakoff syndrome when giving the dextrose to an alcoholic patient with thiamine deficiency; and naloxone, an opioid antagonist, to reverse the effects of opioid intoxication. Flumazenil is a benzodiazepine antagonist that should not be used before obtaining further history because it may theoretically lower the seizure threshold.

483. **(A)** Detoxification from heroin can usually be managed with clonidine. Clonidine, a central alpha-2 agonist, suppresses the sympathetic response to the heroin withdrawal and helps control agitation and autonomic instability, such as elevated blood pressure and heart rate, seen in opioid withdrawal. It does not take away heroin craving. Some centers use methadone for heroin withdrawal, but some authors advise against methadone for detoxification in patients who have never detoxified before because of the success of clonidine detoxification. Propranolol is not used for heroin detoxification. Naloxone would not be appropriate beyond the initial resuscitation efforts. Benzodiazepines may be helpful as adjuncts to control anxiety, but they are not sufficient.

484. **(B)** Bupropion (Wellbutrin, Zyban) is an antidepressant that has been shown to be effective as part of a smoking cessation program. The mechanism of action is unclear, but it is believed to have an effect on dopaminergic transmission. Giving up cigarettes may be extremely difficult for a patient who is also suffering from major depression; however, starting bupropion during the depression may help her quit smoking after she has recovered from her depression.

485. **(C)** Several TCAs have been used to treat chronic pain, including amitriptyline and nortriptyline. Using such an antidepressant in this patient may have the added benefit of reducing the chronic pain. However, TCAs, as compared with SSRIs, are more lethal in overdose and generally have more side effects, particularly anticholinergic and cardiovascular.

486. **(D)** Gabapentin is an anticonvulsant that has been reported to be modestly effective in bipolar disorder as well as in neuropathic pain disorders. Gabapentin has not been studied as extensively as lithium, valproic acid, or even carbamazepine; however, it has been shown to be more efficacious than placebo in a few studies. Additionally, it has been used to treat neuropathic pain, such as

trigeminal neuralgia. In this patient, who is demonstrating hypomanic symptoms, it could potentially treat both disorders.

487. **(C)** Weight gain is a side effect of most neuroleptic medications, traditional and atypical; however, it has been particularly troubling for olanzapine. For most patients, the weight gain can be modest (5 to 15 pounds), but for some it can be particularly troubling, necessitating discontinuation of the medication. Elevated prolactin is a side effect of typical antipsychotics and less common with olanzapine, while agranulocytosis is a rare side effect of clozapine. Olanzapine is likely to cause sedation and is usually administered in the evening. As an antipsychotic with mood-stabilizing properties, it is useful for both psychotic disorders and bipolar disorder. Olanzapine is not associated with increased excitability or cataracts.

488. **(B)** This patient is a candidate for intramuscular injections of long-acting haloperidol, which, after a short loading period, requires administration every 4 weeks. The haloperidol is administered intramuscularly in a suspension, which delays its absorption into the bloodstream. Depot fluphenazine is administered every 2 weeks, but its use would not be appropriate here since the patient has been responding well to haloperidol. Risperidone is an atypical antipsychotic agent that, like the other atypical agents currently on the market, is not available in an intramuscular form.

489. **(D)** Risperidone is an "atypical" antipsychotic agent that has potent $5\text{-}HT_{2a}$ antagonist properties, as well as D_2 antagonism and alpha-1-adrenergic blocking activity. Because of the alpha-1 blocking activity, it may cause orthostatic hypotension. It may cause weight gain, not weight loss. Unlike clozapine, hematologic effects do not require routine monitoring. It does not cause significant anticholinergic effects.

490. **(A)** Atypical antipsychotic agents, like clozapine and risperidone, are considered "atypical" because of their decreased propensity for causing extrapyramidal side effects and presumably a reduced risk of TD. Unfortunately, only clozapine appears to truly obey this rule. The other "atypical" antipsychotic agents all appear to have some degree of extrapyramidal side effects. Risperidone seems to have the greatest propensity for extrapyramidal side effects, and at doses greater than 6 mg/d may cause extrapyramidal side effects comparable to haloperidol.

491. **(B)** Antipsychotic agents, in addition to blocking dopamine receptors in the nigrostriatal system (causing extrapyramidal symptoms) and the mesolimbic system (decreasing hallucinations) may also block dopamine in the tuberoinfundibular system, thereby increasing prolactin levels and causing galactorrhea, especially in women. Risperidone may raise prolactin levels 100-fold. Olanzapine has not been demonstrated to raise prolactin levels significantly.

CHAPTER 6

Psychological Treatment and Management

Greer Richardson, MD

Questions

DIRECTIONS (Questions 492 through 553): Each of the numbered items or incomplete statements in this section is followed by answers or by completions of the statement. Select the ONE lettered answer or completion that is BEST in each case.

Questions 492 through 494

A 34-year-old married man comes into your office complaining of being "overcome" with discrete episodes of palpitations, sweating, shortness of breath, "choking," abdominal discomfort, and feelings of impending doom. He goes on to say that he was a football player in high school and was never scared of anything. Now, he says, he is starting to avoid driving for fear of being locked in the car when he has one of these "attacks" and not being able to get out. All of his friends say that he is "losing it," and he wants to know if you think he is.

492. What would be the most appropriate response?

   (A) "Yes, you are."
   (B) "No, you are not."
   (C) "Why do you want to know?"
   (D) "What do you think?"
   (E) Ask him what he means by "losing it."

493. He goes on to say that he will not take medication for these episodes. What therapy is generally most effective in treating panic disorder?

   (A) psychodynamic psychotherapy
   (B) cognitive–behavioral therapy
   (C) couples therapy
   (D) family therapy
   (E) paradoxical therapy

494. Flooding is an example of what form of psychotherapy?

   (A) family therapy
   (B) couples therapy
   (C) psychodynamic psychotherapy
   (D) behavioral therapy
   (E) hypnosis

495. A 43-year-old man is chastised at work. When he comes home, his friend asks him how his day went. He responds angrily saying that a "real friend wouldn't be so nosy." What is the name of this defense mechanism?

   (A) denial
   (B) displacement
   (C) isolation of affect
   (D) intellectualization
   (E) humor

496. A 20-year-old woman diagnosed with borderline personality disorder thinks of her therapist as "the best person in the world." The next week, the therapist announces that he will be going on vacation. The patient then says that he is "the worst person in the world." What is the defense mechanism that allows people to see others as either "all good" or "all bad"?

    (A) splitting
    (B) intellectualization
    (C) repression
    (D) devaluation
    (E) idealization

497. A 16-year-old boy has just lost his mother and father in a car accident. In your office, he talks philosophically about death and its implications. When asked how he feels about his parents' death, he responds by saying that "it is the nature of things to pass away." This patient's inability to talk directly of his emotional experience concerning personal losses is an example of which defense mechanism?

    (A) lying
    (B) projection
    (C) intellectualization
    (D) denial
    (E) suppression

Questions 498 through 500

A 44-year-old woman with schizophrenia is struggling with paranoia, auditory hallucinations, and delusions. She lives with her mother but has a poor relationship with her. She tells you that everyone wants her to spend a lot of money and buy drugs.

498. Which of the following would be the best response?

    (A) "Well, deciding for yourself is best."
    (B) "If you buy drugs, I'll call the police."
    (C) "Perhaps we should look at what your mother would think about that."
    (D) "Why do you think everyone wants you to do that?"
    (E) "No, they don't."

499. She then asks you why everyone wants to hurt her. She has a long-standing delusion of persecution. What would be the best response?

    (A) "I don't believe everyone wants to hurt you, but I am concerned that you do not feel safe."
    (B) "Why would you think something like that?"
    (C) "Perhaps what you feel is that you actually wish to hurt yourself."
    (D) "It would probably be best not to believe that."
    (E) "What do you want me to say to something like that?"

500. You decide that supportive therapy would be helpful to this patient. Which of the following is a goal of supportive therapy?

    (A) personality change
    (B) correcting faulty ideas
    (C) the reestablishment of psychic homeostasis through the strengthening of defenses
    (D) exploring the feeling of meaninglessness in life
    (E) investigating the freedom of individuals

501. A 32-year-old psychiatry resident is in psychoanalysis. He is lying on the couch and saying whatever comes to mind. This is an example of what analytic technique?

    (A) repression
    (B) speakeasy
    (C) countertransference
    (D) transference
    (E) free association

502. A psychotherapist finds herself getting angry at a patient after the patient reports beating up his little brother. The psychotherapist is exhibiting what phenomenon?

    (A) countertransferance
    (B) transferance
    (C) resistance
    (D) interpretation
    (E) extinction

503. On an acute inpatient psychiatric ward, the resident psychiatrist is in charge of leading a group consisting of patients admitted to the ward. In the morning, she asks each patient in turn to comment on his or her goals for treatment. What is the name of this technique of group psychotherapy?

(A) go-around
(B) free association
(C) feedback
(D) interpretation
(E) resistance

Questions 504 and 505

A 29-year-old health professional entered group therapy wanting to know why he was unable to stay in a long-term relationship with a woman. A handsome man, he said that women found him attractive and he didn't understand why he should restrict himself to one person. However, he was bored with the attention and felt empty inside. At work, he was very competitive with his male colleagues. In the group, members pointed out to him that whenever he was criticized by other men in the group, he made advances toward women in the group. These advances sometimes continued outside the group, but he lost interest when he felt better.

504. What is the name of this defense mechanism?

(A) idealization
(B) acting out
(C) abreaction
(D) ventilation
(E) catharsis

505. Compared with inpatient groups, which of the following is a treatment objective most characteristic of outpatient groups?

(A) crisis intervention
(B) return to previous level of functioning
(C) personality change and reconstruction
(D) stabilization of psychotic symptoms
(E) discussing current feelings regarding alcohol detoxification and heart disease

Questions 506 through 509

You have been assigned to lead various groups that help patients who suffer from personality disorders. In order to accomplish this task, you need to know which personality disorders are appropriate for group psychotherapy. In addition, you need to know which personality disorders benefit from combined individual and group psychotherapy.

506. Patients with which of the following personality disorders are usually excluded from group therapy because of their characteristic lack of empathy, social irresponsibility, deceitfulness, and failure to conform to social norms?

(A) borderline personality disorder
(B) antisocial personality disorder
(C) narcissistic personality disorder
(D) avoidant personality disorder
(E) schizotypal personality disorder

507. Patients with which of the following personality disorders are poor candidates for group psychotherapy because of their guardedness and mistrust of others?

(A) narcissistic personality disorder
(B) borderline personality disorder
(C) avoidant personality disorder
(D) obsessive–compulsive personality disorder
(E) paranoid personality disorder

508. Which of the following personality disorders is best treated with combined individual and group psychotherapy because of intense transferences and countertransferences that develop in a single mode of treatment?

(A) borderline personality disorder
(B) avoidant personality disorder
(C) schizotypal personality disorder
(D) antisocial personality disorder
(E) schizoid personality disorder

509. Patients with narcissistic personality disorder are best treated with combined individual and group psychotherapy. Which of the following reasons is most consistent with why this is true?

   (A) Wounds to self-image while in the group can be examined supportively in individual therapy.
   (B) These patients need as much attention as they can get.
   (C) These patients deplore the attention of others and need exposure to overcome this.
   (D) These patients constantly believe others are conspiring against them.
   (E) These patients need much structure to occupy their time.

Questions 510 through 514

A 29-year-old woman has been depressed for 2 months prior to seeking medical attention. She believes that "nobody" likes her even though she is always cordial, and there is "nothing that [she] can do to change" the way other people perceive her. She adamantly refuses to take antidepressants. You believe that cognitive therapy is indicated for this patient.

510. Cognitive therapy is based on which of the following premises?

   (A) Negative feelings and perspectives are preceded by specific, habitual errors in thinking.
   (B) Supportive, compassionate listening is sufficient to effect a change in psychopathology.
   (C) Oedipal issues are the result of most psychopathology.
   (D) Maladaptive thoughts can change only by changing maladaptive behavior.
   (E) Medications do not work.

511. Which of the following cognitive profiles most reflects the profile seen in depression?

   (A) negative view of self, experience, and future
   (B) fear of being fat and unattractive
   (C) concern about serious, insidious medical disorders
   (D) view of others as biased, manipulative, and devious
   (E) fear of physical or psychological danger

512. According to cognitive psychology, what are automatic thoughts?

   (A) thoughts that impede free association
   (B) thoughts that cannot be changed
   (C) thoughts at the edge of conscious awareness that regularly precede unpleasant feelings
   (D) genetically determined thoughts
   (E) thoughts that every human ought to have

513. According to cognitive psychology, psychopathology can arise because of cognitive distortions. What is the definition of selective abstraction?

   (A) drawing a conclusion in the absence of supportive evidence
   (B) focusing on a detail taken out of context; ignoring other, more salient features of a situation; and conceptualizing the whole experience on the basis of this element
   (C) drawing a conclusion across all situations based on a single experience
   (D) splitting
   (E) overemphasizing the relative importance of events

514. What is the definition of the cognitive distortion personalization?

   (A) the general belief that others always disapprove of personal actions
   (B) relating external events to oneself when there is no basis for doing so
   (C) relating external events to oneself when there is a basis for doing so

(D) splitting

(E) overemphasizing the relative importance of events

Questions 515 through 519

A 45-year-old man presents to the outpatient clinic handicapped by a fear of open spaces. This fear started 4 months prior to this visit. At the beginning of cognitive therapy, he says that his behavior is constantly being scrutinized and criticized by other people. He says that he cannot change his behavior because if he does, others will think that he is a fool.

515. What would be the most appropriate response from the therapist?

(A) "That's silly. People will not think you are a fool."

(B) "Yes, I can see that."

(C) "What makes you think that others are constantly scrutinizing your behavior?"

(D) "How can you possibly think other people care enough about you to constantly scrutinize your behavior?"

(E) "Well, maybe you are a fool. Have you ever thought of that?"

516. Which of the following best describes the therapeutic posture of a cognitive therapist?

(A) actively listening only

(B) actively pinpointing present problems and proposing and rehearsing cognitive techniques

(C) ignoring the patient for his own good

(D) lecturing the patient prior to each session

(E) uninvolved

517. What is one reason that homework is assigned in cognitive therapy?

(A) because no real work can happen during the therapy session

(B) the patient must identify all of the problems because the therapist cannot

(C) to identify maladaptive thoughts prior to each distressing symptom

(D) to give the patient something to do

(E) to contrast this therapy with pharmacotherapy

518. As part of cognitive therapy, which of the following would be indicated to effect change?

(A) asking the patient to change a way that he behaves and having him observe the response from other people

(B) listening to the patient over a series of meetings and then making an interpretation based on defense mechanisms and drive theory

(C) hypnosis

(D) fluoxetine (Prozac)

(E) asking the patient not to behave in a certain way

519. Which of the following statements best describes the view of cognitive therapy regarding the role of cognition in psychiatric disorders?

(A) Cognitive distortions are always the cause of various psychiatric syndromes.

(B) Cognitive distortions are never the cause of various psychiatric syndromes.

(C) Correcting cognitive distortions is always sufficient to correct symptomatology.

(D) Although cognitive distortions are not necessarily the ultimate cause of psychiatric syndromes, correcting distortions can be an effective intervention in psychiatric syndromes.

(E) Correcting cognitive distortions never completely alleviates symptoms.

Questions 520 through 522

An 18-year-old man presents to your office complaining that he cannot pass a movie theater without stopping, going inside, and buying candy. This behavior is troublesome to him and interferes with his daily activities, causing him to be constantly late to other appointments. You decide to help the patient with behavior therapy.

520. Which of the following does behavior therapy attempt to change?

   (A) maladaptive thoughts underlying a maladaptive behavior
   (B) neurobiology
   (C) how a patient perceives the environment
   (D) maladaptive behaviors seen in a particular syndrome
   (E) underlying conflicts in an attempt to change behavior

521. Which of the following best describes behavior therapy?

   (A) a long-term assessment of relational issues
   (B) a set of procedures designed to change maladaptive thoughts
   (C) a set of procedures designed to enhance the learning of adaptive behaviors and the unlearning of maladaptive behaviors
   (D) hypnosis
   (E) a technique used to resolve unconscious conflicts

522. Which of the following therapeutic instructions most influences the success of the therapy?

   (A) a firm, terse command from the therapist to the patient
   (B) a positive belief in the outcome and a suitable rationale for the therapy
   (C) an uninvolved, aloof suggestion to the patient
   (D) a negative belief in the outcome of the therapy
   (E) vague therapeutic instructions about the nature of the therapy

523. According to behavioral therapy, which of the following best describes the term *modeling?*

   (A) feedback as to progress
   (B) changing beliefs that promote behaviors
   (C) an aversive event contingent on the occurrence of a particular behavior
   (D) reproducing behavior after being shown that particular behavior
   (E) displaying clothes while in a fashion show

524. A 39-year-old man presents to your office complaining of headaches, which you diagnose as tension headaches. As part of this patient's treatment, you decide to use behavior therapy. Which of the following behavior techniques is used in the reduction of tension headaches?

   (A) stress reduction
   (B) stimulus control
   (C) systematic desensitization
   (D) aversive stimuli
   (E) negative reinforcement

Questions 525 through 527

A 23-year-old woman broke up with her boyfriend of 8 months 1 month before presenting to your office complaining of depression. Currently, she is just starting to date someone else. Given that her episode meets criteria for a major depressive episode, you decide to use both medication and interpersonal psychotherapy.

525. Which of the following is the major focus of interpersonal psychotherapy?

   (A) character change
   (B) clarifying communication patterns
   (C) interpreting transference
   (D) hypnosis
   (E) pointing out resistance

526. Interpersonal psychotherapy typically lasts for how many sessions?

   (A) 60 to 70
   (B) 3 to 5

(C) 120 to 150

(D) 10 to 12

(E) 25 to 50

527. Which of the following best represents the hypothesis on which interpersonal psychotherapy rests?

    (A) In addition to any biological diathesis, certain interpersonal problems predispose one to depressive disorders, complicate their course, or interfere with recovery.

    (B) Unconscious conflicting psychic processes need to be resolved.

    (C) Maladaptive behaviors may be changed by examining cognitive errors.

    (D) Maladaptive behaviors may be changed by positive reinforcement.

    (E) Maladaptive behaviors may be changed through the power of suggestion.

Questions 528 through 530

A 22-year-old college student presents complaining of having no goals in life, not doing as well as he could in school, and desiring but having no serious long-term romantic relationship. He has not chosen a major and says that his indecision is paralyzing him from moving on with the rest of his life. After discussing various forms of psychotherapy with the patient, you recommend psychoanalysis and he agrees.

528. Typically, how many days a week are required for psychoanalysis?

    (A) 1

    (B) 2 to 3

    (C) 4 to 5

    (D) 6

    (E) 7

529. Why does it take the above number of days per week to have a successful analysis?

    (A) It is difficult for patients to sustain a transference and keep their defenses lowered with fewer sessions.

    (B) Analytic patients are more seriously mentally ill and therefore need more time.

    (C) Analytic patients are typically more seriously mentally ill and therefore need less time.

    (D) Analysis is based on a supportive model of therapy.

    (E) Analysis is a quick therapy.

530. What is the major tool of treatment in psychoanalysis?

    (A) interpretation of transference

    (B) altering maladaptive behaviors

    (C) altering cognitive errors

    (D) interpreting dreams

    (E) solving interpersonal problems

Questions 531 through 534

A 50-year-old man is in psychoanalysis because he feels ineffective in his professional and personal relationships.

531. Which of the following best defines the analytic term *dynamic?*

    (A) the notion that all mental phenomena are the result of a continual interaction of forces that oppose one another

    (B) the notion that mental phenomena reveal themselves at various levels in the psyche

    (C) the notion that personality and its subsequent development has a historical aspect

    (D) the notion that the psyche is organized into functional units called the id, ego, and superego

    (E) fun, interactive, and pleasant

532. Typically, how long does it take to complete psychoanalysis?

    (A) 1 to 3 months

    (B) 8 to 12 months

    (C) 1 to 2 months

    (D) 3 to 5 years

    (E) 10 years

533. How are dreams useful in psychoanalysis?

(A) Dreams are interpreted by the analyst in order to subliminally influence the minds of patients.

(B) Dreams are used to alter cognitive errors.

(C) Dreams provide information about psychic conflicts.

(D) Dreams are used to change behavior.

(E) Dreams represent the conscious framework for behavior.

534. A patient in psychodynamic psychotherapy typically sees the therapist how many times per week?

(A) 1 to 2

(B) 3 to 4

(C) 5

(D) 6

(E) 7

Questions 535 through 538

You are seeing a 50-year-old man who suffers from generalized anxiety disorder (GAD) for cognitive–behavioral therapy. He is having a hard time with the restructuring of maladaptive thoughts. You decide that hypnosis may be helpful as an adjunctive therapy for this patient.

535. Which of the following best defines *hypnosis?*

(A) a state in which critical judgment is suspended and a person experiences alterations in perception, memory, or mood in response to suggestions

(B) an individual psychotherapy directed at changing behavior

(C) a group psychotherapy directed at changing maladaptive thoughts

(D) a procedure that directly accesses repressed memories

(E) an altered brain state that can be mapped by electroencephalogram (EEG)

536. Which of the following is most needed for a successful hypnosis?

(A) a skillful hypnotist

(B) a patient who is highly responsive to suggestion

(C) a quiet room

(D) a skilled induction technique

(E) creative ability

537. Hypnosis is best used as an adjunctive therapy within a psychotherapeutic relationship. In which of the following is hypnosis a relative contraindication?

(A) intractable hiccups

(B) anxiety disorders

(C) pain disorder

(D) treatment of warts (specifically verrucae planae juvenalis)

(E) psychotic disorders

538. The speed and intensity of which of the following characteristic events of psychotherapy is intensified by hypnosis augmentation?

(A) transference and countertransference

(B) interpretation

(C) cognitive restructuring

(D) a change in behavior

(E) guided imagery

Questions 539 through 544

A 14-year-old girl is brought by her mother to see you. The mother says that the patient has been depressed for the last year. You learn that 1 year ago, the patient's mother and father began divorce proceedings and are currently still living together. Also, 1 year ago, the patient's younger brother was born. You suspect that there are significant environmental stressors that are contributing to this patient's depression and decide that a trial of family therapy is warranted.

539. Family therapy is based on which of the following theories?

(A) Individual therapy is inappropriate for someone in a family.

(B) When families are dysfunctional, look for the individual who is causing the trouble.

(C) Families that live together fight together.

(D) The familial dynamic can help explain individual psychopathology.

(E) Role-playing can explore a patient's interpersonal relationships, personality makeup, and conflicts.

540. Which of the following is the first task of the family therapist?

(A) to obtain a proper history

(B) to join the family in order to be privy to its unique experiences and communications style

(C) to prescribe medication

(D) to identify the "problem" family members

(E) to let the family know at the outset that the therapist will function as the new, transient leader of the family

After further questioning, it becomes clear that the patient's mother is also depressed.

541. Which of the following is the greatest risk factor for depression for women with chronic depression?

(A) marital status and satisfaction

(B) being single

(C) age over 30 years

(D) low income

(E) high-fat diet

542. Which of the following treatments for depression in patients with dysfunctional marriages has the best outcome?

(A) antidepressant medication alone

(B) couples therapy alone

(C) combined antidepressant medication and couples therapy

(D) hypnosis alone

(E) St. John's wort

Further history taking reveals that the mother believes that she is an ineffectual person, her environment is always hostile, and things will never change.

543. The symptoms of feeling ineffectual, believing the environment is always a hostile place, and feeling that things will never change represent a triad of symptoms that are associated with which of the following disorders?

(A) depressive disorders

(B) GAD

(C) panic disorder

(D) schizophrenia

(E) dissociative disorder

544. Which of the following treatments would best target the above symptoms?

(A) behavioral therapy

(B) paradoxical therapy

(C) interpersonal therapy

(D) couples therapy

(E) cognitive therapy

Questions 545 and 546

A 9-year-old boy with attention deficit–hyperactivity disorder (ADHD), predominantly hyperactive type, presents to your office accompanied by his mother. He is currently on methylphenidate (Ritalin), and they both wonder if there is something else that can be done to help the patient. You recommend behavior therapy.

545. Which of the following best illustrates how behavioral therapy would help this patient?

(A) reinforcing attention to various tasks necessary for learning and ignoring disruptive behaviors

(B) interpreting a transference

(C) positively reframing a negative experience

(D) focusing on the patient's interpersonal relationships

(E) focusing on maladaptive communication techniques in the family

546. Which of the following represents a behavioral tool that is helpful for patients with ADHD?

(A) a well-timed interpretation of maladaptive behaviors

(B) a report card of various behaviors that can be rewarded at home by parents

(C) clozapine (Clozaril)

(D) methylphenidate (Ritalin)

(E) positively reframing a negative experience

Questions 547 through 549

A 25-year-old man in his fourth year of medical school presents to your office complaining of not being able to remain in a relationship with a girlfriend for longer than 3 months. He says that he would like an insight-oriented therapy, and you agree that this form of therapy would help him. You decide to treat this patient with brief psychodynamic psychotherapy.

547. How many sessions characterize brief psychodynamic therapy?

(A) 5 to 10

(B) 20 to 40

(C) 50 to 70

(D) 80 to 100

(E) 200 to 300

548. Which of the following factors best predicts a positive outcome with brief psychodynamic psychotherapy?

(A) gender

(B) age

(C) motivation for change

(D) marital status

(E) socioeconomic status

549. Which of the following most distinguishes brief psychodynamic therapy from other forms of therapy?

(A) correcting cognitive errors

(B) interpreting many different conflicts

(C) modifying maladaptive behaviors

(D) interpreting resistance

(E) identification of a focal conflict

Questions 550 and 551

A 20-year-old man is currently in college and has completed his first semester of the sophomore year. Halfway into his second semester, his grades drop from A's to F's over a 3-month period. He becomes increasingly isolated and paranoid, believing that the government is after him because he has solved all theological problems through direct communication with God. He is started on olanzapine (Zyprexa) 10 mg PO daily and is tentatively diagnosed with schizophreniform disorder. He recovers after 4 months but has another relapse 6 months later in the absence of elevated, irritable, or depressed mood. He is given a diagnosis of schizophrenia.

550. Which of the following is most indicated for the treatment of this patient's schizophrenia?

(A) psychoeducation alone

(B) medication alone

(C) family therapy

(D) psychoanalysis

(E) a combination of psychoeducation, medication, and family therapy

551. Which of the following therapies is usually not indicated for the treatment of psychotic disorders?

(A) behavioral therapy

(B) psychoanalysis

(C) supportive psychotherapy

(D) family therapy

(E) group psychotherapy

Questions 552 and 553

A 33-year-old woman presents to the emergency department saying that she wants to kill herself. She is hopeless and feels helpless. She has a plan to overdose on pills that she has stockpiled at home.

552. Other than severe hopelessness, which of the following cognitive difficulties do suicidal patients characteristically exhibit?

(A) personalization

(B) begging the question

(C) rigid, black-or-white, either-or thinking that limits problem-solving options

(D) selective abstraction

(E) circular reasoning

553. Which of the following forms of psychotherapy would be most appropriate to help this patient think of alternatives to suicide?

(A) behavioral therapy

(B) cognitive therapy

(C) interpersonal psychotherapy

(D) hypnosis

(E) paradoxical therapy

DIRECTIONS (Questions 554 through 561): Each set of items in this section consists of a list of lettered headings followed by several numbered words or phrases. For each numbered word or phrase, select the ONE lettered option that is most closely associated with it. Each lettered option may be selected once, more than once, or not at all.

Questions 554 through 556

(A) undoing

(B) negative reinforcement

(C) punishment

(D) biofeedback

(E) operant conditioning

(F) Sigmund Freud

(G) Franz Anton Mesmer

(H) Josef Breuer

(I) Jean-Martin Charcot

(J) Friedrich Nietzsche

(K) splitting

554. Who is considered the father of psychoanalysis?

555. Who is considered the father of modern hypnosis?

556. The process of giving a patient information on physiologic variables in order to alter those variables

Questions 557 through 559

(A) conditioning

(B) insight

(C) therapeutic alliance

(D) schema

(E) real relationship

(F) anxiety

(G) posttraumatic stress disorder (PTSD)

(H) projection

(I) transference neurosis or transference

(J) countertransference

(K) projective identification

557. What is the name for an enduring cognitive structure?

558. What is the term used to describe the intense constellation of events in an analysis that gradually places the analyst in a position of unsurpassed dominance in a patient's life?

559. What is the name for the process by which the meaning, significance, pattern, or use of an experience becomes clear?

Questions 560 and 561

(A) punishment

(B) reward

(C) desensitization

(D) avoidance

(E) extinction

(F) conditioned avoidance

(G) flooding

(H) positive reinforcement

(I) reciprocal inhibition

(J) hypnosis

(K) modeling

560. A response opposite to anxiety is evoked in the presence of a feared object or situation; the anxiety response is inhibited and gradually eliminated.

561. A patient with alcoholism is prescribed disulfiram (Antabuse).

Answers and Explanations

492. (E) Although it would be tempting to reassure this patient that he is not "going crazy," it is better to find out what he specifically means by "losing it." He could mention a specific fear that would be important for you to help him clarify or address. Asking the patient why he wants to know or asking "what do you think" is easily interpreted as an insulting and patronizing statement that does nothing to enhance doctor–patient trust.

493. (B) Cognitive–behavioral therapy is actually the combination of two therapies, cognitive therapy and behavioral therapy. Cognitive therapy would help the patient think about his symptoms as misinterpretations. For example, his feelings of impending doom, while frightening, do not actually predict the end of his life. An example of behavioral therapy is exposure. The premise is to expose patients to feared situations while maintaining a safe atmosphere. For example, a therapist could accompany the patient to the car to precipitate symptoms. In the controlled atmosphere, the patient can separate the connection of feared symptoms with the specific environment. In paradoxical therapy, developed by Bateson, the therapist suggests that the patient engage in the behavior with negative connotations (e.g., a phobia or compulsion). The efficacy of cognitive–behavioral therapy is more established than that of paradoxical therapy. Couples therapy is not indicated here because we have no evidence that the root of the patient's disorder is a conflict with a significant other; similarly, family therapy is not indicated. Psychodynamic psychotherapy is a form of therapy informed by psychodynamic processes.

494. (D) Flooding is an exposure technique that is commonly used in behavior therapy. The premise is confrontation with the feared symptom. Couples and family therapy are designed to modify relationships between the patient and others in his or her social constellation. Psychodynamic psychotherapy is a form of therapy informed by psychodynamic processes. Hypnosis is a sleeplike state induced by a therapist that has been of some use in uncovering psychodynamic processes and in behavioral modification such as stopping smoking.

495. (B) Displacement is a defense that transfers a feeling about, or a response to, one object onto another object. Denial is a defense that keeps out of conscious awareness an aspect of external reality or subjective distress that is too uncomfortable for the person to accept. Isolation of affect involves detachment of feelings from a particular idea or experience. Intellectualization is a defense in which the individual favors abstract thinking over dealing with the disturbing feelings of an idea or experience. Humor is considered a defense mechanism that emphasizes the amusing or ironic aspects of the stressor.

496. (A) Splitting occurs when an individual is unable to see others moderately; that is, people's actions are either all good or all bad. Intellectualization is a defense that utilizes excessive abstract thinking or generalizations to control threatening emotions. Repression is a defense that expels disturbing wishes, thoughts, or experiences from conscious awareness. The feeling component may remain but be divorced from the idea. Devaluation is a defense that attributes excessive negative qualities to another. Idealization is a defense that attributes excessive positive qualities to another.

497. **(C)** This is an example of intellectualization, a defense that utilizes excessive abstract thinking or generalizations to control threatening emotions. Lying is not considered a defense mechanism. Denial is a defense that keeps out of conscious awareness an aspect of external reality or subjective distress that is too uncomfortable for the person to accept. Projection is a defense whereby a thought, feeling, or idea that is unacceptable to the person is falsely attributed to another person. Suppression is a defense in which one intentionally avoids thinking of distressing thoughts, feelings, ideas, or experiences.

498. **(D)** The best strategy in any communication is to try to gain clarity. Asking this patient why she believes what she does may lead nowhere, or it may very much help understand this thought. Choice A may be helpful in some situations and certainly has a positive ring to it. However, this patient's comment is an implicit question. She is asking for help and genuinely does not know what to do. Hiding behind pithy maxims is not helpful. Choices B and C are coercive and block communication. Giving supportive guidance is appropriate in this situation, but coercion is never appropriate in a therapeutic relationship. Choice E is not coercive but blocks communication. This may be the content that needs to be heard, but it abruptly terminates communication and could sacrifice a more insightful, empowering response.

499. **(A)** This patient is suffering from a delusion—a fixed false belief. No amount of arguing will change a delusion. Therefore, an appropriate response is to let her know in a nonjudgmental way that you do not believe the thought. This helps the patient know that others do not affirm her belief. Telling her that you are concerned that she does not feel safe communicates that you care about her. Choice B is a pejorative statement and can only harm a relationship. Choice C may have a psychological underpinning but would risk the therapeutic alliance at this juncture. Choice D is futile and potentially inhibits further communication. Choice E may very well be a feeling that the doctor is having but is potentially humiliating to the patient.

500. **(C)** The goal of supportive therapy is not to break down the defenses in order to achieve a more optimal level of functioning. This would be a long-term goal of psychodynamic psychotherapy. Supportive therapy's goal is the strengthening of current defense mechanisms. Through supportive care, the patient can learn to cope with difficult problems using already established abilities. Personality change is a goal of psychodynamic psychotherapy, while correcting faulty ideas is the expressed goal of cognitive therapy. Exploring the feeling of meaninglessness in life and investigating the freedom of individuals are goals of existential psychotherapy.

501. **(E)** This is an example of free association. Freud believed that all mental activity is causally related, meaning that free associations are not truly random. They follow logically, but the missing connection is being "held down" or repressed unconsciously by defenses. Repression is a defense mechanism that expels disturbing wishes, thoughts, or experiences from conscious awareness. Transference, in strict terms, is the reexperiencing of past experiences with the analyst in the setting of psychoanalytic psychotherapy. Countertransference is the analyst's response to this. However, these terms have come to mean the transferring of emotions and feelings that one has from one's past to the physician or care provider in the case of transference and the physician toward the patient in countertransference. A speakeasy was an underground bar during Prohibition.

502. (A) Countertransference is the conscious or unconscious emotional reaction of the therapist to the patient. Transference is the conscious or unconscious emotional reaction of the patient to the therapist based on a past relationship the patient had with a significant other person. Resistance is unconscious opposition to full disclosure of feelings or ideas. Interpretation is insight offered by the therapist regarding patterns of thought or behavior. Extinction is the reduction in frequency of a learned response as a result of the cessation of reinforcement, and is a term frequently used in learning theory.

503. (A) The go-around is a technique frequently used in inpatient groups. By having each patient comment on a plan, theme, mood, behavior, or idea, active participation by all members is ensured, and other members of the group can benefit from various ideas presented. The go-around also helps patients feel that they are not the only ones with difficulties. Free association is used in psychoanalytically oriented groups. These groups are largely outpatient groups whose members can tolerate and effectively use this technique. Members are encouraged to be spontaneous with their thoughts and feelings, and the therapist assists in pointing out common themes and possible connections. Feedback, a cardinal feature of group psychotherapy, comes from peers as well as from the leader. Feedback from peers in the group can be a powerful stimulus for insight and change. Interpretation is the offering of insight that allows patients to gain an understanding of conflicts and motivations that contribute to their behavior. Resistance is the unconscious opposition to full disclosure of thoughts or feelings.

504. (B) Acting out is characterized by behaviors that distract a patient who needs to relieve tension or to gratify needs through activity rather than through verbalization of uncomfortable feelings in the group. Idealization is a defense that attributes excessive positive qualities to another. Abreaction is a process by which repressed material, particularly a painful experience of conflict, is brought back to consciousness. In the process, the person not only recalls the experience but relives the experience, which is accompanied by the appropriate emotional response. Ventilation (also known as self-disclosure) is the expression of suppressed feelings, ideas, or events to other group members; this relieves a sense of sin or guilt. Catharsis is expression of ideas, thoughts, and suppressed material that is accompanied by an emotional response that produces a state of relief in the patient.

505. (C) Personality change and reconstruction are goals of psychoanalytically oriented outpatient groups. This type of significant change is virtually impossible in an inpatient group. Crisis intervention, return to previous level of functioning, and preparation for outpatient therapy are all objectives for inpatient group psychotherapy. Certain outpatient groups can also help with these objectives so that inpatient hospitalization may be averted. If a patient has heart disease and needs alcohol detoxification, inpatient detoxification is indicated.

506. (B) These characteristics comprise antisocial personality disorder. These patients cannot maintain the confidentiality of groups and frequently disregard interpretations. These patients need a group that is very homogeneous and takes place in a highly restrictive setting. For example, penal institutions, which are populated by large percentages of people with antisocial personality disorder, are ideal. Patients with borderline personality disorder are known for their intense personal relationships, self-destructive behaviors, anger management issues, and poor senses of self-image. Narcissistic personality disorder is marked by a grandiose sense of self-worth, entitlement, lack of real empathy, and tendency to use others for one's own ends. Schizotypal patients are known for their quirkiness and seemingly magical thinking styles. Unlike the patient with schizotypal personality disorder, the patient with avoidant personality disorder longs for relationships, yet is morbidly shy and fears them.

507. **(E)** Patients with paranoid personality disorder are guarded and do not trust others. In a group setting, these symptoms are at great risk of being exacerbated but not helped. For example, if the patient has a strong alliance with either the therapist or a member of the group, the patient can receive collective validation from the group about his or her unwarranted suspicions. Patients with borderline personality disorder are known for their intense personal relationships, self-destructive behaviors, anger management issues, and poor senses of self-image. Narcissistic personality disorder is marked by a grandiose sense of self-worth, entitlement, lack of real empathy, and tendency to use others for one's own ends. The patient with avoidant personality disorder longs for relationships, yet is morbidly shy and fears them. Patients with obsessive–compulsive personality disorder are perfectionists, inflexible, and overly demanding of themselves and others.

508. **(A)** Patients with borderline personality disorder develop intense transferences in individual treatment. This can impede the work of psychotherapy. Transference is usually diluted in group psychotherapy because of the number of people. The group can offer stability and moderation to the extreme ways of seeing others that distort borderline perceptions. The combined modes of treatment, individual and group, offer the patient with borderline personality disorder a higher probability for personality change. Patients with borderline personality disorder are known for their intense personal relationships, self-destructive behaviors, anger management issues, and poor senses of self-image. Schizotypal patients are known for their quirkiness and seemingly magical thinking styles. Unlike the patient with schizotypal personality disorder, the patient with avoidant personality disorder longs for relationships, yet is morbidly shy and fears them. Schizoid personality disorder is marked by bizarre behavior and withdrawal.

509. **(A)** This is one of the strongest reasons for combining the two forms of therapy. In individual therapy, patients can reflect on what their feelings are in the group and the responses of others to them from the group. Choice B is true of this personality disorder but is not a reason to combine therapies. Choices C, D, and E are not characteristic of narcissistic personality disorder.

510. **(A)** Cognitive therapy is founded on the premise that many emotional states are preceded by distorted thoughts. Examples of these thoughts are pervasive ways of seeing the world or particular thoughts that stem from misinterpreting others' behavior. Choice B is a belief of supportive therapy. Choices C and E are not espoused by any form of therapy. Choice D is a foundation of behavior therapy.

511. **(A)** The cognitive triad of depression is a belief that oneself is ineffective, the world is a hostile place, and nothing one can do will ever change anything. The other choices are cognitive profiles typical of various psychiatric syndromes. Fear of being fat and unattractive is typical of anorexia nervosa and bulimia nervosa. Concern about serious, insidious medical disorders is typical of hypochondriasis. Seeing others as biased, manipulative, and devious is typical of paranoid states. Fear of physical or psychological danger is typical of anxiety disorders.

512. **(C)** Automatic thoughts are constant ways of perceiving situations and oneself in relation to the environment. They can be thought of as a "given" way of evaluating events. Cognitive therapy aims to identify negative automatic thoughts and then change them so that individuals do not constantly view themselves or their environment in a negative light. Automatic thoughts are not genetically determined. They have not always been present and can be changed. There is no moral imperative from automatic thoughts, and they do not impede free association.

513. (B) This question focuses on specific kinds of logical errors. Drawing a conclusion in the absence of supportive evidence is an arbitrary inference. Drawing a conclusion across all situations based on a single experience is overgeneralization. Splitting is a defense mechanism derived from analytic theory but can also be called dichotomous thinking, which occurs when the patient makes an evaluation based on an either-or, black-or-white style of thinking. Overemphasizing or underemphasizing the relative importance of events is called magnification or minimization, respectively.

514. (B) This is another example of a cognitive error. This is the same as ideas of reference or referential thinking; by definition, there is no basis for the belief. Splitting is a defense mechanism derived from analytic theory but can also be called dichotomous thinking, which occurs when the patient makes an evaluation based on an either-or, black-or-white style of thinking. Overemphasizing or underemphasizing the relative importance of events is called magnification or minimization, respectively.

515. (C) One of the reasons that this is the best of the possible responses is that it is a question. Patients with cognitive distortions often take their view of the world as a given. They do not question their perspectives. Asking a question invites patients to examine their perspectives and thereby become open to the possibility that their thoughts may be inaccurate. Choices D and E are also questions but are authoritarian and punitive, not to mention insulting. In order to have the best outcome in any form of therapy, there must be a good relationship or alliance between the patient and therapist. Choices A and B have not been supported by any evidence. Choice B is ambiguous—to which part of the question are you responding? The patient may not think you are awkwardly trying to be supportive but may believe that you are insulting him. Choice A is dangerous—a patient should not be called "silly."

516. (B) This describes the work that happens in cognitive therapy. Exploring the past can help with understanding how the cognitive error arose in the first place. Actively listening only does not completely describe the stance of the cognitive therapist, although the good cognitive therapist will listen actively. The answer also emphasizes that all good listening is active listening. The therapist that listens always should do so with an ear for testing hypotheses, formulating alternative explanations for behavior, and trying to place the present session in the context of the whole therapy. The other answers describe stances that are not helpful and can be harmful.

517. (C) A large part of the work that happens in cognitive therapy requires the patient to actively pursue outside of the therapy session the insights and ideas identified in the actual session with the therapist. Choice C is an example of a possible homework assignment. Choice A is false. If choice B is correct, the patient probably does not need the therapist in the first place. That is not to say, however, that the patient cannot identify cognitive errors without the help of the therapist. Hopefully, the patient will sufficiently learn the process of cognitive therapy to use the principles to help himself outside of the therapy session.

518. (A) In cognitive therapy, a therapist may give the patient a homework assignment to change his behavior and then observe what happens. The purpose is not to change the behavior but to change the way the patient views the way others perceive him. If the patient can see that he is mistaken and has committed some sort of logical fallacy in his thinking, he can become more comfortable about changing the way he thinks about a particular situation. Choice B may happen in analytic or psychodynamic therapy. *Analytic* and *psychodynamic* are synonyms. Asking the patient not to act in a certain way has no clear cognitively therapeutic effect. Incidentally, cognitive, behavioral, and psychodynamic therapies can all take place in groups.

Cognitive therapy itself does not involve the use of medications such as fluoxetine.

519. **(D)** This question is meant to emphasize that although correcting cognitive distortions may have symptomatic benefit, it should not be inferred that cognitive distortions are the ultimate cause of the psychiatric syndromes. The other choices are wrong because of the "always" or "never" used in the question. The other choices can be true at times but are not always true or false.

520. **(D)** Behavior therapy is focused on behaviors, not on possible underlying factors that cause behaviors. Behavior therapy is a "here and now" approach to maladaptive behaviors. It may utilize information surrounding the emergence of a particular maladaptive behavior to construct a behavior modification plan. Although behavior therapy can and does change neurobiology, this is not its expressed goal. Changing maladaptive thoughts underlying a maladaptive behavior and changing how the patient perceives the environment involve perspectives more appropriate for cognitive therapy. Changing underlying conflicts in an attempt to change behavior is a description of the goals of psychodynamic therapy.

521. **(C)** Behavior therapy is a set of procedures designed to enhance the learning of adaptive behaviors and the unlearning of maladaptive behaviors. In a strict sense, it is not designed to uncover or alter unconscious conflicts using hypnosis or other methods. It is also a short-term therapy.

522. **(B)** A positive yet realistic belief in the outcome of the therapy and an explanation of the rationale used to accomplish the therapy has been shown to significantly improve the outcome of behavior therapy. A relationship of extremes is not helpful; neither vagueness and distance nor an authoritarian stance benefits the therapy.

523. **(D)** Modeling is a behavior technique used to reproduce behavior. The patient is first shown a behavior, and then he or she tries to imitate that behavior. An aversive event contingent on the occurrence of a particular behavior is the definition of punishment. Behavior therapy does not attempt to change beliefs. Obviously, displaying clothes in a fashion show is a lay definition of modeling.

524. **(A)** Stress reduction and biofeedback are used to reduce the frequency and the severity of each headache. They are equally effective in accomplishing this goal. Stimulus control is used in the treatment of insomnia. Stimulus control procedures are used to narrow the stimuli associated with sleep onset. Systematic desensitization is a technique used in asthma, in which the patient becomes relaxed and visualizes typical situations that precipitate asthma attacks. Substance withdrawal syndromes are examples of the aversive stimuli and consequently negative reinforcement that lead to decrease in substance use.

525. **(B)** The major focus of interpersonal psychotherapy is communication analysis. Indirect, unclear interpersonal communication patterns are identified in the course of therapy. These communication patterns are then altered, for instance, by role-playing or asking the patient to try out different forms of communication during the session. Interpreting transference, pointing out resistance, and character change are more the focus of psychodynamically oriented psychotherapy. Hypnosis is a sleeplike state induced by a therapist, which has been of some use in uncovering psychodynamic processes and in behavioral modification such as stopping smoking. It is not part of interpersonal psychotherapy.

526. **(D)** Interpersonal psychotherapy typically lasts for 10 to 12 sessions. There are no correlations to other forms of therapies with the other answers.

527. **(A)** Interpersonal psychotherapy focuses on the patient's role and communication style within important relationships, and how that role may be causing or complicating the ill-

ness, such as depression. If one or two specific ways of communicating can be altered so that a relationship improves, the depressive illness will also be improved. This therapy also has the added benefit of durability; once a communication pattern is improved and the patient better understands how his or her role in a relationship may create distress, the depressive illness will not be as likely to recur. While other processes such as those in the remaining answers may be used, choice A best reflects the foundation of the therapy.

528. **(C)** Generally, it takes 4 to 5 days a week to successfully complete an analysis.

529. **(A)** It takes 4 to 5 days a week to successfully complete an analysis because it is difficult for patients to sustain a transference and keep their defenses lowered with fewer sessions. There is no correlation between severity of mental illness and length of therapy. Psychoanalysis tends to be among the longest therapies, and involves the process of free association in which the patient lies on a couch, facing away from the therapist, and says whatever comes to mind. Psychoanalysis is based on an expressive or exploratory model of therapy, as opposed to a supportive model aimed at stabilizing crisis and reestablishing a baseline level of function.

530. **(A)** Psychoanalysis may accomplish many tasks, including changing maladaptive thoughts and behaviors and "solving" interpersonal problems, but these are the consequences of analysis, not the instrument of change. Altering cognitive errors is more in the domain of cognitive therapy. The major tool of psychoanalysis is the careful interpretations of the transference neurosis. Certainly, interpreting dreams can lead to deep insights into a patient's thoughts and feelings, but it is an adjunctive tool.

531. **(A)** The term *dynamic* or *psychodynamic* refers to the notion that all mental phenomena are the result of a continual interaction of forces that oppose one another. Choices B, C, and D

are related ideas; specifically, the notion that the psyche is organized into functional units called the id, ego, and superego was a construction formulated by Freud. Fun, interactive, and pleasant is close to a lay definition of *dynamo*.

532. **(D)** There is no rule that requires that psychoanalysis take 3 to 5 years. It appears, however, that to execute and sustain real psychic change, and a change in personality structure (a pervasive way of relating to others), 3 to 5 years is typically necessary.

533. **(C)** Dreams provide information about psychic conflicts. Dreams can lead to a change in behavior, but they are not used per se in analysis in order to change behavior or cognitive errors. Dreams are used to uncover psychic conflicts, which, when interpreted appropriately (not subliminally), can lead to a productive change in behavior. According the psychoanalytic theory, dreams represent the unconscious workings of the mind, not the conscious ones, and may be symbolic in content.

534. **(A)** Psychodynamic psychotherapy uses the content of psychoanalysis as a model for the approach to psychopathology. However, the use of interpretation of the transference neurosis is not as powerful as in psychoanalysis. Meeting only once or twice a week, the patient usually cannot sustain as robust a transference to the therapist. However, the psychoanalytic psychotherapist can offer the patient significant insight on psychic frustrations and conflicts, which, when resolved, can lead to symptom alleviation.

535. **(A)** Hypnosis is a state in which critical judgment is suspended and a person experiences alterations in perception, memory, or mood in response to suggestions. Hypnosis is not a psychotherapy. It is better understood as a procedure that may be used as an adjunct to psychotherapy. Hypnosis should not be used if the therapist is not willing or able to treat the patient with a psychotherapy, because it seems to help some patients talk about events

that are otherwise too emotionally laden to be expressed. The judgment of whether these thoughts are "repressed memories" is controversial. Hypnosis cannot be tracked or mapped with an EEG.

536. **(B)** Far and away the most important factor in hypnosis is a patient who is highly responsive to suggestion. Some people are able to alter their subjective experience in response to suggestion more than others; a patient can be taught self-hypnosis. Needless to say, a skillful hypnotist and induction technique are helpful. Neither a quiet room nor creative talent is a factor.

537. **(E)** Hypnosis should not be used in psychotic disorders. Patients with schizophrenia often have cognitive disorders or paranoid symptoms that make the use of hypnosis problematic. Often, these patients do not remember the changes that were supposed to be induced through the hypnosis, and there is controversy over the extent to which patients with schizophrenia can be hypnotized. Hypnosis has been used successfully for the treatment of anxiety disorders and pain. There is also literature indicating its efficacy in the treatment of warts.

538. **(A)** Transference and countertransference are tremendously intensified with hypnosis. These factors become more difficult to interpret because of the active role of the therapist, as opposed to the passive role of the therapist in psychodynamic therapy. This can aid the therapy if the therapist is able to handle the rapid rate of change and the intensity. If performing hypnosis for a patient, one should be well aware of the potential dangers involved. None of the other choices are intensified by hypnosis.

539. **(D)** Family therapy is based on the idea that the interactional dynamics of the family can help explain individual psychopathology. Individual psychotherapy can be very useful in conjunction with family therapy. Role-playing can explore a patient's interpersonal relationships, personality makeup, and conflicts.

However, this is not the basis for family therapy; it is the basis for psychodrama.

540. **(B)** Certainly, obtaining a proper history is extremely important. However, the first priority of the family therapist is to join the family so that, for instance, an intimate history may be obtained. In all psychotherapy, if there is not a trusting relationship between patient and therapist, the work will be extremely compromised. The problem is with the family as a family, not with individuals. Identifying individuals as "problems" is often more hurtful than helpful. The therapist is not the new, transient leader of the family. Prescribing medications is a difficult task for the family therapist.

541. **(A)** A dysfunctional marriage is a greater risk factor for depression than being single. Certainly, many people are content and single. The other three answers are not correlated risk factors for depression. Some studies have shown age greater than 45 to be a risk factor for depression in general. Others have shown age greater than 65.

542. **(C)** A combination of antidepressant medication and couples therapy has been shown to have the best outcome for patients with dysfunctional marriages. In fact, there is a growing impression that a combination of psychotherapy and medication is the best way to treat most forms of depression. European trials have shown St. John's wort to be moderately helpful in milder forms of depression; further studies regarding its efficacy have been mixed. Hypnosis should be combined with psychotherapy and is more appropriate for individual therapy.

543. **(A)** These symptoms are known as "Beck's triad." Beck, who developed the Beck Depression Inventory, is a seminal thinker with respect to cognitive therapy. His triad of symptoms has been very helpful in the diagnosis and treatment of major depressive disorder (MDD). This particular triad is not characteristically seen in other disorders.

544. (E) These symptoms are Beck's triad of depressive symptoms (see answer 543). Cognitive therapy can help alter these negative ways of perceiving the self and the environment. In paradoxical therapy, developed by Bateson, the therapist suggests that the patient engage in the behavior with negative connotations (e.g., a phobia or compulsion). Behavioral therapy is focused on behaviors, not on possible underlying factors that cause behaviors such as cognitive errors. Couples therapy would be less efficacious than cognitive therapy, given this patient's symptoms. The major focus of interpersonal psychotherapy is communication analysis and one's role in relationships.

545. (A) Behavioral therapy helps patients who suffer from ADHD to derive satisfaction from learning and ignoring disruptive behaviors. The other answers can also be very helpful; however, they are not examples of behavioral therapy.

546. (B) A behavioral tool that is used quite effectively is a report card. This tool can function as a bridge between school and home. In addition, a report card can serve as a positive incentive to good behavior when the report is good and is therefore rewarded. The rewards can be adjusted for the degree of good behavior obtained. So, a 40% increase in a desired behavior gets rewarded with a proportional prize. Methylphenidate (Ritalin) is also effective in treating ADHD but is not a behavior therapy. Clozapine, a newer-generation antipsychotic, is not effective in treating the disorder. Interpretive strategies such as a well-timed interpretation of maladaptive behaviors and positively reframing a negative experience are not helpful behavioral tools.

547. (B) A brief psychodynamic therapy usually lasts about 20 sessions. However, it can last for as long as 40 sessions. This is obviously much shorter than a psychoanalysis.

548. (C) Motivation for change goes beyond a desire for removal of symptoms and includes a willingness to tolerate discomfort and to take risks in a search for understanding. Demographics do not play a role.

549. (E) Brief psychodynamic therapy identifies a single, focal area of conflict and spends the time of the therapy actively interpreting transferences as they pertain to this identified focal conflict. Interpretations of resistance certainly take place in brief psychodynamic therapy. However, the resistance would be interpreted in light of the identified focal conflict. Many types of therapy correct cognitive errors and modify maladaptive behaviors, although cognitive therapy and behavioral therapy, respectively, are specifically concerned with these outcomes.

550. (E) The treatment of the devastating illness of schizophrenia needs to involve not only the patient but also the family who will care for the patient. This includes education of the patient and his family, medication of the patient, and family therapy to help the family accommodate the patient and his new illness. Recent evidence supports reducing high levels of expressed emotion in the family in order to decrease psychotic relapses. Psychoanalysis is not useful in the treatment of schizophrenia and is generally considered contraindicated in the treatment of patients with psychotic disorders.

551. (B) Psychoanalysis is usually not indicated in patients who have difficulty with reality testing. The introspection and self-examination required in psychoanalysis is usually overwhelming to psychotic patients and actually may cause more harm than good. All of the other treatments can be helpful.

552. (C) Patients who are suicidal characteristically have severe hopelessness and think about events in rigid, black-and-white ways. They see very few options and become overwhelmed with the hopelessness that is exacerbated by seeing "no way out." Personalization is a patient's tendency to relate events to himself without any reason for doing so.

553. **(B)** Cognitive therapy is the psychotherapy that would be most appropriate to help the patient solve problems more productively. Behavioral therapy is focused on behaviors, not on possible underlying factors that cause behaviors. Interpersonal therapy is aimed at understanding communication patterns and roles in relationships. Hypnosis is a sleeplike state induced by a therapist, which has been of some use in uncovering psychodynamic processes and in behavioral modification such as stopping smoking. In paradoxical therapy, developed by Bateson, the therapist suggests that the patient engage in the behavior with negative connotations (e.g., a phobia or compulsion).

554. **(F)** Certainly, Sigmund Freud is one of the most well-known figures of the twentieth century. He is generally credited with the modern form of psychoanalysis that is practiced today. However, Freud did not work in a vacuum; he was influenced by an array of people and ideas, including the internist Joseph Breuer and the neurologist Jean-Martin Charcot. Incidentally, Freud began his career as a neurologist. Just as there have been many changes in physics since Aristotle, there have been many changes in psychoanalysis since Freud.

555. **(G)** Franz Anton Mesmer is considered the father of modern hypnosis; the word *mesmerism* is derived from his name.

556. **(D)** Biofeedback is the process of giving a patient information on physiologic variables in order to alter those variables and ultimately the corresponding behavior. Patients with migraine headaches receive information on muscle tension or temperature. They use this information to decrease the intensity of the headaches by directly trying to relax and alter the known parameters. Undoing is a concept described by Freud in which a patient with obsessive–compulsive disorder will perform a compulsive act to prevent or undo the consequences from a feared impulse. Negative reinforcement describes the delivery of an averse stimulus based on a given response. Punishment is the administration of an unpleasant stimulus based on a given response, while reward describes a pleasant stimulus delivered to a given response. In operant conditioning, a response is rewarded or punished each time it occurs, so that over time the response increases or decreases in frequency. Friedrich Nietzsche was a nineteenth-century philosopher. Splitting, characteristic of patients with borderline personality disorder, occurs when an individual is unable to see others moderately; that is, people's actions are either all good or all bad.

557. **(D)** Piaget is the person credited with the popularization of the term *schema*, which refers to enduring categories of cognitive structure.

558. **(I)** *Transference* and *transference neurosis* are synonyms. Transference can also be understood as a general phenomenon in which the person displaces onto all aspects of living the emotions and forgotten memories of one's past (particularly the earliest years of one's life).

559. **(B)** When a patient gains insight, the meaning, significance, pattern, or use of an experience becomes clear. Conditioning is the manner in which the frequency of responses is increased or decreased according to the relationship between the response and a reinforcement schedule. The therapeutic alliance is of the utmost importance in the patient–therapist relationship. Real relationship is a nonsense term. PTSD is characterized by a history of a traumatic event, intrusive memories of trauma, avoidance of reminders, and hypervigilance. Projection is the attribution of impulses and feelings, usually undesirable, onto another person. Countertransference occurs within the analyst, and refers to the analyst's emotional response to the patient. Projective identification is a process in which object representations or self-representations are denied and instead attributed to others. Anxiety is a state of apprehension, tension, or uneasiness occurring in anticipation of internal or external danger.

560. **(I)** Joseph Wolf, a South African psychiatrist, used this term to describe gradual decreases in abnormal behavior of cats when they were fed in a cage that had previously delivered a shock. Feeding the cats in the same cage and not shocking them gradually lessened the agitated behavior displayed by the cats.

561. **(F)** A patient with alcoholism who drinks alcohol while taking disulfiram will likely avoid this combination in the future. The goal of disulfiram therapy is to give patients negative associations with alcohol. Nevertheless, patients learning to not drink while on disulfiram still illustrates the principal of conditioned avoidance. Punishment is the administration of an unpleasant stimulus based on a given response, while reward describes a pleasant stimulus delivered to a given response. Desensitization refers to a behavioral modification technique of increasing exposure to an unpleasant or phobic stimulus with the goal of minimizing negative effects. Avoidance is learned cessation of behavior. Extinction is a learned response to removal of a stimulus. Positive reinforcement is the process by which certain consequences of behavior raise the probability that the behavior will occur again. Modeling is a process by which behavior is changed simply by observation. Flooding is an exposure technique that is commonly used in behavior therapy. The premise is confrontation with the feared symptom. Hypnosis is a sleeplike state induced by a therapist, which has been of some use in uncovering psychodynamic processes and in behavioral modification such as stopping smoking.

CHAPTER 7

Legal and Ethical Issues in Psychiatry and Medicine

Vladimir Coric, MD, and Louis Sanfilippo, MD

Questions

DIRECTIONS (Questions 562 through 615): Each of the numbered items or incomplete statements in this section is followed by answers or by completions of the statement. Select the ONE lettered answer or completion that is BEST in each case.

Questions 562 and 563

The case manager of an 18-year-old man that you are treating notifies you that your patient has been acting strangely lately. You learn from the case manager that the patient makes provocative sexual comments toward her on a daily basis. During your session, the patient expresses concern that his case manager is somehow conspiring against him, and he plans to do something about it. On further questioning, he becomes increasingly anxious and abruptly storms out of your office. You hear him in the hallway, exclaiming, "That woman, I'm going to stab her and she won't bother me anymore."

562. Your first course of action should be to

- (A) respect the patient's confidentiality and wait until your next scheduled appointment with him to discuss his feelings
- (B) contact the patient's family and let them know about his threats toward the case manager
- (C) inform the police of the content of your previous sessions and his recent threat toward the case manager

- (D) notify the case manager of the potential danger
- (E) attempt to contact the patient over the next several hours to discuss the intent of his parting comments

563. The legal precedent that guides the appropriate course of action in this case is

- (A) *Rogers v. Commissioner of the Department of Mental Health*
- (B) *Tarasoff v. Regents of University of California*
- (C) *Durham v. United States*
- (D) *Zinerman v. Burch*
- (E) *Kansas v. Hendricks*

564. In medical malpractice cases, the plaintiff must establish

- (A) burden of proof beyond a reasonable doubt
- (B) clear and convincing evidence of wrongdoing
- (C) harm or damage
- (D) criminal intent
- (E) criminal mischief

Questions 565 and 566

An 80-year-old widow with a history significant for bipolar I disorder has recently been diagnosed with end-stage hepatic cancer. She is concerned about the disposition of her estate and does not want her family to receive any of her money; she plans to donate her entire estate to the local humane society.

565. Which of the following is most important in establishing a legally valid will?

(A) mens rea
(B) informed consent
(C) lack of mental illness
(D) testamentary capacity
(E) conservatorship of estate

566. The patient's family hires an attorney to challenge the integrity of her will. Which of the following items, if present, would undermine this patient's competence to make a will?

(A) paranoid delusions regarding the patient's family
(B) the presence of a diagnosable Axis I disorder
(C) the patient's explanation of why she wants to donate her estate to the local humane society
(D) inability to read and write
(E) refusal to undergo treatment with chemotherapy

567. As opposed to fact witnesses, expert medical witnesses

(A) are familiar with a particular body of evidence no more so than laypersons
(B) are not allowed to charge a fee
(C) can provide only factual information
(D) can testify only for the defense
(E) may provide opinion testimony

Questions 568 through 570

A 23-year-old man with no prior psychiatric history is charged with murdering his next-door neighbor. His friends note that he became increasingly isolative and suspicious of others in the weeks prior to the crime. The examining psychiatrist found him to be having paranoid delusions regarding his neighbor and noted that his thought processes were too disorganized to complete the examination.

568. Which of the following legal standards is the current basis for establishing an insanity defense?

(A) M'Naghten rule
(B) American Law Institute test (Model Penal Code)
(C) Durham rule
(D) extreme emotional disturbance
(E) irresistible impulse rule

569. The burden of proof in an insanity defense rests on

(A) the defendant
(B) the prosecution
(C) clear and convincing evidence
(D) establishing habeas corpus
(E) the preponderance of evidence

570. Criminal responsibility requires demonstration of the criminal act along with which of the following elements?

(A) actus reus
(B) diminished mental capacity
(C) mens rea
(D) product test
(E) "wild beast" test

Questions 571 and 572

An obese 54-year-old woman presents to the emergency department by ambulance complaining of severe substernal chest pain lasting 40 minutes, profuse sweating, and nausea. Her vital signs are blood pressure 195/96, heart rate 63, respiratory rate 18, temperature 98.8°F. An electrocardiogram (ECG) reveals 3-mm ST segment elevations in leads V4, V5, and V6. Cardiac enzymes and laboratory workup are pending. You suspect a lateral wall myocardial infarction and recommend immediate thrombolytic therapy. The patient states, "You're crazy if you think I'm gonna let some intern care for me . . . my family will drive me across town to the private hospital." The patient then jumps from the gurney and begins walking toward the exit.

571. The appropriate next step is to

   (A) sedate the patient and begin thrombolytic therapy

   (B) allow the patient to leave against medical advice

   (C) admit the patient to the cardiology service on a physician emergency certificate

   (D) detain the patient until the results of the cardiac enzymes are available

   (E) detain the patient until you can assess her ability to provide informed consent

572. On further evaluation, the patient demonstrates a thorough understanding of the information you have given to her and appreciates the consequences of not being treated immediately. The appropriate next step is to

   (A) sedate the patient and begin thrombolytic therapy

   (B) allow the patient to leave against medical advice

   (C) admit the patient to the cardiology service on a physician emergency certificate

   (D) detain the patient until the results of the cardiac enzymes are available

   (E) detain the patient until you can assess her ability to provide informed consent

573. A 19-year-old man with a history significant for bipolar I disorder is charged with assaulting a police officer. The patient has been able to work with his attorney in preparation for his defense. Which of the following items would be consistent with the assertion that the patient is competent to stand trial?

   (A) comprehension of the court proceedings

   (B) ability to read and write

   (C) presence of a diagnosable mental illness

   (D) testamentary capacity

   (E) capability to provide informed consent

574. A 35-year-old man is admitted to the locked psychiatric unit of the emergency department after threatening to unload his 9-mm pistol into his "blood brother's" chest. Urine toxicology is negative for cocaine, phencyclidine (PCP), or opioids, and his blood alcohol level is 0.04. You learn from the patient's family that he has been threatening to assault his brother for several days and has even written notes about executing his plan. On Mental Status Exam (MSE), the patient's speech is loud, pressured, and very threatening toward the emergency department staff. Family history is significant for bipolar disorder. The patient states that he hasn't done anything wrong and wants to be released immediately. The next appropriate step is to

   (A) notify the police about the patient's homicidal threats

   (B) warn the patient's "blood brother" about the threats

   (C) arrange for a police hold given the patient's potential for violence

   (D) involuntarily admit the patient to a locked psychiatric ward

   (E) medicate the patient with a mood stabilizer and arrange for outpatient follow-up

575. Individuals found not guilty by reason of insanity

   (A) have to serve their original criminal sentence once deemed sane

   (B) are barred from using the defense in the future

   (C) typically serve less time than those found guilty

   (D) generally spend at least the same amount of time or more than those found guilty

   (E) are immediately released without further psychiatric evaluation

576. Criteria for involuntary admission to the hospital include

   (A) medication noncompliance

   (B) inability to care for self

   (C) permission from the conservator of person

   (D) presence of at least one diagnosable mental disorder

   (E) clinical decompensation

Questions 577 and 578

A 9-year-old girl is brought to the pediatric emergency department by her parents for evaluation of persistent cough. She is withdrawn and complains of a "scratchy throat." Vital signs are stable and the patient is afebrile. On exam, the lungs are clear to auscultation bilaterally and the posterior oropharynx is clear. There are multiple bruises on her buttocks and back. A chest x-ray demonstrates several rib fractures in different stages of healing. Her parents report that their daughter is quite active with her younger siblings and often gets into fights with them. The patient agrees with her parents.

577. The most likely diagnosis in this case is

    (A) somatization disorder

    (B) sexual abuse

    (C) major depressive disorder (MDD)

    (D) age-appropriate "rough play"

    (E) physical abuse

578. The next appropriate step is to

    (A) discharge the patient with follow-up in 1 week to reevaluate her bruises

    (B) refer for family therapy to address the issue of "rough play"

    (C) treat the patient with penicillin 2.5 million units IM

    (D) notify child protective services

    (E) confront the siblings about their behavior

Questions 579 and 580

A 17-year-old girl presents to your office complaining of a burning vaginal discharge. She informs you that she has been involved in a consensual sexual relationship with her boyfriend and is worried that she has contracted a sexually transmitted disease (STD). You start the patient on antibiotics. Three days later, you discover that the culture of her vaginal discharge grew *Neisseria gonorrhoea*.

579. A few days later, you receive a call from the patient's parents demanding to know why their daughter was seen in your office. Since the patient is a minor, the appropriate next step would be to

    (A) explain to the parents that their daughter has contracted an STD and requires immediate antibiotic treatment

    (B) maintain confidentiality by disclosing no information, but encourage the patient to discuss this issue with her parents

    (C) ask the parents about their daughter's sexual history

    (D) alert the parents that their daughter is at risk for human immunodeficiency virus (HIV) and should be tested

    (E) find out the boyfriend's name and telephone number to confirm the history

580. At the patient's next follow-up visit, she requests to be tested for HIV. She reports that her boyfriend recently tested negative, but given her promiscuity, she wonders if she has contracted HIV. Before administering the HIV test, you should

    (A) notify her parents about the HIV test

    (B) directly inform the patient's boyfriend that he is at risk for HIV

    (C) obtain a complete blood cell count to determine if the test is necessary

    (D) explain how the test is performed and interpreted, along with information on confidentiality and how you will proceed if the result is positive

    (E) perform a pregnancy test

581. A 44-year-old man with insulin-dependent diabetes mellitus and end-stage renal failure has been on dialysis several years while awaiting a kidney transplant. He feels as though he has "waited long enough" and does not want to continue "living tied to a machine." After several family meetings and consultations with other physicians, he informs you that he no longer wishes to be dialyzed. You obtain a psychiatric consult that concludes no evidence of mood or thought disorder. The family is upset with the patient's decision and demands that you continue to administer dialysis until a transplant is available. The most appropriate next step is to

    (A) respect the patient's wishes and discontinue dialysis

(B) coerce the patient into continuing treatment

(C) continue dialysis until you convince the ethics committee to support the family's decision

(D) tell the patient you're sure a transplant will arrive soon and encourage him to remain in treatment

(E) place the patient on a physician's emergency certificate since he is a danger to himself

582. A 40-year-old surgical attending is admitted to the medical unit after developing severe right flank pain. Further workup confirms a diagnosis of nephrolithiasis. One of the surgical residents asks you about the attending's diagnosis so that coverage can be arranged. The most appropriate next step is to

(A) reveal only the estimated length of stay

(B) inform the chief surgical resident of the attending's condition and length of stay

(C) tell the surgical resident that you won't say anything, but she could take a look in the attending's chart

(D) tell the resident to address the questions directly to the attending

(E) arrange a conference between your medical attending and the surgical house staff

583. A 43-year-old man is referred for continued treatment of depression after release from jail. The court mandated psychiatric treatment while he is on probation. The patient's probation officer calls you for information regarding his condition, progress, and treatment compliance. You should

(A) discuss the case with the probation officer since the treatment is court mandated

(B) limit your discussion with the probation officer to only treatment compliance since the rest of the information is confidential

(C) obtain a confidentiality waiver from the patient before speaking to the probation officer

(D) ignore the request altogether since psychiatric treatment bears no relation to law enforcement

(E) correspond with the probation officer only through written documents

584. A 55-year-old woman is admitted for intravenous (IV) antibiotic treatment for acute hematogenous osteomyelitis. The nurse informs you that the patient was accidentally given the wrong antibiotic but has suffered no adverse reaction. Which of the following best applies in this case?

(A) the "no harm, no disclosure" rule

(B) informing the patient that she was given the wrong medication

(C) first reporting the mistake to the hospital advisory committee

(D) notifying the patient's family of the mistake

(E) encouraging the patient to seek legal action because a critical mistake has occurred

585. A 38-year-old woman is admitted to the oncology unit with severe aplastic anemia. She appears pale and weak. Vital signs indicate a blood pressure of 110/75 and a pulse of 90. Hematocrit is equal to 18. On MSE, cognition is intact and there is no evidence of a mood or psychotic disturbance. The patient states that she is a Jehovah's Witness. She refuses any blood transfusion on the basis of her religious beliefs. Which of the following best applies to your next step in the treatment of this patient?

(A) administering packed red blood cells

(B) persuading the patient that she must accept the transfusion

(C) explaining the implications of nontreatment but respecting the patient's refusal for treatment

(D) utilizing a "confrontation method" to secure lifesaving treatment

(E) referring the patient for involuntary psychiatric treatment based on her life-threatening decision

586. The parents of a newborn with Down syndrome find their daughter to be lethargic and minimally responsive. Medical evaluation is significant for the following cerebrospinal fluid findings: opening pressure of 100 mm Hg, white blood cell count of 5,000 (predominantly neutrophils), protein > 40 mg/dL, glucose content < 40 mg/dL, and Gram stain positive for bacteria. You suspect group B streptococcal meningitis and recommend IV antibiotic therapy. The parents feel as though their Down child will ultimately have a poor quality of life and request that treatment be withheld. You should

(A) respect the parent's wishes since they are the primary decision makers

(B) refer the case to the ethics committee for review at their next scheduled meeting

(C) inform the parents that after reviewing the lab data you realize the patient has viral meningitis and care will be mostly supportive

(D) start ampicillin and cefotaxime against the parents wishes

(E) repeat the lumbar puncture to verify the diagnosis

587. You are called by a local news station to offer a specific psychiatric diagnosis on a prominent politician. There is considerable information in the print and television media that suggests the politician has bipolar I disorder. Which of the following best applies?

(A) Stating your opinion publicly is legitimate as long as the politician is not your private patient.

(B) Offering a psychiatric diagnosis in such instances is unethical.

(C) Comment in written form only.

(D) Agree to an "off-the-record" or anonymous interview.

(E) State your diagnosis, but indicate that other problems may account for the symptoms.

588. An 84-year-old widowed man with severe dementia, for whom you have been the primary care physician for years, is diagnosed with hepatocellular carcinoma. The patient does not have an advance directive and never designated a power of attorney. Psychiatric consultation concludes that the patient is unable to make an informed decision regarding treatment options, and you turn to his family for guidance. The patient's oldest son is adamant that his father receive chemotherapy, while the two younger daughters feel that he should not suffer the adverse effects of chemotherapy "especially because he's so demented." The next appropriate step is to

(A) ask the patient which family member he would like to designate power of attorney

(B) let the patient decide whether or not to proceed with treatment

(C) abide by the son's wishes since he is the oldest

(D) abide by the daughters' wishes since the patient's quality of life is already poor

(E) seek the hospital ethics committee's opinion

Questions 589 and 590

A 25-year-old woman is referred to you for evaluation of insomnia, frequent crying spells, and weight loss. She informs you that her symptoms began several weeks ago after she lost her job and that she now experiences bouts of helplessness and hopelessness. On MSE, she describes her mood as "depressed" and notes that she occasionally has thoughts of taking an overdose of aspirin.

589. The most significant predictor for suicidal behavior would be

(A) prior serious suicide attempt

(B) current alcohol use

(C) current diagnosis of MDD

(D) physical pain

(E) recent loss of a family member

590. Which category of mental disorders is most common in individuals who have completed suicide?

(A) affective disorders

(B) psychotic disorders

(C) alcohol-related disorders

(D) anxiety disorders

(E) toxic metabolic states

591. Which of the following statements is most accurate in regard to sexual relations with medical/surgical patients?

(A) Sexual relations with a former patient is unethical.

(B) Sexual relations with a former patient is permitted as long as the physician does not exploit his or her past position of authority.

(C) Sexual relations with a current or former patient is ethical.

(D) Terminating the physician–patient relationship is not required prior to dating a patient.

(E) Sexual relations between consenting adults is not bound by any professional code of ethics.

592. Which of the following statements is most accurate in regard to sexual relations with psychiatric patients?

(A) Sexual relations with a former patient is unethical.

(B) Sexual relations with a former patient is permissible as long as the physician does not exploit his or her past position of authority.

(C) Sexual relations with a current or former patient is ethical.

(D) Terminating the physician–patient relationship is not required prior to dating a patient.

(E) Sexual relations between consenting adults is not bound by any professional code of ethics.

593. A 52-year-old man for whom you have been the primary care physician for the last 20 years was recently diagnosed with amyotrophic lateral sclerosis. The disease has rapidly progressed, and he has experienced multiple respiratory complications that likely will require a tracheotomy. Severe muscle weakness and atrophy are apparent in all limbs. The patient states that there is no meaning in continuing without his physical capacities. He asks for your help in ending his life in a humane and dignified manner. MSE is at baseline, and there is no evidence of any psychiatric disorder. You discuss the patient's request with his family, and they unanimously support his desire to "end the suffering." The most appropriate course of action would be to

(A) respect the patient's wishes by helping him end his life in a painless and respectful manner

(B) refuse to participate in assisting the patient with suicide and focus on responding to the patient's end-of-life issues

(C) provide the patient with plenty of medication refills to provide a lethal dose

(D) provide the patient with information regarding how to effectively end his life

(E) ignore the patient's request

594. Antisocial personality disorder is estimated to exist in what percentage of the male prison population?

(A) 80 to 100%

(B) 55 to 75%

(C) 30 to 50%

(D) 10 to 20%

(E) less than 10%

Questions 595 and 596

You receive a subpoena from an attorney representing a party that has filed a lawsuit against one of your patients. The subpoena pertains to releasing the medical records of your patient.

595. The appropriate next step is to

   (A) contact the attorney who obtained the subpoena to discuss the process of releasing the medical information
   (B) release the medical records upon receiving the subpoena
   (C) sign a release of information form and turn over the records
   (D) not release the information and contact your patient regarding the subpoena
   (E) release the medical records directly to the presiding judge

596. A court hearing has been organized by your patient's attorney to quash the subpoena you have been issued. At the hearing, the judge rules that you should release the medical records even though your patient has not consented to the release of information. Which of the following statements is most accurate regarding the release of this patient's records?

   (A) Disclosing this patient's medical records is unjustifiable.
   (B) Releasing a patient's medical records is always unethical regardless of court orders.
   (C) It would be appropriate to release this patient's records.
   (D) Disclosing a patient's medical records when there is potential harm to the therapeutic alliance is unethical.
   (E) Work out a plan of legal action with your patient.

597. A 12-year-old boy has a 1-year history of vandalism, violating parental curfews, starting fights, and stealing. Which of the following personality disorders is this patient most likely to develop?

   (A) borderline personality disorder
   (B) narcissistic personality disorder
   (C) oppositional defiant disorder
   (D) antisocial personality disorder
   (E) paranoid personality disorder

598. A 28-year-old woman with dysthymic disorder has been seeing you in weekly psychotherapy and has failed to pay her bill for 2 months. The appropriate next step is to

   (A) contract with a billing collector to demand immediate payment
   (B) terminate the treatment
   (C) contact the patient's family to determine if the patient is financially stable
   (D) inquire as to the reasons she has been avoiding payment at the patient's next visit
   (E) inform the patient that you will not see her if she doesn't pay for her treatment

599. A wealthy 46-year-old male banker is in psychotherapy with you for treatment of a single episode of depression. After significant improvement in his symptoms, he offers you the opportunity to take part in one of his financial ventures. The investment appears to be sound. The most appropriate comment to make to the banker is

   (A) "Thanks for thinking about me . . . I'd be honored to invest with you."
   (B) "Since your depression is improved, it would be appropriate for us to be business partners."
   (C) "I can invest with you only when our treatment is nearing its end."
   (D) "It is probably a bad idea since I'm already committed in other investments."
   (E) "I have to decline since it potentially may interfere with our treatment relationship."

600. A 23-year-old Caucasian Catholic woman with a history of schizophrenia presents to your office after getting into an argument with her husband. She is unemployed and has been staying home taking care of the couple's children. She notes feeling sad and reports thoughts of killing herself. She has a past history of an overdose attempt with aspirin. Which of the following places this patient in a high-risk category for suicide?

(A) age

(B) past history of suicide attempt

(C) gender

(D) marital status

(E) terminal medical illness

Questions 601 through 603

A 36-year-old man with a history of bipolar I disorder is brought to the emergency department by police after stabbing a patron in a barroom brawl. His blood alcohol level was 0.320 upon arrival, and the patient required IM droperidol (Inapsine) for agitation. The patient has no recollection of the event, and the victim died 2 hours later. The patient has a history of assault while psychotic and is currently in weekly psychotherapy. His lawyer has chosen to assert an insanity plea in defense of the patient.

601. Which factor may undermine this patient's assertion of the insanity defense?

(A) voluntary intoxication

(B) mental disease or defect

(C) inability to recall the event

(D) involuntary intoxication

(E) prior conviction of a violent crime

602. You are asked by the patient's lawyer to provide a psychiatric evaluation. The first topic that should be addressed is to

(A) determine whether the patient committed the crime

(B) discuss your fee for testifying

(C) explain that confidentiality covers only those topics unrelated to the event

(D) assess whether the patient understands the charges against him and can work with his attorney

(E) explain the limitations on confidentiality in court-mandated or forensic evaluations

603. A psychiatrist called as an expert witness is primarily responsible for

(A) obtaining a not guilty by reason of insanity verdict

(B) rendering an opinion based on reasonable medical certainty

(C) establishing reasonable doubt

(D) evaluation, diagnosis, and initiation of treatment of the accused

(E) countering evidence of criminal responsibility

Questions 604 and 605

A 48-year-old man is involuntarily admitted to the hospital after an acute manic episode. The patient is pressured, demanding, and increasingly talkative on the unit. He becomes intrusive, not able to be redirected, and demands immediate release. You explain to him that you feel he is gravely disabled and unable to care for himself. He respectfully disagrees with you and demands "due process."

604. The patient's request for a hearing is based on which of the following legal principles?

(A) parens patriae

(B) actus reus

(C) habeas corpus

(D) rights under the 4th Amendment

(E) mens rea

605. The court agrees that the patient is severely disabled and in need of acute medical management. You load the patient with valproic acid (Depakote) 20 mg/kg, and 3 days later his symptoms of mania are markedly diminished. The patient requests immediate discharge and agrees to follow up with a partial hospital program. You feel that he would benefit from further inpatient treatment but is no longer gravely disabled or a threat for self-harm. The next appropriate step would be to

   (A) file for another court hearing to detain the patient further
   (B) ignore the patient's request since he has been committed by the court
   (C) release the patient to the partial hospital program
   (D) persuade the patient to stay for a few more days
   (E) appease the patient by increasing smoking privileges

606. Which of the following is most important in discussing informed consent?

   (A) raising alternative treatment options
   (B) involving family members in this discussion
   (C) petitioning a court to establish the patient's competence
   (D) capacity to read and write
   (E) absence of mental illness

607. Which of the following best characterizes the intent of a living will?

   (A) establishing personal preferences regarding end-of-life issues
   (B) requesting physician-assisted suicide if the patient were to become terminally ill
   (C) arranging for funeral services and distributing the estate to loved ones
   (D) preventing patients from changing their minds about life support as they become ill
   (E) absolving personal responsibility

608. It is unethical for a physician to

   (A) refuse to see nonemergent patients
   (B) own or operate a pharmacy
   (C) use a collection agency to solicit delinquent patient bills
   (D) charge patients for missed appointments
   (E) participate in court-ordered executions

609. A 28-year-old man involved in a motor vehicle accident brings a lawsuit against the driver. Emergency department records do not show any physical injuries, but the patient is claiming to suffer from posttraumatic stress disorder (PTSD). You are asked to evaluate the patient's symptoms. He complains of distressing dreams of the accident, having flashbacks while awake, and avoiding the intersection where the accident occurred. His symptoms have lasted for 3 months. Past psychiatric history is significant for major depression, impulsivity, and violent behavior. He has been incarcerated numerous times, showing a blatant disregard for the law. On MSE, the patient is likable and cooperative. His mood is reported as being depressed, and he currently denies any hallucinations or delusions. Which of the following items from your evaluation of the patient raises your suspicion regarding a diagnosis of malingering?

   (A) history of major depression
   (B) lack of physical injuries
   (C) flashbacks while awake
   (D) antisocial personality disorder
   (E) duration of symptoms

Questions 610 through 612

A 35-year-old woman is referred by her plastic surgeon for a psychiatric evaluation in preparation for sexual reassignment surgery. The patient recalls dressing in her brother's clothes since she was 4 years old and has always preferred opposite-sex playmates. She insists that she is "a man trapped inside of a woman's body." She has fully assumed the male gender role for the last 15 years. On MSE, there is no evidence of psychosis, delusions, or cognitive impairment. She does report a mildly dysphoric mood, which she attributes to her lack of male genitalia. Complete blood count, serum electrolytes, folate, vitamin B_{12} level, and liver function tests are within normal limits; rapid plasma reagin/Venereal Disease Research Laboratory (RPR/VDRL) are nonreactive. Karyotype analysis demonstrates XX genotype.

610. The most appropriate diagnosis in this case is

(A) homosexuality

(B) transvestite fetishism

(C) frotteurism

(D) schizophrenia

(E) gender identity disorder

611. Which of the following best characterizes your response to the plastic surgeon's request for psychiatric consultation?

(A) "There is currently no evidence of a psychotic process or other major psychiatric illnesses that would interfere with this patient's ability to provide informed consent."

(B) "It is unethical to perform a psychiatric exam that would endorse sexual reassignment surgery."

(C) "The competency of this individual is compromised by delusions of being the opposite sex."

(D) "Sexual reassignment surgery is a personal decision that does not require a psychiatric examination."

(E) "I cannot authorize surgery in this case."

612. The plastic surgeon and patient decide to proceed with the surgery. Which of the following is most important in obtaining informed consent?

(A) contingency analysis

(B) discussing potential complications of the procedure

(C) establishing the lack of any mental illness

(D) seeking approval from family members

(E) exploring the patient's dreams and desires

613. One of your patients consistently misses appointments without giving you advance notice. After numerous failed attempts at resolving this issue with the patient, you realize that the patient's behavior is not changing and you decide to discharge the patient from your care. Which of the following most appropriately describes the discharge process?

(A) Write a letter to the patient notifying her that she has been discharged due to her failure to comply with treatment.

(B) Notify your staff that the patient is not to be given further appointments.

(C) Contact the patient's family/friends to request their help in improving the patient's attendance.

(D) Write a letter to the patient stating that she will be discharged in 60 days.

(E) Notify the patient's insurance company that she is discharged from your care.

614. You are asked by the court to provide a forensic evaluation for a child custody case. The most important factor in determining which parent should get custody is that he or she

(A) is the biologic parent

(B) can provide for the best interests of the child

(C) is most financially stable

(D) has the highest level of education

(E) is in the best mental/physical health

615. You discover that one of the physicians in your hospital is abusing narcotics. The appropriate course of action is to

(A) notify the local police

(B) contact the Drug Enforcement Administration to rescind his license

(C) do nothing so as to avoid personal liability

(D) admonish him for using but do not report

(E) notify the hospital's committee for impaired physicians

DIRECTIONS (Questions 616 through 621): Each set of items in this section consists of a list of lettered headings followed by several numbered words or phrases. For each numbered word or phrase, select the ONE lettered option that is most closely associated with it. Each lettered option may be selected once, more than once, or not at all.

Questions 616 through 621

For each definition, select the most accurate corresponding term.

(A) American Law Institute test
(B) conservatorship of person
(C) diminished mental capacity
(D) *Durham v. United States*
(E) *Dusky v. United States*
(F) extreme emotional disturbance
(G) irresistible impulse standard
(H) mens rea
(I) M'Naghten rule
(J) parens patriae
(K) *Tarasoff v. Regents of University of California*
(L) testamentary capacity
(M) testimonial privilege
(N) wild beast test

616. Modern standard for the insanity defense

617. Right to preserve confidentiality when subpoenaed without patient consent

618. Legal precedent establishing the "duty to protect" third parties

619. Legal concept excusing criminal responsibility based on one's inability to control behavior

620. Insanity defense based on the inability to distinguish between right and wrong ("right–wrong test")

621. Legal precedent establishing the "product test"

Answers and Explanations

562. **(D)** A physician or therapist has a duty to protect identifiable victims from imminent danger. This obligation may be fulfilled by directly contacting the party at risk, notifying the police, or taking other appropriate measures to protect the victim. Contacting the patient's family fails to protect the intended victim. Although notification of the police is an acceptable intervention in this case, disclosing unrelated confidential information about the patient is inappropriate. When notifying third parties, care should be taken to release only information necessary to protecting the potential victim. The remaining choices fail to protect the potential victim.

563. **(B)** *Tarasoff v. Regents of University of California* is the landmark legal precedent establishing liability to third parties. It states "when a psychotherapist determines . . . that his patient presents a serious danger of violence to another he incurs an obligation to use reasonable care to protect the intended victim against such danger." Therefore, the physician may ethically break confidentiality in cases involving imminent harm to others. In the *Tarasoff* case, a student at the University of California (Prosenjit Poddar) expressed intentions to kill a fellow student (Tatiana Tarasoff) to his therapist. Poddar tragically followed through on his threat and murdered the young woman at her home. *Tarasoff v. Regents of University of California* holds legal precedent only in the state of California; however, the case has been adopted by physicians/therapists as the standard of care and has led to nationwide legislative changes. There have been two rulings regarding the *Tarasoff* case. The

original decision, *Tarasoff I* (1974), established a "duty to warn." The California Supreme Court revised its previous holding in Tarasoff II (1976) with a "duty to protect." In *Rogers v. Commissioner of the Department of Mental Health,* the court expounded opinions regarding the treatment of involuntarily committed patients. *Durham v. United States* held that an individual "is not criminally responsible if the unlawful act was the product of mental disease or mental defect." The holding of this case has become known as the "product test" for determining an insanity defense and ultimately was replaced by the American Law Institute standard. *Zinerman v. Burch* and *Kansas v. Hendricks* involve court decisions regarding civil commitment.

564. **(C)** The 4 D's of establishing medical malpractice cases involve proving that a dereliction of duty directly causes damage. The plaintiff must establish the presence of a fiduciary relationship (a duty), negligence (dereliction of duty), and damages directly caused by that negligence. Typically, the burden of proof in medical malpractice cases (i.e., civil cases) is by a preponderance of the evidence (greater than 50%). Proof beyond a reasonable doubt refers to criminal cases, while clear and convincing evidence is reserved for special cases decided by the court. Neither criminal intent nor criminal mischief is required to prove medical malpractice.

565. **(D)** Testamentary capacity refers to the level of competence required to make a legally valid will. Case law and statutes differ across states. However, the central elements of testamentary capacity include: (1) comprehension of the act of writing/signing a will, (2) knowledge of potential heirs, (3) understanding the extent of one's assets, (4) lack of undue influence, and (5) the absence of delusions compromising rational thought. Mens rea refers to criminal intent and has nothing to do with drafting a will. Informed consent is the process of obtaining permission for medical treatment. Important elements include the ability to make a voluntary decision regarding treatment, explanation of risks/benefits, and competency to make an informed decision. The presence or absence of a mental illness does not necessarily impair an individual's competency to make a will. Therefore, the lack of mental illness is incorrect. Conservatorship of estate refers to an individual's ability to manage his or her finances.

566. **(A)** Paranoid delusions regarding the patient's family may significantly undermine this patient's assertion that she was competent to make a will. The absence of delusions, which may compromise rational decision making, is one of several criteria required for testamentary capacity. The presence of a diagnosable Axis I disorder, the inability to read and write, and refusal to undergo treatment with chemotherapy do not automatically undermine a patient's competence to make a will as long as the criteria for testamentary capacity are met. An explanation of why the patient wants to donate her estate to the local humane society does not undermine the patient's competence to make a will unless such an explanation demonstrates that the patient is unable to meet any of the specified criteria.

567. **(E)** An expert medical witness may be called to testify in both civil and criminal trials. Expert witnesses have a familiarity with a body of knowledge that exceeds that held by laypersons and are often called to provide opinion testimony, making choices A and C incorrect. Choices B and D are incorrect because expert witnesses commonly charge a fee for their services and provide testimony for either defense or plaintiff.

568. **(B)** The American Law Institute test is the modern standard for the insanity defense. It holds that a person with a mental disease/defect should not be held criminally responsible for an act if the person (1) could not appreciate the wrongfulness of the conduct and (2) could not conform the conduct to the requirements of the law. The American Law Institute test expanded upon the 1843 M'Naghten rule, which held that an individual was not guilty by reason of insanity if, as a result of a mental defect, the person did not know the nature of what he or she was doing or did not know that what he or she was doing was wrong ("right–wrong test"). The Durham rule arose from a 1954 District of Columbia case in which the court held that "an accused is not criminally responsible if his unlawful act was the product of a mental disease or mental defect." This is also known as the "product test." Extreme emotional disturbance and the irresistible impulse rule are not modern standards for proving an insanity defense. Extreme emotional disturbance is an affirmative defense used to render the accused less culpable for the crime (i.e., reduce the charge from murder to manslaughter). The irresistible impulse rule, established in England in 1922, states that an individual is not responsible for a criminal act if he was unable to resist that act due to a mental illness.

569. **(A)** Throughout the United States, the burden of proof in an insanity defense rests on the defendant. Habeas corpus and the prosecution are incorrect. The standard of proof in criminal cases is beyond a reasonable doubt.

570. **(C)** Criminal responsibility requires (1) criminal intent (mens rea) and (2) a criminal act (actus reus). Diminished mental capacity serves to avoid criminal responsibility; certainly, it is not required to prove criminal responsibility. The product test and the wild beast test are antiquated standards of the insanity defense.

571. **(E)** Before discharging or transferring the patient, it is important to determine whether she can make an informed decision regarding her care. Informed consent requires that the patient (1) comprehend the issues and/or choices furnished by the physician, (2) appreciate the consequences of making a certain decision, and (3) arrive at a voluntary decision after weighing the facts. At this point in the vignette, there is not enough information to establish the patient's ability to make an informed decision regarding her care. Exceptions to informed consent include incompetence, emergency situations (i.e., comatose, unresponsive patient), a competent patient's waiver of informed consent, and therapeutic privilege. The other choices are incorrect because this patient's ability to make an informed decision has not been assessed.

572. **(B)** A competent patient has the right to refuse treatment, even if the consequences are life threatening. In the extension of this vignette, the patient has adequately demonstrated the elements of an informed decision. The other choices are incorrect because they would prevent a competent patient from making an informed decision in her treatment.

573. **(A)** In *Dusky v. United States*, the Supreme Court ruled that competency to stand trial requires the ability to (1) rationally consult with one's attorney and (2) understand the proceedings in both factual and rational terms. Illiteracy does not constitute grounds for incompetency. A person can suffer from a mental illness and be competent to stand trial. Testamentary capacity refers to the level of competence required to make a valid will. Informed consent is important in making decisions related to medical treatments but has little bearing on one's competency to stand trial.

574. **(D)** Involuntary commitment is used when a physician believes that an individual is a threat to self or others or is gravely disabled. Medicating the patient and arranging for outpatient treatment when the patient is actively

homicidal is an improper course of action. Notification of the police or warning the patient's "blood brother" is not immediately necessary as this patient is well contained on a locked unit. Arranging a police hold is incorrect. Police holds are issued when an individual who is arrested requires a psychiatric evaluation. If the arrested individual does not require inpatient psychiatric care, he is released back into the custody of the police.

575. **(D)** Contrary to popular opinion, the insanity defense (1) is seldom asserted, (2) is usually unsuccessful, and (3) typically leads to a greater number of years of incarceration. Individuals found not guilty have no obligation to serve a criminal sentence. There is no limit to the number of times one may assert the insanity defense. Releasing an individual found not guilty by reason of insanity without an appropriate psychiatric evaluation/treatment would be unethical and fails to protect society.

576. **(B)** Involuntary admission to the hospital is justified when the patient is judged to be (1) a danger to self or others or (2) gravely disabled. The criteria for involuntary commitment derive from the doctrines of "police power" (state as protector of public safety) and "parens patriae" (the "state as parent" for those unable to care for themselves), respectively. State laws differ on the length of time a person can be committed to the hospital on the basis of either criteria. Permission from the conservator of person is not required for involuntary commitment. The other choices may be important factors, but are not requisite elements for involuntary hospitalization.

577. **(E)** Typical signs of physical abuse include burns with peculiar patterns (i.e., cigarette marks, geometric designs, bilateral immersion patterns), bruises in low-trauma areas (i.e., buttocks, genital areas, or back), retinal hemorrhages, and multiple fractures at different stages of healing. Although there is a high rate of comorbidity between physical and sexual abuse, there is no evidence to suggest sexual abuse in this particular case. Sexual or physical abuse may predispose an individual to the development of other psychiatric disorders such as depression, PTSD, and borderline personality disorder. Although the differential in this case should include depression and somatization disorder, history and mental status do not provide sufficient evidence to diagnose either. Age-appropriate "rough play" is not relevant.

578. **(D)** Each state requires mandatory reporting of abuse or neglect to child protective services. In cases in which there is a reasonable suspicion of abuse, a report should be filed even if the patient and family deny the allegations. In cases of suspected abuse, steps to ensure the safety of the minor should be taken immediately. Discharging the patient with follow-up in 1 week to reevaluate her bruises would disregard her safety and potentially subject the minor to continued abuse. Considering the extent of physical injuries, it is unlikely that they were inflicted by the patient's younger siblings. Consequently, confronting the siblings about their behavior would serve no purpose.

579. **(B)** Confidentiality in the treatment of minors should be maintained unless specifically prohibited by state law (i.e., in cases of abortion) or when the parent's involvement is necessary to make complicated or life-threatening treatment decisions. The other choices all constitute violations of confidentiality to your patient.

580. **(D)** Informed consent for HIV testing involves a thorough explanation of the test's interpretation, information regarding confidentiality, and further evaluation needed if the test is positive. The patient should be aware of the risk of false positives and negatives, and the need for confirmatory testing if the test result is positive. Choices A and B are incorrect because they violate patient confidentiality. When a patient tests positive for HIV, state laws may require notification of the sexual partner (this is usually done without revealing the patient's identity). There is no

reason to first perform a complete blood count or a pregnancy test before administering an HIV test.

581. **(A)** The patient's desire to stop dialysis should be respected since competent adults are able to determine which treatment to accept or deny. The American Medical Association (AMA) Code of Ethics notes that there is no ethical distinction between withdrawing and withholding medical treatment. The remaining choices undermine the patient's right to make an informed decision.

582. **(D)** Physician–patient confidentiality should be maintained except in certain cases (i.e., duty to protect others, mandatory reporting, or emergencies). The remaining choices violate physician–patient confidentiality.

583. **(C)** Confidentiality between patient and physician should be respected even in cases of court-mandated treatment. In such cases, issues around disclosure to a probation officer can be used to explore the patient's attitudes toward probation and incarceration. Obtaining a confidentiality waiver from the patient should be done in a thoughtful manner and is essential before releasing any information to the probation officer. Ignoring the probation officer's request would be inappropriate in such circumstances. The other choices are incorrect because they violate physician–patient confidentiality.

584. **(B)** The patient should immediately be informed that she was accidentally given the improper medication. The physician should also evaluate for potential adverse reactions. The fact that the patient did not suffer harm is no reason to conceal the medication error. Although many hospitals require documentation of such errors, or reporting of them to the appropriate person/committee, this should not be the first course of action. Evaluating the patient for any adverse reaction and explaining the mistake is the appropriate first step. Notifying the patient's family of the mistake is a breach of confidentiality and inappropriate. Encouraging the patient to seek le-

gal action is both alarmist and inappropriate in such a case.

585. **(C)** Explaining the implications of nontreatment but respecting the patient's refusal for treatment is the most appropriate course of action. This allows the patient to make an informed decision with regard to her treatment. The elements integral to informed consent include (1) competency to make a decision; (2) an adequate explanation of the risks, benefits, rationale for treatment, and alternative treatments (including no treatment at all); and (3) a voluntary decision. In this vignette, there is no evidence that the patient suffers from a condition that might impair her competency. Further, her stated religious belief is consistent with a Jehovah's Witness's refusal of human blood products. Administering packed red blood cells infringes on the patient's right to refuse a blood transfusion and consequently is incorrect. Strongly persuading the patient to arrive at a decision for treatment or utilizing a confrontation method to secure lifesaving treatment is coercive in nature and could prevent the patient from making a voluntary decision. It would be inappropriate to involuntarily hospitalize this patient if she has arrived at her decision in compliance with the elements of informed consent.

586. **(D)** According to the AMA Code of Medical Ethics, treatment decisions must be made in the best interest of the child or neonate regardless of the desires of the parents. Treatment can be withheld or withdrawn only in cases in which the risks far outweigh the benefits, there is low potential for success, or when treatment will only extend the child's suffering without potential for a joyful existence. The lumbar puncture results unequivocally demonstrate bacterial meningitis. In this particular case, the neonate suffers from a serious, but treatable, central nervous system infection, and treatment should not be withheld. Withholding treatment until the next regularly scheduled ethics meeting would likely result in the neonate's demise.

587. **(B)** It is unethical to offer specific psychiatric diagnoses for individuals that you have not personally examined. Moreover, commenting on an individual that you have evaluated would be a breach of confidentiality.

588. **(E)** Family and/or close associates should be consulted to aid in reaching treatment decisions if there is no advance directive or designated power of attorney. Consultation with the ethics committee should be sought when the patient's prior wishes are unclear or family members are unable to agree on treatment options. Ethics committee consultations are also useful when the power of attorney's decision is unreasonable or contrary to the patent's prior wishes. It would be inappropriate to allow a severely demented patient to designate a power of attorney or make treatment decisions. Choosing sides in a family conflict would be arbitrary; consultation with the hospital ethics committee would help clarify issues in a complicated case such as this.

589. **(A)** The most significant predictor of suicidal behavior is a prior serious suicide attempt. The other choices are all associated risk factors for suicidal behavior but are not the most significant predictor of it.

590. **(A)** Affective disorders (i.e., MDD, bipolar I/II disorder) account for 40 to 70% of completed suicides. Alcohol-related disorders account for 20 to 30% of completed suicides. Psychotic and anxiety disorders are less frequently associated with completed suicides, as are toxic metabolic states. However patients with schizophrenia are at high risk for suicide.

591. **(B)** The AMA Code of Medical Ethics cautions that sexual and/or romantic relations with former patients may be influenced by the previous physician–patient relationship; care should be taken to not exploit the power derived from the professional relationship. Sexual relations with current patients is unethical and constitutes sexual misconduct. At the very least, current physician–patient relationships should be terminated prior to initiating any romantic or sexual relationships.

592. **(A)** Sexual or romantic relationships between current and former psychiatric patients are considered unethical, making the other choices incorrect.

593. **(B)** According to the AMA Code of Medical Ethics, "physician-assisted suicide is fundamentally incompatible with the physician's role as healer," and the physician should aggressively respond to a patient's end-of-life needs rather than assist in suicide. The term *physician-assisted suicide* is defined as the act of facilitating a patient's death by "providing the necessary means and/or information to enable the patient to perform the life-ending act." Simply ignoring the patient's request would be inappropriate because it fails to recognize and address potential end-of-life issues. End-of-life issues that should be addressed with the patient include adequate pain control, emotional/family support, comfort care, respect of patient autonomy, and appropriate multidisciplinary referrals (hospice, counseling, religious issues). The remaining choices are consistent with the definition of physician-assisted suicide and are therefore unethical.

594. **(C)** The rate of antisocial personality disorder in the male prison population has been estimated at 30 to 50%.

595. **(D)** When a physician is served a subpoena to release medical information, the appropriate first step is to contact the patient to find out if he or she consents to the release. Discussing the implications of the lawsuit with your patient and clarifying whether the patient has the proper legal counsel for the lawsuit also are important. Contacting the attorney of the party requesting the subpoena and releasing the medical records without consent from the patient constitute unethical breaches of physician–patient confidentiality. The confidentiality privilege belongs to the patient, not the physician. Releasing the medical information directly to the judge at this stage makes no sense and would likewise be a breach of confidentiality.

596. **(C)** Turning over medical records to comply with a direct court order is ethical. Working out a plan of legal action is not the role of the physician, but rather the patient's attorney. The other choices are incorrect because there are cases in which disclosing the patient's medical records without consent is ethically permissible (e.g., in certain criminal proceedings, malpractice cases initiated by the patient, contestation of a will).

597. **(D)** Antisocial personality disorder is an Axis II psychiatric disorder (i.e., personality disorder) characterized by a pervasive disregard for the rights of others, which often develops out of the symptoms described in this patient. Behaviors associated with antisocial personality disorder include repeated unlawful acts, lying, stealing, contempt for the safety of others, and lack of remorse for having hurt or mistreated others. A diagnosis of antisocial personality disorder requires evidence of conduct disorder with onset before 18 years of age. Conduct disorder describes the clinical picture of the patient presented in the vignette; further, it is not classified as a personality disorder. Oppositional defiant disorder is an Axis I disorder characterized by a pattern of hostile, defiant, or negative behaviors, generally of less severity than that of conduct disorder. Narcissistic and paranoid personality disorders might develop in this patient but are not as likely to occur as antisocial personality disorder.

598. **(D)** Inquiring about possible reasons the patient may be avoiding payment may help uncover important treatment issues. Such inquiry often leads to how the patient feels about the therapy and/or the therapist. These feelings can be utilized to address factors related to her symptoms. Exploring such issues should be done in a sensitive manner to avoid alienating the patient. Requesting that the billing collector demand immediate payment and terminating treatment would be far too aggressive at this point. Contacting

the patient's family violates physician–patient confidentiality. At this point, informing the patient that you will not see her if she doesn't immediately pay her bill may be perceived as confrontational and threatens the therapeutic alliance.

599. **(E)** Becoming involved in the business venture of a psychotherapy patient could have significant adverse effects on the patient's transference (feelings and memories experienced by the patient that are aroused by the therapist) as well as on the physician's countertransference (feelings aroused in the physician while working with the patient); therefore, it should be avoided. Anger, distrust, and guilt are some of the feelings that may occur if a business venture such as the one described were to fail. Further, a physician's business involvement with a patient might affect the neutral stance essential to effective psychotherapy. A central problem is that involvement in a business venture might interfere with treatment. This is best explained to the patient honestly.

600. **(B)** Suicide risk factors include:
- Increasing age (> 40)
- Gender (M > F)
- Marital status (separated or divorced > married)
- Past history of suicide attempt or threat
- Race (Native Americans/Alaskan natives > whites > blacks/Hispanics)
- Religion (Catholics are lowest risk)
- Employment status (unemployed or retired > employed)
- Support system (living alone > living with others)
- Health status (serious medical condition or terminal illness > good health)

601. **(A)** An individual who commits a crime while voluntarily intoxicated cannot assert an insanity defense because the basis of such behavior stems from a rational decision to drink. Involuntary intoxication may be used effectively as an insanity defense if the individual had no choice in becoming intoxicated (i.e., the person was drugged). A mental dis-

ease or defect or inability to recall the event might be used to enhance an insanity defense, not undermine it. Prior conviction of a crime in itself should have no bearing on an insanity defense. However, if prior violent behavior has been associated with mental illness and the inability to appreciate the criminality of one's conduct or conform to the law, this might be used to strengthen an insanity defense.

602. **(E)** In contrast to the traditional physician–patient relationship in which confidentiality is maintained except in special cases (e.g., emergencies, mandatory reporting statutes, duty to protect), information acquired during forensic or court-mandated evaluations can be expected to be brought before the court through testimony or a written report. This should be explained to the patient at the very outset of the evaluation so that the individual is fully aware that what he says may not be confidential. All material covered in the evaluation can potentially be used in court. Typically, the objective of a forensic psychiatric evaluation is not to determine whether an individual committed a crime. Discussing one's fee is important, but not before the issue of confidentiality has been thoroughly explained to the patient. Evaluating whether the patient understands the charges against him and can work with his attorney is a vital component of a forensic psychiatric evaluation but is not the first topic that should be addressed.

603. **(B)** Medical expert witnesses are called to present their professional opinions based on reasonable medical certainty. Expert witnesses are expected to perform an impartial evaluation and testify as to their findings; it is not the responsibility of the expert to ensure a particular outcome for either side. Unlike the traditional physician–patient relationship, the expert witness does not typically initiate treatment of patients and has limits on confidentiality.

604. **(C)** Habeas corpus refers to the U.S. Constitution's 4th Amendment's clause that the state shall not "deprive any person of life, liberty, or property, without due process of law." Under habeas corpus, citizens have the right to petition the court when detained in order to decide whether they are being held lawfully. Parens patriae refers to the state's function as "parent" for those unable to care for themselves. This is often used for justification of involuntary commitment. Establishing criminal responsibility requires the presence of both actus reus and mens rea. Actus reus refers to the voluntary act of committing a crime, and mens rea refers to criminal intent. They are both incorrect because they have nothing to do with the patient's right to due process. The 4th Amendment is incorrect; it protects citizens from unreasonable searches and seizures.

605. **(C)** It would be unethical to involuntarily detain a patient in treatment if he or she is no longer deemed to be gravely disabled or a threat to self/others. In this case, the patient should be promptly discharged to the partial hospital program. Ignoring the patient's request since the court has committed him is incorrect. Filing for another court hearing would be appropriate only if the patient were still gravely disabled or a danger to self/others. Persuading the patient to stay a few more days even though he wishes to leave the hospital and no longer meets criteria for involuntary commitment is inappropriate. Appeasing the patient by increasing smoking privileges fails to address the key issue in this question.

606. **(A)** The key elements to informed consent include competency to make a decision; a voluntary choice; and an adequate explanation of the rationale, risks, benefits, and alternative treatment options. The remaining choices are not necessary for informed consent.

607. **(A)** Living wills, or advance directives, preserve patient autonomy by establishing personal preferences regarding end-of-life issues. If patients lose capacity in the future, advance directives outline what procedures they do or do not desire without relying on physician or family member opinions. The

remaining choices are not characteristics of a living will.

608. **(E)** According to the AMA Code of Ethics, it is unethical for a physician to participate in a legally authorized execution. Participation in an execution is defined by the AMA as any action that would directly cause, assist, or supervise the death of the condemned. Physicians have a right to choose whom they treat with the major exception being patients who are in need of emergent care or who are unable to get care elsewhere. Physicians may own/operate their own pharmacy but should not refer patients to the pharmacy. Additionally, physicians should disclose their financial interests in health care facilities/operations that are likely to be utilized by their patients. When a patient does not pay his or her bill after repeated notices, it is ethical for the physician to contract with a collection agency to collect overdue payments. Care should be taken to release only that information necessary to collecting the bill without divulging sensitive information (i.e., diagnosis, type of treatment, length). Charging for missed appointments is ethical as long as the patient is made aware of the physician's policy ahead of time.

609. **(D)** Malingering is characterized by intentional feigning of symptoms for secondary gain (i.e., financial remuneration, disability benefits, avoiding criminal prosecution or military duty). A diagnosis of malingering should be suspected when there is the presence of one or more of the following factors: (1) litigation (especially when the patient is referred by a lawyer), (2) discrepancy between objective findings and patient's complaints, (3) a diagnosis of antisocial personality disorder, and (4) a failure to comply with the evaluation and recommended treatments. A past history of major depression does not raise one's suspicion of malingering. The lack of physical injuries or the presence of flashbacks in a claim of PTSD is not sufficient to raise suspicions of malingering. PTSD occurs in individuals exposed to actual or threatened death/injury and consequently may

have no physical injuries. Classic symptoms of PTSD include flashbacks, distressing dreams, intrusive memories, avoidance of trauma-related stimuli, and increased autonomic activity. The duration of symptoms in this case has no bearing on a diagnosis of malingering.

610. **(E)** Gender identity disorder is characterized by a persistent desire/claim to be the opposite sex, a desire to participate in games/play of the opposite sex, preference for opposite-sex playmates, wearing cross-gender clothing, and the desire to change one's physical characteristics to conform with his or her gender identification. Generally, homosexuals lack the desire to assume the opposite gender role. Rather, they are attracted to members of the same sex. Transvestite fetishism is characterized by cross-dressing behaviors for sexual excitement without an underlying desire to assume the opposite gender identity. Frotteurism is the act of rubbing or touching nonconsenting individuals for sexual excitement. Psychotic disorders such as schizophrenia are associated with disorganized speech/behavior, hallucinations, delusions, or impaired reality testing. In this case, the patient's desire to become a male is not delusional in nature. She acknowledges that she is genetically a female but identifies herself as the opposite gender without evidence of psychosis.

611. **(A)** The reason for psychiatric consultation in surgical cases is generally to determine whether or not the presence of a psychiatric illness would interfere with a patient's ability to provide informed consent. In this case, the clinical scenario is consistent with a diagnosis of gender identity disorder, and there is no evidence of a major psychiatric illness impairing the patient's ability to make an informed decision. There is nothing unethical about performing a psychiatric exam in cases involving sexual reassignment surgery. In fact, most surgeons will not proceed with sexual reassignment until a thorough psychiatric evaluation is performed. There is no evidence of delusions in this case. The psychia-

trist's role in this case is to provide the surgeon with an assessment of the patient's current mental status as it relates to her decision-making abilities. In general, consultants do not authorize or decline procedures performed by another physician.

612. **(B)** Elements essential to informed consent include (1) voluntary decision making, (2) explanation of risks and benefits of treatment, (3) discussion of alternative treatment options (including consequences of withholding treatment), (4) ability to understand/appreciate the information presented, and (5) absence of any condition that would impair an individual's competency to make a decision. Contingency analysis is not relevant to informed consent. The presence of a mental illness does not necessarily preclude one from making an informed decision. The severity of impairment caused by a mental illness is vital in determining whether the patient is capable of providing informed consent. Although the patient may desire to discuss the issue with members of her family, the physician is not obliged to take into consideration their opinions in seeking an informed decision. Exploring a patient's dreams and desires, while perhaps useful in understanding possible reasons behind any decision, is not an essential element in determining informed consent.

613. **(D)** According to the AMA Code of Medical Ethics, physicians are obligated to provide continuity of care for their patients. When discharging a patient from your care, advance notice of the pending discharge must be given with sufficient time to obtain another physician. Contacting the patient's family breaches confidentiality and is not the appropriate procedure for discharging the patient. Notifying the insurance company fails to inform the patient of her discharge and does not provide her time to obtain a new physician. The remaining choices fail to provide the patient with sufficient notice to obtain proper medical follow-up.

614. **(B)** The prevailing concept in determining child custody is based on which individual(s)

can provide for the best interests of the child. Factors that can be used to determine the best interests of the child include assessing the individual's biologic relation, financial stability, level of education, and health; however, it is the aggregate best interest, rather than any single factor, that determines what is in the best interest of the child.

615.   (E) Physicians are ethically obliged to report impaired colleagues. Reporting procedures vary from state to state. However, the AMA Code of Medical Ethics suggests initial reporting to a hospital's in-house impaired physician program. If no such program exists, the chief of staff or clinical service director should be notified. For physicians without hospital privileges, an impaired physicians program run by a medical society or the state board licensing committee should be made aware of the impaired physician. The other choices do not meet the AMA guidelines and fail to initiate proper treatment and supervision of the impaired physician.

616.   (A) The American Law Institute test (also known as the Model Penal Code) is currently used to determine criminal responsibility. The test states "a person is not responsible for his criminal conduct if at the time of such conduct as a result of mental disease or defect, he lacks substantial capacity to appreciate the criminality of his conduct or to conform his conduct to the requirements of the law." The American Law Institute test combines the earlier M'Naghten rule and the irresistible impulse standard.

617.   (M) Testimonial privilege is the right to maintain confidentiality when a physician is served a subpoena for medical information. The confidentiality privilege belongs to the patient and can be waived with his or her consent.

618.   (K) The landmark legal precedent, *Tarasoff v. Regents of University of California*, establishes the therapist's "obligation to use reasonable care to protect the intended victim against . . . danger."

619.   (G) The irresistible impulse standard expanded on the earlier M'Naghten rule to include an individual's mental state in determining criminal responsibility ("if some controlling disease was, in truth, the acting power within him which he could not resist, then he will not be responsible . . .").

620.   (I) The M'Naghten rule, also known as the right–wrong test, is a standard for determining criminal responsibility based on an individual's ability to distinguish between right and wrong ("at the time of committing the act, the party accused was laboring under such a defect of reason, from disease of the mind, as not to know the nature and quality of the act he was doing; or if he did know it, that he did not know he was doing what was wrong"). The M'Naghten rule focused on the cognitive act of differentiating right from wrong and has been criticized as being too narrow an insanity standard; consequently, alternative insanity standards have emerged over the years, including the irresistible impulse standard, the product test, and, more recently, the American Law Institute test.

621.   (D) The product test is an insanity standard based on whether or not the criminal act "was the product of mental disease or defect." *Durham v. United States* (1954) is the legal precedent endorsing the product test.

CHAPTER 8

Differential Diagnosis and Management

William Roman, MD, and Elizabeth Walter, MD

Questions

DIRECTIONS (Questions 622 through 714): Each of the numbered items or incomplete statements in this section is followed by answers or by completions of the statement. Select the ONE lettered answer or completion that is BEST in each case.

Questions 622 through 624

A 37-year-old male presents to your office complaining of auditory hallucinations that have worsened over the last several months. He notes that the devil has been telling him that he is "no good," and that he won't "amount to anything." During the last several months, the patient also reports feeling "depressed" and has been sleeping poorly. He has no desire to get out of bed and has lost interest in even watching sports (normally one of his favorite activities). The patient states that even when his mood is improved, he still can't "get the voices out of my head." He denies using any drugs or alcohol.

622. Which diagnosis best accounts for this patient's symptoms?

    (A) major depression

    (B) schizophrenia

    (C) schizoaffective disorder

    (D) bipolar II disorder

    (E) schizoid personality disorder

623. What medication combination could be used to adequately treat this patient's symptoms?

    (A) mirtazapine (Remeron) and citalopram (Celexa)

    (B) fluoxetine (Prozac) and diazepam (Valium)

    (C) ziprasidone (Geodon) and sertraline (Zoloft)

    (D) haloperidol (Haldol) and perphenazine (Trilafon)

    (E) valproic acid (Depakote) and lorazepam (Ativan)

624. You decide to prescribe haloperidol for this patient's psychotic symptoms. On his next visit to your office, he reports that his hallucinations have improved but that he "can't sit still" and feels like he needs to be constantly in motion. The patient intermittently stands up and walks around your office as you interview him. This patient most likely has

    (A) acute dystonic reaction

    (B) akathisia

    (C) neuroleptic malignant syndrome (NMS)

    (D) mania

    (E) none of the above

Questions 625 through 627

A 20-year-old single female presents to your office complaining of "episodes of complete terror." She states that "totally out of nowhere" she became extremely anxious, experienced heart palpitations, felt short of breath, began sweating profusely, and believed that she was going to die. She reports that these episodes last approximately 10 minutes and that they have occurred several times over the last 3 months. She constantly worries that they will occur again.

625. What general medical condition should be considered in the differential diagnosis for this patient's cluster of symptoms?

(A) hypothyroidism
(B) systemic lupus erythematosus
(C) pheochromocytoma
(D) folate deficiency
(E) hypertension

626. The most likely diagnosis for this patient's symptoms is

(A) generalized anxiety disorder (GAD)
(B) social phobia
(C) panic disorder
(D) obsessive–compulsive disorder (OCD)
(E) agoraphobia

627. The patient is in college and reports that she has an important oral presentation in 2 weeks. She requests a treatment that will not take several weeks to begin to work. Which of the following medications is likely to have the most immediate effect in alleviating her symptoms?

(A) imipramine (Tofranil)
(B) paroxetine (Paxil)
(C) haloperidol (Haldol)
(D) buproprion (Wellbutrin)
(E) alprazolam (Xanax)

Questions 628 through 630

A 64-year-old woman is brought to the emergency department by her neighbor, who says "my friend isn't acting right." The patient requires the support of a nurse while walking to an examination table. Examination reveals that she cannot correctly identify the season or the town she's in. She does not recognize her neighbor. She is inattentive and seemingly apathetic to the activity around her. She dozes off repeatedly during the interview, but each time is arousable and resumes answering questions. Her answers are illogical and inconsistent.

Vital signs are within normal limits, and she is neither tremulous nor diaphoretic. Neurologic exam finds bilateral 6th nerve palsy and horizontal nystagmus. Urine toxicology screen and blood alcohol level are negative.

628. What is the most likely diagnosis?

(A) subdural hematoma
(B) alcohol withdrawal
(C) Wernicke's encephalopathy
(D) folic acid deficiency
(E) normal pressure hydrocephalus

629. What is the most important first step in managing this patient?

(A) administration of a benzodiazepine
(B) computed tomographic (CT) scan of the head
(C) administration of folic acid
(D) administration of thiamine
(E) intravenous (IV) fluids and observation

630. After appropriate treatment and admission to the hospital, the patient's 6th nerve palsy almost completely resolves. However, the nystagmus persists, and her gait improves but remains wide-based. She accurately describes her husband, who died 10 years ago, and can name the last five presidents. Immediate memory and attention are normal. Each morning, she is alert and engages in conversation with the medical team, although careful examination reveals she has no memory of them from the day before. How can these symptoms be explained?

(A) alcoholic dementia
(B) Korsakoff's syndrome
(C) stroke
(D) delirium
(E) Alzheimer's disease

Questions 631 through 633

A 29-year-old man with no psychiatric history is brought in by police to the emergency department after threatening a neighbor with a knife. He says that people in his neighborhood have organized against him in an effort to ruin his life. According to the patient, people are tape-recording his telephone conversations and videotaping him with cameras concealed in his house, and have recently recruited the police in their efforts. While he is intensely distraught over this invasion of his privacy, he is performing well at his job, exercising daily, eating and sleeping well, and is engaged to be married. He is well-groomed and well-related in his conversation. His thinking seems otherwise logical.

631. What is the most likely diagnosis?

(A) schizophrenia
(B) brief psychotic disorder
(C) delusional disorder
(D) paranoid personality disorder
(E) major depressive disorder (MDD) with psychotic features

632. What would be the most appropriate treatment?

(A) fluoxetine (Prozac)
(B) alprazolam (Xanax)
(C) olanzapine (Zyprexa)
(D) electroconvulsive therapy (ECT)
(E) lithium

633. Which statement regarding this illness is true?

(A) Auditory hallucinations are common.
(B) The delusions are usually bizarre.
(C) Negative symptoms predominate.
(D) The delusion is plausible but unlikely.
(E) Persecutory delusions are relatively rare.

Questions 634 through 638

A 29-year-old man with a history of chronic paranoid schizophrenia comes to the emergency department with a temperature of 102.9°F, labile blood pressure rising to 210/110, a pulse of 110, and a respiratory rate of 22 breaths/min. This patient's medications include haloperidol (Haldol), benztropine (Cogentin), and clonazepam (Klonopin). He cannot correctly identify the day, date, or year, and believes himself to be in a city from which he moved 10 years ago. A family member indicates that 3 days ago he was healthy and completely oriented and that he has no significant medical or surgical history.

634. What is the most likely diagnosis?

(A) infection
(B) delirium
(C) malignant hyperthermia
(D) hypertensive encephalopathy
(E) drug intoxication or withdrawal

635. Physical examination of this patient reveals that he is in acute distress with hypertonicity. Laboratory examination reveals a creatine phosphokinase (CPK) of 45,000, a white blood cell (WBC) count of 14,000 and no left shift, a sodium of 145, and a creatinine of 2.5. Lumbar puncture produces clear fluid with a slightly elevated protein count. What is the most likely diagnosis?

(A) anticholinergic syndrome
(B) malignant hyperthermia
(C) central nervous system (CNS) infection
(D) prolonged immobilization
(E) NMS

636. Where should this patient be treated?

(A) psychiatric unit
(B) medical unit
(C) medical unit with close monitoring by psychiatry consult/liaison service
(D) medical intensive care unit
(E) remain in the emergency department for observation

637. What therapy is most important initially for this patient?

(A) start anticholinergic medication
(B) stop all neuroleptics
(C) start broad-spectrum IV antibiotics
(D) start bromocriptine
(E) stop anticholinergic medications

638. With appropriate treatment, the patient recovers completely and returns home. In a month's time, he comes to the emergency department stating that the "voices in the walls" are telling him to kill himself. He has taken no medications since he left the hospital. His vital signs are stable and a medical workup is negative. Initial therapy may include

(A) ECT

(B) haloperidol depot injections

(C) olanzapine (Zyprexa)

(D) safety monitoring only

(E) physical restraints

Questions 639 through 641

A 39-year-old woman comes to the emergency department and complains that since her boyfriend broke up with her 3 months ago, she has been sleeping and eating poorly, has lost all interest in her work, and feels guilty that she drove her boyfriend away. In the past month, she has begun to feel hopeless, helpless, and that "life may not be worth it." In the past 2 weeks, she has developed a belief that a rare disease is rotting her heart, and in the past week, a voice in her ear tells her she is no good and that she should take an overdose of a heart medication she is prescribed.

639. What is the most likely diagnosis?

(A) adjustment disorder

(B) brief psychotic disorder

(C) bipolar disorder

(D) MDD

(E) delusional disorder

640. What would be the most appropriate treatment?

(A) medication and discharge to a close family member

(B) referral to an outpatient psychiatrist

(C) admission to a psychiatric unit

(D) admission to a medical unit

(E) restraints and medication in the emergency department

641. What medication(s) would be most appropriate?

(A) tricyclic antidepressant (TCA) only

(B) lithium and a selective serotonin reuptake inhibitor (SSRI)

(C) an SSRI and a neuroleptic

(D) a benzodiazepine only

(E) lithium only

Questions 642 through 645

A 21-year-old man is brought to the emergency department by police after an episode in which he ransacked the office where he works looking for "evidence." He started this job 2 months ago after graduating from college. He lives with four roommates, and he believes they are jealous of him because of his job and have been poisoning his food. His family reveals that once before, when he went away to college, he went through a period of "acting crazy" but got better without treatment and has done well since. In the emergency department, he is shouting that he's been up for a week writing a "classic" book about accounting, and someone at the office stole it from him. He needs to be physically restrained by emergency department security. Physical examination and complete laboratory workup and toxicology screen prove to be negative.

642. What is the most likely diagnosis?

(A) bipolar II disorder

(B) bipolar I disorder with psychotic features

(C) bipolar I disorder without psychotic features

(D) adjustment disorder with disturbance of conduct

(E) schizophrenia

643. Initial medications should include

(A) lithium

(B) a neuroleptic and a benzodiazepine

(C) an SSRI

(D) carbamazepine (Tegretol)

(E) buspirone (BuSpar)

644. Three months later, the patient sees his doctor for follow-up. He is taking lithium and haloperidol (Haldol). He is doing well, except he complains of muscle stiffness. His lithium level is 0.8 mEq/L. A reasonable intervention would be to

(A) increase the lithium dose
(B) decrease the lithium dose
(C) start baclofen (Lioresal)
(D) discontinue the haloperidol
(E) increase the haloperidol dose

645. A year after treatment is initiated, the patient is brought to the emergency department by a friend. Earlier in the week, he had a respiratory tract infection and fever, and now he is confused and complains of blurred vision. He has a generalized tonic–clonic seizure in the emergency department. His lithium level is 2.5 mEq/L, and his thyroid-stimulating hormone (TSH) is 4.2 mU/L. A reasonable intervention would be

(A) dialysis
(B) to decrease the dose of lithium
(C) to initiate immediate treatment for hypothyroidism
(D) hydration only
(E) intramuscular (IM) injection of an anticholinergic medication

Questions 646 through 650

A 29-year-old woman tells her doctor that about 3 weeks ago a child she was caring for ran into the street and was killed by a bus. Since then, she cannot get the image of the accident out of her mind. Even in sleep, she dreams about it. While she used to take a bus to work, she now drives, because she cannot bear to be near buses. In the past week, she has begun missing work because she is uncomfortable leaving her house. She feels guilty, believing the accident was her fault.

646. What is the most likely diagnosis?

(A) posttraumatic stress disorder (PTSD)
(B) acute stress disorder
(C) MDD

(D) panic disorder with agoraphobia
(E) adjustment disorder

647. In considering the patient for short-term treatment with a benzodiazepine, what is the most important consideration?

(A) the patient's liver function
(B) the patient's kidney function
(C) the patient's age
(D) the presence of a history of drug or alcohol abuse
(E) the half-life of the selected benzodiazepine

648. The patient decides against any medication and follows up with psychotherapy. A year later, while she is no longer having distressful symptoms relating to the accident, she complains she feels sad and tearful most of the time, is having trouble eating, has lost interest in gardening, and wakes up at 4:00 every morning, unable to get back to sleep. What is the most likely diagnosis?

(A) PTSD
(B) acute stress disorder
(C) MDD
(D) panic disorder with agoraphobia
(E) adjustment disorder

649. In considering pharmacologic treatment as an adjunct to psychotherapy, the psychiatrist should obtain

(A) blood for laboratory investigation
(B) an electrocardiogram (ECG)
(C) a head CT scan
(D) a neurologic consultation
(E) a chest x-ray

650. Which of the following medications would be appropriate first-line treatment?

(A) amitriptyline (Elavil)
(B) paroxetine (Paxil)
(C) haloperidol (Haldol)
(D) clonazepam (Klonopin)
(E) clonidine (Catapres)

Questions 651 through 655

A patient is admitted to a psychiatric hospital. Her medications include an SSRI and a benzodiazepine, which are both discontinued on admission. A neuroleptic and a mood stabilizer are started. Two days after her admission, she calls the nursing staff to her bed. She is extremely frightened and complains excitedly that she cannot stop looking up. On exam, her eyes are noted to be deviated upward bilaterally.

651. This is most likely

(A) a reaction to discontinuing the benzodiazepine
(B) a reaction to discontinuing the SSRI
(C) akathisia
(D) refractory psychosis
(E) a reaction to initiating neuroleptic treatment

652. This specific reaction is called

(A) torticollis
(B) trismus
(C) oculogyric crisis
(D) retrocollis
(E) NMS

653. Which statement best characterizes this condition?

(A) It occurs most commonly weeks to months after initiation of the offending medication.
(B) It can occur in any muscle group.
(C) It most commonly occurs when low-potency neuroleptics are used.
(D) It is a benign side effect of medication with minimal therapeutic consequences.
(E) It occurs most frequently in elderly females.

654. What is the initial concern in managing this condition?

(A) airway obstruction
(B) malignant hypertension
(C) autonomic instability
(D) acute renal failure
(E) future compliance with pharmacologic treatments

655. What is the initial treatment of choice?

(A) beta blockers
(B) muscle relaxants
(C) anticholinergics
(D) aggressive hydration
(E) anxiolytics

Questions 656 and 657

A 59-year-old woman with a long history of GAD tells her primary care doctor that in a crowded supermarket 2 days previously she felt dizzy, with associated heart palpitations, pressure on her chest, and a frightening sense of doom. Shortly thereafter, she fell unconscious and woke up minutes later with a crowd around her. She felt somewhat better and rejected others' advice that an ambulance be called. She quickly made her way home.

656. What is the most likely diagnosis?

(A) cardiovascular disease
(B) panic attack
(C) GAD
(D) acute stress disorder
(E) anxiety disorder due to cardiovascular disease

657. What is the most appropriate intervention?

(A) short-acting benzodiazepines
(B) an SSRI
(C) cognitive–behavioral therapy
(D) ECG
(E) reassurance that her condition is benign

658. A 41-year-old woman you have been following for depression comes for a follow-up visit. She has taken increasing doses of an SSRI over the past 10 weeks, is now at the recommended maximum dose, and has shown little, if any, improvement. She is having no side effects to the medication. What is the appropriate next step in her treatment?

(A) add lithium

(B) stop the SSRI and try a second antidepressant

(C) add a second antidepressant

(D) continue at the current dose and follow up in 2 weeks

(E) discontinue all antidepressant treatment

Questions 659 through 662

A 19-year-old college junior goes to the university health care office because she has stopped menstruating. Physical exam reveals a lean, athletic woman in no apparent distress, but is notable for poor dentition and erosion of the enamel of her teeth. With respect to her body habitus, age, and height, her weight is less than average, but within normal limits. She admits to being "a little weird" about her weight and exercises vigorously in response to "pigging out."

659. Which of the following statements regarding this patient is true?

(A) It is unlikely she has an eating disorder.

(B) It is unlikely she has an affective or mood disorder.

(C) Her amenorrhea requires no further workup.

(D) It is likely that she has anorexia nervosa.

(E) It is likely that she has bulimia nervosa.

660. Associated laboratory and physical exam findings of this patient might include

(A) low serum amylase

(B) salivary gland atrophy

(C) hyperkalemia

(D) hypermagnesemia

(E) normal thyroid function

661. Which of the following statements regarding eating disorders is true?

(A) Binge eating and purging may be seen in both anorexia and in bulimia.

(B) The patient who binges on food and then vigorously exercises and fasts would not receive a diagnosis of bulimia.

(C) Laxative abuse is rare.

(D) Approximately 30% of eating disorders are diagnosed in men.

(E) Amenorrhea may or may not be present in anorexia nervosa.

662. Which of the following statements regarding the treatment of this patient is true?

(A) A reasonable intervention would be prescribing an SSRI, with follow-up in 1 month's time.

(B) Anorexia nervosa tends to be more responsive to pharmacotherapy than is bulimia nervosa.

(C) Hospitalization is rarely indicated.

(D) Treatment is necessary because she is at risk for seizures.

(E) Cognitive–behavioral therapy will be of little value.

Questions 663 through 665

A 19-year-old man with no previous psychiatric history is noted by his college roommate to be acting bizarrely for the past month and a half, talking to people who are not there, walking around the dorm room naked, and accusing the roommate of calling the FBI to have him monitored. The patient's vital signs are all within normal limits, and the neurologic exam shows no deficits or abnormalities.

663. The most important first test would be

(A) a noncontrast CT scan of the brain

(B) a toxicology screen

(C) an erythrocyte sedimentation rate (ESR)

(D) a complete blood count (CBC)

(E) liver function tests

664. If this test were negative, the most likely diagnosis would be

(A) major depression with psychotic features

(B) delusional disorder

(C) schizophreniform disorder

(D) chronic paranoid schizophrenia

(E) substance-induced psychosis

665. The most appropriate medication would be

(A) lorazepam (Ativan)

(B) clozapine (Clozaril)

(C) benztropine (Cogentin)

(D) haloperidol (Haldol)

(E) lactulose

Questions 666 through 668

You have been asked by the surgery team to evaluate a 35-year-old man who had surgery to repair his fractured right wrist 24 hours ago and is now complaining of anxiety. The patient has been in the hospital for 2 days. His heart rate is 120, and his blood pressure is 160/106. He is afebrile and reports that he has never suffered anything like this before. He is not in any pain and has no previous psychiatric history. His medication includes only acetaminophen for pain control. You note that he is diaphoretic and tremulous.

666. The most likely diagnosis is

(A) alcohol abuse

(B) cocaine withdrawal

(C) cannabis withdrawal

(D) alcohol withdrawal

(E) opiate withdrawal

667. The most appropriate single-agent therapy is

(A) clonidine (Catapres)

(B) methadone

(C) lorazepam (Ativan)

(D) carbamazepine (Tegretol)

(E) naltrexone (ReVia)

668. Without this treatment, he is at risk for developing

(A) fatty liver

(B) abdominal pain

(C) seizures

(D) muscle cramps

(E) appendicitis

Questions 669 through 672

You are working in the psychiatric emergency department of a large metropolitan hospital. A 20-year-old man with unknown psychiatric history is brought in by police after being found stumbling naked around a local college campus. He is markedly agitated, pacing, and appears to be responding to internal stimuli. On examination, you note that he is tachycardic with a heart rate in the 110s, he has tics or spasms in his face, and he has vertical nystagmus.

669. Your initial diagnosis is

(A) phencyclidine (PCP) intoxication

(B) chronic paranoid schizophrenia

(C) cocaine intoxication

(D) amphetamine intoxication

(E) brief psychotic disorder

670. The test most likely to be diagnostic is

(A) a noncontrast head CT

(B) a magnetic resonance image (MRI) of the brain

(C) an electroencephalogram (EEG)

(D) a CBC

(E) a toxicology screen

671. The most appropriate treatment is

(A) placing the patient in a low-stimulus environment

(B) phenytoin (Dilantin)

(C) methylphenidate (Ritalin)

(D) benztropine (Cogentin)

(E) propranolol (Inderal)

672. The treatment plan for this patient will most likely include

(A) a long-term psychiatric hospitalization

(B) return to previous level of functioning without hospitalization

(C) a short hospitalization to evaluate his schizophrenia

(D) a short hospitalization on the neurology service to evaluate a movement disorder

(E) immediate discharge from the psychiatric emergency department

673. A 40-year-old divorced woman is brought in to the emergency department after being found sleeping in a pile of leaves. Initially, she is difficult to arouse and has trouble answering your questions, but she appears to be in no respiratory distress. You also notice that her pupils are pinpoint. After a few hours, she becomes more interactive and is complaining of diffuse, crampy abdominal pain and symptoms of "the flu." Her pupils are now slightly dilated, and she is yawning. Her vital signs are a temperature of 99.3°F, a heart rate of 99, and blood pressure of 142/90. After the second interview, your diagnosis is

(A) cannabis abuse
(B) opiate withdrawal
(C) cocaine withdrawal
(D) cocaine intoxication
(E) opiate intoxication

Questions 674 through 676

A 70-year-old widow is admitted for an evaluation of depression and anxiety. She tells you that for the past 15 years her family doctor has prescribed "some pills" that have helped her sleep and feel less nervous. She says that she ran out of them yesterday and since that time has felt increasingly anxious and jittery. She also notes that she's now having tremors in her hands that have not been there before.

674. Your initial concern would be greatest if you found that the medication was

(A) nortriptyline (Pamelor)
(B) triazolam (Halcion)
(C) thioridazine (Mellaril)
(D) fluphenazine (Prolixin)
(E) imipramine (Tofranil)

675. The most worrisome side effect of abruptly stopping this medication would be

(A) autonomic hyperactivity
(B) seizures
(C) hallucinations
(D) worsening anxiety
(E) vomiting

676. The best way to determine if the patient is withdrawing from this medication is

(A) to check vital signs
(B) an ECG
(C) an EEG
(D) Wada's test
(E) a phenobarbital challenge

Questions 677 and 678

A 73-year-old man is admitted to the hospital for community-acquired pneumonia and dehydration. On day 2 of hospitalization, you are asked to evaluate the patient for depression as the staff has noted that he seems very withdrawn. He is not eating or sleeping well. Last night, the nursing staff reports, he was angry and requesting to leave the hospital. You talk with the patient's family and find that the patient has no previous psychiatric history. Prior to the onset of this illness 5 days ago, he had no depressive symptoms and no difficulties with cognition. On exam, his vital signs are temperature 98.2°F, heart rate 87, blood pressure 130/86, and a peripheral oxygen saturation of 95% on room air. He is drowsy and oriented only to person. His Mini-Mental Status Exam (MMSE) score is 24/30.

677. The most likely diagnosis is

(A) MDD
(B) anxiety disorder
(C) dementia
(D) delirium
(E) factitious disorder

678. The medical team asks for medication recommendations if the patient becomes agitated. You recommend

(A) lorazepam (Ativan)
(B) benztropine (Cogentin)
(C) thioridazine (Mellaril)
(D) diphenhydramine
(E) haloperidol (Haldol)

Questions 679 through 681

A 75-year-old widow is brought to the hospital by her son, who says that his mother has been having progressive difficulty with her memory since her husband died 3 years ago. The memory difficulties, however, have worsened in the last week. Prior to a week ago, the patient and her family noted that she had difficulty remembering new names, often could not remember where she had left her purse, and was having more problems paying her bills. One week ago, however, her family noted that she was having difficulty dressing and feeding herself. On exam, her vital signs are significant for a blood pressure of 170/100, a heart rate of 80, a temperature of 98.8°F, and a peripheral oxygen saturation of 99% on room air. She is alert, pleasant, and oriented to person, place, and time. She scores a 24/30 on the MMSE.

679. The next step in the diagnosis would be a

(A) physical exam
(B) noncontrast head CT
(C) lipid profile
(D) carotid ultrasound
(E) transesophageal echocardiogram

680. The most concerning part of the history and exam is the

(A) history of progressive memory difficulties
(B) recent sudden decline in function
(C) hypertension
(D) fact that she is fully oriented
(E) low score on the MMSE

681. The most likely diagnosis is

(A) personality change
(B) depression
(C) dementia
(D) bereavement
(E) pseudodementia

Questions 682 and 683

A 65-year-old woman with a past medical history of non–insulin-dependent diabetes mellitus and depression is admitted with increasingly depressed mood over the last month. She is unable to complete her crossword puzzles because of difficulty concentrating. She has difficulty falling asleep and also wakes up in the middle of the night. She denies suicidal ideation, but does feel guilty that she is depressed. Prior to this episode, she was doing well and was actively engaged in community volunteer groups. In the last month, she has lost 13 pounds due to poor intake. When you ask why she isn't eating, she tells you that she's worried that she will become infected with bacteria. She has been to her primary physician for an evaluation, but she says everything was normal. Her husband confirms that the patient has been very worried about "getting a disease" to the point where she will eat only food in sealed containers. He also confides in you that she has been worried that she might have cancer and despite reassurances from her primary care physician, she continues to voice her concerns to her husband that "my intestines are not working."

682. The diagnosis that best describes her illness is

(A) somatization disorder
(B) MDD without psychotic features
(C) dysthymia
(D) MDD with psychotic features
(E) OCD

683. The treatment of choice is

(A) sertraline (Zoloft)
(B) sertraline and perphenazine (Trilafon)
(C) lithium and sertraline
(D) valproic acid (Depakote)
(E) nortriptyline (Pamelor) and lorazepam (Ativan)

Questions 684 through 688

An 18-year-old man is brought to the psychiatric emergency department by his parents for evaluation of his behavior. Three months ago, the patient started classes at the state university in a different city, but he comes home each weekend. His parents have noticed that over the past 2 months the patient has become increasingly withdrawn and doesn't seem to be taking care of himself. The parents were called by the patient's roommate who says that the patient has not been going to classes for the last 2 months, has not been eating or bathing, and has been talking about how people in his classes are trying to kill him. On exam, the patient's vital signs are all within normal parameters. He is pacing and appears to be responding to internal stimuli. His mood is euthymic and his affect is flat. He denies any drug use and is not on any medication. He is fully oriented. He says that he hears a number of people talking to him, "maybe in my head." They seem to be saying bad things about him. He looks frightened and asks, "What is happening to me?"

684. You explain to the patient and family that the current diagnosis is

(A) delusional disorder
(B) chronic undifferentiated schizophrenia
(C) schizophreniform disorder
(D) brief psychotic disorder
(E) substance-induced psychotic disorder

685. If this condition had been occurring for less than 1 month, your diagnosis would be

(A) delusional disorder
(B) chronic undifferentiated schizophrenia
(C) brief psychotic disorder
(D) schizophreniform disorder
(E) substance-induced psychotic disorder

686. The most helpful laboratory test to make this diagnosis is

(A) toxicology screen
(B) EEG
(C) noncontrast head CT
(D) a CBC
(E) electrolytes

687. The most appropriate treatment is

(A) psychotherapy
(B) clozapine (Clozaril)
(C) ECT
(D) haloperidol (Haldol)
(E) lithium

688. Two hours after you give this medication, the patient says that his muscles feel stiff and he is having trouble talking because his tongue feels thick. To treat this condition, you choose

(A) lorazepam (Ativan)
(B) benztropine (Cogentin)
(C) haloperidol (Haldol)
(D) ketorolac (Toradol)
(E) meperidine (Demerol)

Questions 689 through 691

A 35-year-old woman with no previous personal or family psychiatric history is brought to the emergency department by her husband, who reports that his wife was attempting to kill herself by cutting her wrists. Her husband tells you that 6 months ago the patient's grandmother died. Since that time, her husband thinks the patient has been becoming more depressed. She has difficulty falling asleep and has lost 15 pounds in 2 months. She was recently fired from her job as a paralegal because she was unable to concentrate. She feels guilty that she can't feel better and endorses feelings of hopelessness and worthlessness. She believes that her only way out of this is to kill herself.

689. You explain to her that she is suffering from

(A) dysthymia
(B) bipolar disorder
(C) depressed personality disorder
(D) adjustment disorder with depressed mood
(E) MDD

690. You choose to treat her with

(A) flumazenil (Romazicon)
(B) fluoxetine (Prozac)
(C) fluphenazine (Prolixin)
(D) triazolam (Halcion)
(E) phenelzine (Nardil)

691. A common side effect of this class of medication that may mimic a symptom of depression is

(A) insomnia

(B) nausea

(C) constipation

(D) akathisia

(E) diarrhea

Questions 692 through 695

A 25-year-old man is brought to the emergency department by his fiancé, who says that over the last week the patient has been increasingly angry. He has been yelling about minor things like taking out the trash. His behavior has become so erratic that his boss is going to fire him unless he gets some help. He has not slept more than 3 hours a night for the past week, instead staying up buying over $50,000 worth of stocks. On exam, his vital signs are within normal limits. His speech is rapid, and you are having great difficulty following his conversation because he jumps from topic to topic. He reports increased energy, but also endorses a depressed, anxious mood and suicidal ideation.

692. Your diagnosis is

(A) bipolar disorder, current episode manic

(B) bipolar disorder, current mixed

(C) cyclothymia

(D) MDD

(E) hypomania

693. The most helpful test in this person would be

(A) an ESR

(B) a noncontrast head CT

(C) a Veneral Disease Research Laboratory (VDRL) test

(D) a toxicology screen

(E) serum electrolytes

694. You choose to begin treatment with

(A) valproic acid (Depakote) only

(B) haloperidol (Haldol) only

(C) haloperidol and valproic acid

(D) valproic acid and lorazepam (Ativan)

(E) lorazepam only

695. Before starting this medication, you should evaluate his

(A) liver function tests

(B) blood urea nitrogen (BUN)

(C) creatinine

(D) electrolytes

(E) ECG

Questions 696 and 697

You are asked to see an 18-year-old woman with no previous psychiatric or medical history because the head of her college is concerned about her and worried that she may be depressed. The patient tells you that despite being far away from her home for the first time, she was enjoying school and her new friends until 2 months ago, when she learned that her parents were getting divorced. Since that time, her grades have gone from A's and B's to B's and C's because she is worried about her parents and her sister at home. She says she feels "bummed out" most of the time, and her friends note that she seems unhappy and occasionally becomes tearful when talking about her family. She denies difficulty sleeping or changes in appetite or weight and continues to enjoy daily trips to the gym to work out.

696. The diagnosis that best captures her symptoms is

(A) generalized anxiety disorder

(B) acute stress disorder

(C) MDD

(D) bereavement

(E) adjustment disorder with depressed mood

697. For treatment, you recommend

(A) risperidone (Risperdal)

(B) fluoxetine (Prozac)

(C) psychotherapy

(D) nortriptyline (Pamelor)

(E) alprazolam (Xanax)

Questions 698 and 699

A 26-year-old woman with no previous psychiatric history is referred to you by her primary care physician for evaluation of an episode of anxiety. She tells you that approximately 2 months ago she began having episodes lasting 10 or 15 minutes during which, she says, "I feel like I'm going to die." During these episodes, her heart races, she feels as though she can't catch her breath, she is dizzy and worried she may pass out, and has tingling and tremors in her hands. She is concerned because she is now having problems leaving her house because she is worried these episodes will occur and make it impossible for her to get home. She cannot identify any triggers leading to the episodes. She is not on any medication and has no medical problems.

698. You diagnose her with

    (A) GAD
    (B) panic disorder with agoraphobia
    (C) separation anxiety disorder
    (D) social phobia
    (E) panic disorder without agoraphobia

699. You initiate treatment with

    (A) sertraline (Zoloft)
    (B) alprazolam (Xanax)
    (C) lithium
    (D) propranolol
    (E) tranylcypromine (Parnate)

Questions 700 and 701

A 36-year-old woman with no former psychiatric history is referred to you by a dermatologist for evaluation of her chronically chapped hands. She says she's been seeing her dermatologist for about 5 years for this problem and treated with a variety of topical agents with limited success. Over the past 3 weeks, her hands have become worse, to the point where they are always cracked and bleeding. Reluctantly, she confides in you that she's had a fear of germs, but since her colleague has been sick, she's been washing her hands at least 40 times a day because she is afraid of contracting the disease. She also refuses to touch anything that might infect her without using a handkerchief. She also admits to being very tidy at home as well. She tells you that she spends about 2½ hours in the morning getting showered. She realizes her fears of contamination are irrational, but every time she tries to stop she becomes increasingly anxious.

700. You discuss which of the following diagnoses with the patient?

    (A) MDD
    (B) GAD
    (C) OCD
    (D) panic disorder
    (E) somatization disorder

701. Which of the following treatments do you recommend for the patient?

    (A) cognitive–behavioral therapy
    (B) risperidone (Risperdal)
    (C) ECT
    (D) lithium
    (E) psychodynamic psychotherapy

702. A 47-year-old secretary comes to your office complaining, "I'm always worried." She says that she worries about her job, her kids, her housework, and her husband. She is seeking help now because she has been having an increasingly difficult time concentrating at work and has been more irritable with people around her. Her sleep has been "okay," but she doesn't feel rested when she gets up in the morning. She has been more aware of these feelings over the last 2 years, and they occur almost every day. She denies any discrete episodes of increased anxiety. You discuss which of the following diagnoses with the patient?

    (A) GAD
    (B) OCD
    (C) social phobia disorder
    (D) panic disorder
    (E) schizophrenia

703. A 28-year-old woman with no previous psychiatric or medical history is admitted to the neurology service for evaluation of acute onset of numbness and weakness of the right side of her face and right arm and leg. Physical exam shows symmetrical 2/4 reflexes in all distributions, downgoing plantar reflexes bilaterally, and 2/5 strength in the right upper and lower extremity in all muscle groups. No atrophy or fasciculations are noted. Her gait is ataxic and staggering, with extreme exaggerated movements of her arms; however, she does not fall when ambulating without assistance. Extensive neurologic workup is negative. Given the severity of her deficits, she seems unconcerned by her level of disability. The diagnosis that best captures the patient's symptoms is

(A) factitious disorder
(B) undiagnosed neurologic disease
(C) conversion disorder
(D) malingering
(E) somatization disorder

704. A 54-year-old woman with a past medical history of hypothyroidism is admitted with a septic right knee. The surgery team asks you to evaluate the patient because they found that the fluid aspirate from the knee was growing a pathogen found primarily in the human mouth. They suspect the patient was injecting saliva into her knee. You evaluate the patient and find her to be pleasant and cooperative. She tells you that she's had a very tough time lately because her husband has recently been sick. Fortunately, she is a nurse and has been able to care for him at home. Lately, she admits to feeling overwhelmed and not appreciated. She has no idea what has caused the problem with her knee. You talk to the family and they tell you she is in no financial difficulty and she continues to enjoy work as a nurse. After working with you for a few weeks, she admits to injecting her knee, but she cannot understand why she did. You tell the surgery team that you have diagnosed her with

(A) malingering
(B) somatization disorder

(C) hypochondriasis
(D) conversion disorder
(E) factitious disorder

Questions 705 and 706

An 18-year-old woman in her first year in college comes to see you for evaluation of "depression." Her roommates also encouraged her to see someone. She reports difficulty falling asleep and early morning awakenings, poor concentration, fatigue, and anxiety over the past month since she arrived for the fall semester. She tells you that her parents are very strict and she is worried that she won't get straight A's. On exam, she is a calm, thin woman dressed in a very baggy jogging suit. You comment on her thinness, and she tells you she prides herself on her appearance and tries to stay slim by exercising about 4 hours a day along with a good diet. She denies problems with eating too much or too little and says just diet and exercise help her control her weight. Despite your concerns about her thinness, she tells you she would like to lose a few more pounds. She tells you she has not had a regular menstrual period for over a year. Before you proceed with therapy, you discuss the need for further testing today.

705. The test that would help most in making the diagnosis would be

(A) serum potassium level
(B) weight and height
(C) ECG
(D) serum amylase
(E) serum magnesium level

706. Even before this test is completed, your working diagnosis is

(A) bulimia nervosa
(B) body dysmorphic disorder
(C) MDD
(D) anxiety disorder
(E) anorexia nervosa

Questions 707 and 708

A 5-year-old boy is referred to you by his pediatrician for evaluation of aggressive behavior. A pediatric neurologist's extensive workup was negative.

Interview with parents and the patient reveals a restless boy who is able to engage in conversation. He tells you he gets angry and frustrated in school and thinks it is "boring." His parents report that he has never been a strong student. He is currently repeating kindergarten due to poor performance and difficulty socializing with other children. His mother tells you that she still has to help him pick out his clothes for school and get dressed. Aggressive outbursts at school seem to occur at times when he does not understand the schoolwork. His family history is positive for two paternal uncles with learning disabilities.

707. You recommend that which of the following tests be done first in the evaluation?

(A) Kohs Block Test
(B) Minnesota Multiphasic Personality Inventory-2 (MMPI-2)
(C) Wechsler Intelligence Scale for Children (WISC)
(D) Peabody Vocabulary Test
(E) Goodenough Draw-a-Person Test

708. A score of 69 on this test is consistent with

(A) borderline intellectual functioning
(B) mild mental retardation
(C) moderate mental retardation
(D) severe mental retardation
(E) profound mental retardation

Questions 709 through 711

A 12-year-old boy is brought in by his mother for evaluation of hyperactivity. She has been told by teachers and has observed herself that her son has marked difficulty sitting still and concentrating. On exam, you note a well-developed boy who is highly distractible, walking around the room playing indiscriminately with toys for a few seconds, then moving to the windows and the chairs. His mother has a hard time getting him to sit down so that you may talk with him. When he does sit down, he swings his legs and has poor eye contact. He frequently clears his throat, sniffs, and blinks his eyes. Further exam reveals that he suffers from frequent episodes of counting numbers in his head that don't stop until he does it six times. He is very "fussy" about his clothes, requiring them to feel "just right." He often feels the need to touch smooth surfaces "to see how they feel." He admits these habits are bothersome, but he cannot stop them because when he does he gets very anxious. His mother reports that his father has a number of mannerisms similar to her son's, such as clearing his throat and blinking his eyes, but they are noticeable only when he is under stress.

709. The most likely diagnosis is

(A) Tourette's disorder
(B) attention deficit disorder (ADD)
(C) OCD
(D) normal 12-year-old behavior
(E) childhood schizophrenia

710. The patient and his mother agree to begin treatment with

(A) pimozide (Orap)
(B) paroxetine (Paxil)
(C) clozapine (Clozaril)
(D) lorazepam (Ativan)
(E) methylphenidate (Ritalin)

711. Prior to starting this medication and while on therapy, you will need to monitor

(A) liver function
(B) CBC
(C) serum dopamine levels
(D) BUN
(E) ECG

712. A 17-year-old boy with a history of attention deficit–hyperactivity disorder (ADHD) presents with odd behavior, confusion, a blood pressure of 128/85, and a heart rate of 68. His parents reported that at times they have observed him repetitively touching his stomach and rapidly blinking his eyes. On your exam, he appears dazed and unable to concentrate. The most likely diagnosis is

(A) somatization disorder
(B) hypoglycemia
(C) amphetamine toxicosis
(D) epilepsy
(E) MDD

713. A 50-year-old man with a long history of IV drug use is brought to the hospital by police after a local homeless shelter worker noted him to be confused and "walking funny." While at the shelter, he became very suspicious of the workers and accused them of taking his belongings. On exam, you observe that he has a left pupil that accommodates but does not react, depressed deep tendon reflexes in all distributions, and loss of position sense at the great toes bilaterally. Although the patient was treated with antipsychotic medications in the past, he denied currently taking any medication. Which of the following items best accounts for all of this patient's neurologic symptoms?

(A) Wernicke's encephalopathy
(B) Korsakoff's psychosis
(C) NMS
(D) neuroleptic-induced dykinesia
(E) neurosyphilis

714. A 57-year-old woman with no previous psychiatric history complains of increasing anxiety over the last 2 months. Today, she reports, it became "very bad." She also notes that with these periods of anxiety she gets a pounding headache and once fainted. She continues to feel "shaky." When you check her vital signs, her heart rate is 170 and her blood pressure is 230/130. She is diaphoretic and tremulous. Which of the following conditions is most likely given this patient's physiologic symptoms?

(A) hypothyroidism
(B) hypercalcemia
(C) pheochromocytoma
(D) acute alcohol intoxication
(E) posterior circulation stroke

DIRECTIONS (Questions 715 through 726): Each set of items in this section consists of a list of lettered headings followed by several numbered words or phrases. For each numbered word or phrase, select the ONE lettered option that is most closely associated with it. Each lettered option may be selected once, more than once, or not at all.

Questions 715 through 720

(A) systemic lupus erythematosus (SLE)
(B) human immunodeficiency virus (HIV)
(C) hepatic encephalopathy
(D) conversion disorder
(E) pheochromocytoma
(F) somatization disorder
(G) hypoglycemia
(H) hyperthyroidism

715. You are asked to see a 55-year-old man who was admitted to the hospital today. Initially, he was cooperative, but now he is very agitated and wants to leave. His wife reports that he has periods during which he becomes very upset. She also tells you that he's a completely different person from a year ago and is becoming very forgetful. On exam, you observe that he has significant memory impairment, asterixis, palmar erythema, and a large ecchymotic area on his right scapula.

716. A 52-year-old man with a long history of IV drug use is brought to the emergency department for evaluation after a worker at a homeless shelter found the patient having a difficult time trying to figure out how to use his eating utensils. The worker, who has known the patient for the last 10 years, says that she has seen a drastic change in the patient over the last year. He previously was jovial and interactive with the staff, but now seems disengaged and subdued. She also says that he has been increasingly forgetful. She is concerned about other health issues as she says he has lost at least 40 pounds in the last 6 months and has complained about feeling weak and losing his balance. On exam, he is withdrawn and on MMSE he scores a 20/30.

717. A 33-year-old woman is brought to the emergency department by her husband, who tells you that in the last week his wife has been increasingly tearful and easily upset. Over the last few months, she has been increasingly irritable and has a hard time sitting still. Additionally, she had told him she was having some difficulty doing her usual tasks like paying her bills and balancing her checkbook. She has occasional "hot flashes." On exam, she is alert and oriented, but continuously changes position in her seat and gets up frequently. Her speech is normal rate, volume, and production. She has difficulty with simple arithmetic and short-term memory. Her deep tendon reflexes are brisk symmetrically throughout. She has a fine resting tremor of her hands and has difficulty rising from a seated position.

718. A 33-year-old woman presents with a 1-year history of headaches. She was diagnosed with tension headaches by a neurologist after an extensive evaluation that was negative. Her headaches are worsening, and now she also reports blurry vision. Despite a repeat negative neurologic evaluation, the patient is concerned that she has not been treated appropriately. She volunteers that she has been sick most of her life. The real trouble began for her at age 16 when she had surgery for presumed endometriosis, which has left her unable to have sexual relations. Since the surgery, she has intermittent abdominal cramping, bloating, and diarrhea. Three months ago, she saw a rheumatologist for knee, back, and eye pain.

719. A 30-year-old woman is brought to the hospital by her fiancé. He says that over the last 2 weeks, she has been "a totally different person." She has not been eating or sleeping and has been irritable and angry. Earlier in the month, she complained of headaches, pain in her hands and feet, and a fever. On exam, she looks tired; she is fully oriented but has difficulty relating the events of the last month. Occasionally, she seems to become confused.

720. You are asked to evaluate a 42-year-old woman in the emergency department because she appears confused and will not allow any blood to be drawn. She is not oriented to time or place. She knows she takes medications for "a condition," but cannot elaborate further. The only set of vital signs that were taken show a heart rate of 140 and a blood pressure of 172/98. Physical exam is remarkable for a fine tremor of her hands bi-

laterally and diaphoresis. Five minutes after you leave the room, a nurse calls to tell you that the patient has just had a seizure.

Questions 721 through 726

(A) cocaine withdrawal
(B) PCP intoxication
(C) cannabis abuse
(D) opiate intoxication
(E) 3,4 methylenedioxy–methamphetamine (MDMA) intoxication
(F) alcohol withdrawal
(G) opiate withdrawal
(H) alcohol intoxication

721. A 35-year-old woman with no significant past medical or psychiatric history is brought to the hospital by police after crashing her car. You notice that she is slurring her speech, her gait is unsteady, and she demands her car keys so she can drive home. On cognitive exam, she has difficulty paying attention, and tests of her memory show difficulty on immediate recall. Her vital signs are all within normal limits. The physical and neurologic exam is unremarkable.

722. A 25-year-old graduate student is brought to the emergency department by his roommate, who says that since a big party this weekend he's been acting unusual. This morning he's been walking around the room "in a trance" and hasn't been eating or going to class. He is quite disheveled, and periodically makes odd facial grimaces. His exam shows mild increased muscle tone, vertical nystagmus and a large laceration on his upper arm that the patient reports is not painful. Vital signs are remarkable for a blood pressure of 145/95 and a heart rate of 105. Just after you leave the room, he starts screaming at someone and throwing chairs.

723. A 32-year-old woman with a history of poly-substance abuse refers herself to the hospital because she is feeling depressed and intensely suicidal and is worried she may hurt herself. While in the emergency department she asks for something to eat and then falls asleep for the next 4 hours. Upon awakening, the patient is no longer suicidal, but does report intense, unpleasant dreams.

724. A 17-year-old boy is brought to the emergency department by his parents. They are concerned because he was previously an A student and is now failing all of his classes. They are worried because the patient's uncle was diagnosed with schizophrenia at about the same age. You find the patient difficult to engage in conversation but otherwise without evidence of psychosis. He tells you he has been "partying" more in the past few months but denies drug use. He has marked conjunctival injection. He also asks if he will be able to leave soon because he is very hungry. His only complaint is a dry mouth.

725. A 46-year-old woman complains of diffuse muscle pain and vague abdominal cramps. She continuously yawns, blows her nose, and has "goose bumps."

726. A 16-year-old boy is brought to the emergency department by friends after being out all night partying. The patient is found to be diaphoretic and exquisitely sensitive to tactile sensations. Vital signs are HR 98, BP200/100, and temperature of 103°F. The patient is also noted to be wearing a pacifier.

Answers and Explanations

622. **(C)** The most likely diagnosis in this case is schizoaffective disorder. The patient has prominent psychotic symptoms, including auditory hallucinations and paranoid ideation, but also has concurrent mood symptoms, including depressed mood, decreased sleep, anhedonia, and decreased motivation. Also important, the patient's hallucinations have occurred in the absence of mood symptoms, and his mood symptoms appear to have been present for a substantial portion of the total duration of his illness. The presence of prominent psychotic symptoms in the absence of mood symptoms makes major depression unlikely. A diagnosis of schizophrenia alone would not adequately account for this patient's mood symptoms. Bipolar II disorder is not a valid choice since there is no clear history of a hypomanic episode. Schizoid personality disorder is unlikely because that diagnosis would not account for the patient's psychotic and mood symptoms.

623. **(C)** In schizoaffective disorder, it is important to treat both the mood and psychotic symptoms. Because the patient's symptoms mainly consist of depression and psychosis, a combination of an antipsychotic and antidepressant medication would be a reasonable approach. Mirtazapine (Remeron), citalopram (Celexa), fluoxetine (Prozac), and sertraline (Zoloft) are antidepressant medications, while ziprasidone (Geodon), haloperidol (Haldol), and perphenazine (Trilafon) are antipsychotic medications. Lorazepam (Ativan) and diazepam (Valium) are benzodiazepines. Valproic acid (Depakote) is the only mood stabilizer listed.

624. **(B)** This patient most likely has akathisia, which is a neuroleptic-induced side effect. Patients generally experience subjective feelings of restlessness and can be seen swinging their legs, rocking back and forth while sitting, pacing, and rapidly alternating between sitting and standing. Acute dystonias are characterized by contraction of muscles resulting in abnormal movements or postures, such as spasms of the jaw, abnormal positioning of the head, or difficulty swallowing. The onset of acute dystonia usually develops within the first week of initiating a neuroleptic medication. NMS is a life threatening complication involving muscle rigidity and dystonia as well as autonomic symptoms such as elevated temperature, increased heart rate, and increased blood pressure. Akathisia can sometimes be mistaken for anxiety or mania, but in this case there are no other signs (such as delusions of grandeur, decreased need for sleep, increased energy, hypersexuality, etc.) that would indicate a manic episode.

625. **(C)** Hyperthyroidism, hyperparathyroidism, pheochromocytoma, cardiac arrhythmias, and substance abuse should all be considered in the differential diagnosis of panic disorder. *Pheochromocytomas* can produce similar symptoms to panic disorder, such as flushing, sweating, trembling, and tachycardia. Cardiac arrhythmias should obviously be considered in a patient complaining of palpitations. Substance abuse with caffeine, cocaine, or amphetamines can cause symptoms similar to a panic attack, as can withdrawal from alcohol, barbiturates, or benzodiazepines. Hypertension, folate deficiency, hypothyroidism, and lupus are not generally thought of as causing an anxiety-like syndrome.

626. **(C)** The most likely diagnosis in this case is panic disorder. This patient reports some classic symptoms of a panic attack, namely an intense fear in a very short amount of time, associated with palpitations, sweating, shortness of breath, and a feeling of being unable to breathe. The patient has also related past multiple episodes and that she spends a lot of time worrying she will have another episode. These symptoms fit criteria for a panic disorder, and not GAD, social phobia, or OCD. Agoraphobia is the fear of crowded spaces.

627. **(E)** TCAs, SSRIs, benzodiazepines, and cognitive–behavioral therapy are all effective in the treatment of panic disorder. The benzodiazepines have the quickest onset of action but may be associated with sedation and have abuse potential. The maximal anxiolytic effect of SSRI and TCA medications can take 4 to 6 weeks. SSRI medications are preferred for the long-term treatment of panic disorder due to their favorable side effect profile, safety in overdose, and lack of abuse potential.

628. **(C)** This patient presents with the signs of Wernicke's encephalopathy, which results from thiamine (vitamin B_1) deficiency: bilateral abducens nerve palsy, horizontal nystagmus, ataxia, and a global confusion accompanied by apathy. Each of the other choices are possible and should be actively ruled out. Alcohol withdrawal usually presents with unstable vital signs, tremulousness, and agitation. Folic acid deficiency presents with diarrhea, cheilosis, and glossitis; neurologic abnormalities are usually not seen. Normal pressure hydrocephalus is associated with the classic triad of dementia, incontinence, and gait disturbance.

629. **(D)** If Wernicke's is suspected, emergent administration of IV thiamine is essential, because many sequelae of thiamine deficiency

are reversible with this treatment; mistaken administration of thiamine is rarely harmful. A CT scan of the head should be ordered immediately in this case; optimally, the IV thiamine would be started as the CT was being arranged. The remaining choices do not address the urgent need to replete thiamine.

630. **(B)** This patient demonstrates a typical response to thiamine, namely, near complete resolution of her 6th nerve palsy, persistent nystagmus, and some improvement in her gait. However, as her acute delirium and apathy clear, an underlying inability to learn and retain new information emerges. This is known as Korsakoff's psychosis; the amnestic state is best described as anterograde amnesia. Korsakoff's psychosis is also caused by thiamine deficiency but is usually hidden by the acute delirium of Wernicke's encephalopathy. Immediate memory and attention are normal; this would not be true in delirium. Some degree of alcoholic dementia and Alzheimer's disease may be present as well, but the clinical setting most strongly points to Korsakoff's.

631. **(C)** The encapsulated, fixed delusion seen here is typical of delusional disorder. The delusion in this illness is most often of the persecutory sort, as in this case, but may well be somatic, jealous, grandiose, and so on. While this delusion is plausible, albeit unlikely, the delusions encountered in schizophrenia and brief psychotic disorder tend to be more bizarre and impossible, such as believing that others are controlling one's thoughts. Paranoid personality disorder does not present as a fixed, isolated delusion; rather, you would see a more pervasive paranoia permeating many aspects of the patient's life. Patients with MDD with psychotic features suffer from delusions or other psychotic symptoms that are mood congruent (e.g., "my organs are rotting").

632. **(C)** This patient is clearly psychotic and the delusion has progressed sufficiently far as to render the patient potentially dangerous to others. Therefore, most clinicians would pre-

fer to address his delusional thinking with an antipsychotic, in this case olanzapine, a newer atypical antipsychotic. Although alprazolam, a short-acting benzodiazepine, might provide temporary relief from the stress of the delusion, it would provide little long-term benefit. ECT, lithium, and SSRIs have been shown to be helpful in some cases of delusional disorder, but they would not be a first choice in this patient with severe psychosis.

633. **(D)** While tactile and olfactory hallucinations may be present, the presence of auditory hallucinations would suggest a diagnosis such as schizophrenia. In delusional disorder, the delusions are not bizarre (logically impossible); usually, they have some internal logic and could conceivably be possible. As in this case, negative symptoms are not generally a part of the presentation. The most common delusions are of the persecutory type.

634. **(B)** This patient presents initially with a delirium. Delirium is characterized by an acute change in mental status, a waxing and waning sensorium, and difficulty attending; it is most commonly induced by metabolic derangement, infection, or drug intoxication or withdrawal. While each of the other choices in this question may cause delirium, diagnosis may not be reasonably limited to any one of these with the information initially presented.

635. **(E)** NMS is characterized by severe ("lead pipe") rigidity, change in mental status, autonomic instability, elevated CPK, and elevated white blood count; a slight elevation in cerebrospinal fluid protein count is possible. NMS may be induced by any neuroleptic, including the newer atypicals. No one symptom is necessary for the diagnosis; instead, a constellation of symptoms and their severity, in a setting of neuroleptic exposure, makes the diagnosis more or less likely. Anticholinergic syndrome, resulting from overdosing on anticholinergic medications, does not produce rigidity and an elevated CPK. Malignant hyperthermia, an acute muscular patho-

logic process, resembles NMS, but follows the administration of inhaled anesthetic agents, as in general surgery. A diagnosis of CNS infection would be better supported by findings on the lumbar puncture and CT or MRI scan; an elevated CPK would be possible if the CNS infection caused seizures. Prolonged immobilization could result in an elevated CPK, but would not account for the other findings.

636. **(D)** NMS is a life-threatening illness with a significant mortality. The rhabdomyolysis induced by NMS may cause acute renal failure. This patient's CPK may be trending upward; his elevated creatinine suggests at least early renal insult. He should be closely monitored and hydrated in the medical intensive care unit; once stable, he could be transferred to a general medical unit or a psychiatry unit experienced in NMS.

637. **(B)** While there is some evidence that dopamine agonists, such as bromocriptine (Parlodel) and amantadine (Symmetrel), may be beneficial in NMS, if NMS is suspected, the treatment of choice is to stop all neuroleptics and to manage the various symptoms supportively. After recovery, should restarting a neuroleptic be indicated, the recommendation is to try a lower-potency neuroleptic from a different class, in a monitored setting. Recurrence of NMS is possible but usually does not occur. Treating the patient with antibiotics is not helpful, as the cause of the elevated WBC count and temperature is the NMS, not an infection. Anticholinergic medications can exacerbate delirium.

638. **(C)** Command auditory hallucinations are a psychiatric emergency, and most clinicians would agree that this patient should be restarted on a neuroleptic. Because they are long-acting (i.e., hard to stop), depot injections of a neuroleptic would not be a first choice. As the patient is not violent, physical restraints should be avoided. ECT has some efficacy in treatment-resistant schizophrenia but is not a first-line therapy.

639. (D) With her anhedonia, decreased sleep and appetite, suicidal ideation, and feelings of worthlessness, this patient meets criteria for MDD. In this case, the depression is accompanied by psychotic features. Adjustment disorder is the development of behavioral or emotional symptoms in response to a particular stressor. The fact that she meets criteria for MDD, and the intensity of her symptoms, rule out adjustment disorder. While we may be seeing the depressive phase of a bipolar illness, and she in fact may have bipolar illness, we are given no direct clues for this in the history. Delusional disorder would not be accompanied by the extent of affective symptoms seen in this case, nor would a brief psychotic disorder.

640. (C) Command auditory hallucinations to perform suicidal attempts such as overdosing on medications are a psychiatric emergency, and in virtually all cases would require a psychiatric admission. We are given no clues that there is a necessity to admit the patient to a medical unit; however, she will need a complete medical workup to rule out organic causes of depression. This can usually be accomplished on a psychiatric unit. We are given no indication, such as violent behavior, that this patient needs to be restrained.

641. (C) This patient requires an antidepressant. Treating her depression will likely relieve her psychotic symptoms as well, but the antidepressant cannot be expected to start taking effect for at least a week, and likely longer. Therefore, many clinicians would add a neuroleptic, a class of drugs that is relatively quick acting, to treat her auditory hallucinations. A TCA would not be the first choice. First, there is a suggestion that this patient has some cardiac history, and the tricyclics can have a proarrhythmia effect. Second, unlike SSRIs, tricyclics can be lethal in overdose, and this patient has risk factors for overdose. Lithium does have some antidepressant effects, but in the absence of convincing evidence that this patient has a bipolar disorder, lithium would not be used. (If this patient has only a partial response to the SSRI,

lithium may at some point in the future be added for augmentation.) While a benzodiazepine may help this patient's irritability, as a sole agent it would be a poor choice for treating her depression and psychosis.

642. (B) This patient's grandiosity, sleeplessness, intense involvement in goal-directed activity, agitation, and anger all suggest he is in the manic phase of severe bipolar I disorder. The history offered by the family indicates he may have had an earlier episode. It is common for stressful life events, such as graduating from college and getting a new job, to incite a mania. His disorganized behavior and delusional thinking would place his illness at the severe end of the spectrum and would qualify it as bipolar disorder with psychotic features. Bipolar II disorder is characterized by MDD alternating with hypomania. Because this patient's symptoms cause marked impairment in his functioning and include psychotic features, he is in the midst of a manic, not hypomanic, episode. Adjustment disorder would be ruled out because of the psychosis and other severe symptoms seen in this patient. This patient's mood-congruent delusions and mania make a diagnosis of schizophrenia less likely than bipolar disorder.

643. (B) Initial medications in this case would be aimed at the target symptoms of agitation, delusional thinking, and disruptive behavior and could reasonably include a neuroleptic and a benzodiazepine. While he clearly needs a mood stabilizer such as lithium or carbamazepine as well, these would not be expected to start showing an effect for at least a week and are not the critical medications to start emergently in the emergency department. SSRIs must be used with extreme caution in bipolar illness, as they can incite or exacerbate mania. Buspirone is an anxiolytic used mostly in GAD. It is of extremely limited use in bipolar disorder and would not adequately address the target symptoms seen in this case.

644. (D) When the patient returns for his first follow-up visit, his lithium level is therapeutic at 0.8 mEq/L and is not in need of adjustment. However, his muscle stiffness is a parkinsonian side effect of haloperidol. This is normally treated by lowering the dose of the neuroleptic or with anticholinergic medication, not with a muscle relaxant such as baclofen. However, once an acute manic episode is in remission, as in this case, a trial of discontinuing the neuroleptic may be a safe way to address the parkinsonian side effect. The patient would have to be followed closely for reemergence of psychotic symptoms.

645. (A) The patient is showing signs of lithium toxicity. Lithium toxicity often occurs in a setting of dehydration, as is probably the case here, in which the patient recently was ill and febrile. Any lithium level greater than 2.5 mEq/L is considered toxic and may well cause a generalized convulsion, in addition to delirium, cardiovascular collapse, and even death. This is a medical emergency and is best treated with dialysis to decrease the lithium level. While this patient's TSH level suggests hypothyroidism (a common sequela of lithium treatment), it is not severe enough to account for any of the symptoms seen here.

646. (B) Acute stress disorder is a reaction that causes clinically significant disruption or distress in a patient who witnesses or somehow participates in a traumatic event. The event must be quite horrible, invoking in the patient intense fear, and usually involves death or threatened death. The typical symptoms include hyperarousal states, dissociative states, and intrusive reexperiencing of the event (e.g., flashbacks and avoidance behaviors). PTSD is similar in most respects to acute distress disorder, but in PTSD the symptoms persist for at least 4 weeks following the trauma; a shorter duration suggests a diagnosis of acute distress disorder. The patient does not appear to be suffering from any of the typical criteria for MDD or adjustment disorder, except for guilt. While she is

suffering from agoraphobia, a symptom consistent with an acute stress reaction, there is no evidence of panic disorder.

647. (D) In initiating benzodiazepine treatment, one of the most important considerations is the presence of current or past drug or alcohol abuse. Because of their affinity for gamma-aminobutyric acid (GABA) receptors (the same receptors bound by alcohol), all benzodiazepines have a potential for abuse and should be used in extreme caution in patients with significant drug use history. While half-life and drug metabolism issues (e.g., aging and liver function) are important, these can be addressed through appropriate selection of the benzodiazepine, dose, and frequency of dosing. For example, in a patient with compromised kidney function, one would not choose a benzodiazepine cleared principally by the kidney.

648. (C) While MDD, panic disorder with agoraphobia, and adjustment disorder are all in the differential diagnosis at the initial presentation and should be carefully considered, MDD does not emerge as a clear diagnosis until the third question in this case. At this time, the principal symptoms of the acute stress disorder have remitted, and the classic symptoms of depression—feelings of sadness, loss of interest, a change in sleep habits, tearfulness, and change in appetite—are apparent. These outweigh the earlier working diagnoses.

649. (A) MDD may be rooted in a medical condition that can be unearthed through routine blood work. A search for vitamin B_{12} or folate deficiency, hypothyroidism, and electrolyte disturbances should be undertaken as part of the workup. While an ECG, a head CT scan, neurologic consultation, and chest x-ray may also each reveal a finding that could be contributing to or causing the depression, without a specific indication, these are less often routinely obtained.

650. (B) The first choice in pharmacologic treatment in MDD is an SSRI such as paroxetine.

Amitriptyline, a TCA, is likely to be equally efficacious as the SSRIs in depression but has more side effects, is more dangerous in overdose, and is less often used as first-line therapy. The remaining choices each target symptoms other than depression. In some cases, each of these may be used to address some symptoms that frequently accompany depression, but only as an adjunct to the antidepressant. Haloperidol is an antipsychotic. Clonazepam is a long-acting benzodiazepine used for anxiety. Clonidine is an alpha-adrenergic antagonist used for hypertension that has shown some usefulness in addressing hyperactivity and stress disorders.

651. **(E)** This is a description of an acute dystonic reaction, an intense muscle spasm induced usually by a high-potency neuroleptic. It is thought to be related to the imbalance in blockage of dopamine receptors versus cholinergic receptors. (High-potency neuroleptics block dopamine receptors to a greater extent than cholinergic receptors.) Akathisia is a subjective, uncomfortable feeling of restlessness induced by neuroleptic treatment. While abrupt discontinuation of benzodiazepines and SSRIs both may result in withdrawal symptoms, these symptoms do not include the so-called oculogyric crisis (spasm of the muscles of extraocular motion) seen in this case.

652. **(C)** Oculogyric crisis is a specific example of an acute dystonic reaction in which there is spasm of the muscles of extraocular motion. Torticollis and retrocollis refer to muscle spasms that cause abnormal positioning of the head. Trismus is a spasm of the jaw muscles. NMS, also a reaction to neuroleptic medications, is characterized by dystonia, autonomic instability, and usually some degree of delirium.

653. **(B)** Most cases of acute dystonias will occur within days of initiation of neuroleptic therapy. Young men are the most commonly affected population of acute dystonias, more commonly in reaction to high-potency (rather than low-potency) neuroleptics. Acute dystonias can occur in any muscle group. Besides

muscles of extraocular motion and muscles that position the head and jaw, it can affect muscles controlling swallowing, speech, and limb and trunk positions.

654. **(A)** The most concerning aspect of acute dystonic reactions is the possibility of laryngeal muscle spasm, which can result in airway obstruction. This must always be immediately assessed in all cases. Acute dystonic reactions are extremely uncomfortable, often giving rise to compliance problems with neuroleptic medications afterward, but this is not the primary concern at the time of presentation. Malignant hypertension, autonomic instability, and acute renal failure are not associated with acute dystonic reactions, but are associated with NMS.

655. **(C)** The treatment of choice is immediate administration of an anticholinergic or antihistaminergic medication. Beta blockers, muscle relaxants, and hydration are not directly helpful. An anxiolytic may be helpful as adjunctive therapy to anticholinergic or antihistaminergic medications but does not directly address the problem.

656. **(A)** Regardless of a patient's past psychiatric diagnosis, organic causes of physical signs and symptoms must always be ruled out. The anxiety disorders, while intensely distressing and uncomfortable to patients, rarely, if ever, result in unconsciousness. Many aspects of the patient's story seem to be related to anxiety and could in fact occur during a panic attack, but this patient's presentation is more consistent with ischemic heart disease and should prompt a cardiac workup.

657. **(D)** Benzodiazepines, SSRIs, and cognitive–behavioral therapy each have a place in treatment of the anxiety disorders. In this case, however, these should not be considered until an organic cause is ruled out.

658. **(B)** Most clinicians agree that after 10 weeks at a reasonable dose, if one SSRI isn't working, it's time to stop the medication and try a new one. Monoamine oxidase inhibitors

(MAOIs), however, require a 2-week washout period before initiation. Lithium is usually used only as augmentation to antidepressant medication when at least a partial response is obtained from the antidepressant. In the absence of evidence that the depression has remitted, there is no advantage gained in discontinuing all medications.

659. **(E)** This woman's binge eating and purging behaviors, as well as her amenorrhea and eroded dental enamel, strongly argue for an eating disorder. The fact that her weight is above the 85th percentile rules out a diagnosis of anorexia nervosa. While amenorrhea is not part of the diagnostic criteria for bulimia (as it is for anorexia), many bulimic patients will present with dysfunction of the menstrual cycle. Regardless of the clinical presentation, other causes of amenorrhea must be ruled out. More than half of patients with eating disorders will have a comorbid diagnosis of an affective or anxiety disorder.

660. **(E)** Despite the tremendous toll binge eating and purging takes on the body, thyroid function tends to remain intact. However, each of the other choices offers the opposite trend in what one tends to find in bulimia. Laboratory abnormalities include hypokalemic, hypochloremic alkalosis; high serum amylase; and hypomagnesemia. The salivary and parotid glands and the pancreas tend to enlarge.

661. **(A)** Binge eating and purging may be seen in both anorexia and in bulimia. The principal difference is, if the binge eating and purging occur in a setting of low body weight (less than 85% expected), the diagnosis shifts toward anorexia. The diagnosis of bulimia can be made if any extraordinary measure—vomiting, laxative or diuretic abuse, fasting, or vigorous exercising—is employed in the service of negating the binge-eating behavior. Laxative abuse should always be asked about, because it is commonly employed and frequently hidden, as are most purging behaviors. Ninety percent or more of eating disorders are diagnosed in women. Amenorrhea

is a necessary criterion of the diagnosis of anorexia nervosa for all postmenarchal and premenopausal women.

662. **(D)** The fluid shifts and electrolyte imbalances introduced by excessive vomiting may cause seizures. Because of the life-threatening nature of severe bulimia, hospitalization is often required. Medications have been of limited success in the treatment of anorexia. However, many studies have documented the benefits of SSRIs and TCAs in controlling bulimic behaviors. Simply prescribing an SSRI to this patient, however, would be a woefully inadequate intervention. Typically, bulimic patients are steered toward a combination of pharmacotherapy and some form of talk therapy (e.g., cognitive–behavioral therapy, group therapy).

663. **(B)** The key points in this case presentation are the absence of a previous psychiatric history and the duration of symptoms. Before diagnosing a mental illness, it is necessary to rule out the effects of a substance. A urine toxicology screen usually includes opiates, cocaine, and PCP. Amphetamines, cocaine, and PCP intoxication can mimic symptoms of schizophrenia. While a CT scan is helpful to rule out a mass lesion or bleeding, it is not likely in this age group, nor is it likely, given the nonfocal neurologic exam, to provide further information influencing treatment. Liver function tests, CBC, and ESR are unlikely to aid in the diagnosis.

664. **(C)** Delusions, hallucinations, and disorganized behavior are some of the hallmark symptoms of schizophrenia. As the symptoms have been present for more than 1 month but less than 6 months, and there is no previous psychiatric history, the most appropriate diagnosis is schizophreniform disorder. There is no history suggestive of a mood disorder, and thus major depression with psychotic features is not correct. The toxicology screen is negative, so the diagnosis of substance-induced mood disorder is less likely. Delusional disorder usually manifests

in a person who is functional in society, with the exception of a circumscribed delusion, which can be of the jealous, erotomanic, grandiose, persecutory, or somatic type. The patient is also suffering hallucinations, which in combination with delusions exclude the diagnosis of delusional disorder.

665. **(D)** The appropriate medication would be a neuroleptic such as haloperidol or clozapine. Clozapine is an atypical antipsychotic, and due to the 1% risk of agranulocytosis, it is reserved for people with treatment-resistant schizophrenia or neuroleptic-induced tardive dyskinesia. Haloperidol would therefore be the treatment of choice. Lorazepam could be used as an adjunctive medication for agitation in psychotic individuals but is not used as monotherapy to treat psychosis. Benztropine is commonly used with high-potency neuroleptics such as haloperidol to minimize the likelihood of extrapyramidal side effects and dystonic reactions. Lactulose is commonly used as a laxative and has no role in the treatment of psychotic illness.

666. **(D)** In this setting, the patient's subjective description of anxiety combined with tremulousness, diaphoresis, and elevated vital signs while afebrile strongly suggest alcohol withdrawal. Cannabis withdrawal may occur in long-term users, but the drug is considered psychologically, not physiologically, addictive. Similarly, opiate withdrawal is highly uncomfortable, but autonomic instability with elevated vital signs is not common.

667. **(C)** Benzodiazepines are the treatment of choice for alcohol withdrawal. Any benzodiazepine can be used—the choice depends on the desired route of delivery or the presence of liver dysfunction. With abnormal liver function tests, lorazepam or oxazepam (Serax) would be chosen because they are primarily metabolized and eliminated renally instead of through the liver as are the other benzodiazepines. Additionally, lorazepam may be chosen because it can be given intravenously, intramuscularly, or orally. Methadone or cloni-

dine may be used for opiate withdrawal. Carbamazepine in conjunction with propranolol has been advocated in some settings for alcohol withdrawal, but carbamazepine is not used as single-agent therapy. Naltrexone has been used to help maintain abstinence from alcohol but has no efficacy in withdrawal.

668. **(C)** Alcohol withdrawal can be life threatening. Tremors begin about 6 to 8 hours after cessation, followed within 8 to 12 hours by psychotic and perceptual abnormalities (hallucinosis). Seizures may follow anywhere from 12 to 72 hours after cessation. Delirium tremens (DTs) may occur any time in the first week of abstinence. Untreated DTs have a mortality rate of approximately 20%. Fatty liver is a long-term consequence of alcohol abuse. Abdominal pain and muscle cramps can be symptoms of opiate withdrawal.

669. **(A)** There are a few classical features of PCP intoxication in this case, including ataxia, nystagmus (either vertical or horizontal), agitation, tachycardia, psychosis, and hyperthermia (helps to explain why patient was found naked). Additionally, abnormal movements such as grimacing, head rolling, and stroking have also been described. While there is some overlap with stimulant or cocaine intoxication, nystagmus, ataxia, and unusual movements are unique to PCP intoxication. Brief psychotic disorder and chronic paranoid schizophrenia are not appropriate diagnoses in this setting as it is most important to rule out a substance-induced psychotic disorder.

670. **(E)** A toxicology screen would be the best way to diagnose this condition. Often, a urine toxicology screen will include opiates, cocaine, and PCP, but this may vary depending on individual institutions. There is no indication for an EEG at this time because no seizure history is elicited and the patient does not appear postictal. While structural brain lesions can cause psychotic symptoms, substance-induced symptoms are more common in this age group. A nonfocal neurologic

exam would further decrease the likelihood that imaging studies would alter the diagnosis or treatment plan in this case.

671. **(A)** Unless the patient is extremely agitated and at risk for hurting himself or others, the best choice for treatment would be to place him in a quiet, dark (low stimulation) room. If the patient is violent and/or psychotic, a combination of neuroleptics and benzodiazepines could be used to keep the patient safe. Methylphenidate is a stimulant; benztropine, used to prevent extrapyramidal symptoms associated with neuroleptic use, might worsen the patient's delirium. Since the patient is not suffering a seizure or at risk for seizures, phenytoin is not indicated.

672. **(B)** The most likely outcome is that the patient will completely recover in the next 24 to 48 hours. However, some patients can remain psychotic for periods as long as 2 weeks after being intoxicated with PCP. In this setting, the patient could be monitored for 1 to 2 days in the emergency department and discharged home. In the less likely event that the patient's symptoms do not resolve, then a brief inpatient hospitalization may be required. There is no need for further neurologic evaluation at this time. Long-term psychiatric hospitalization is unlikely in this setting.

673. **(B)** The first part of the vignette illustrates some of the features of opiate intoxication, namely pupillary constriction, drowsiness, impaired attention and memory, and slurred speech. In the second interaction, the patient shows signs and symptoms of opiate withdrawal. Yawning, muscle aches, diarrhea, lacrimation or rhinorrhea, and fever are all typical of opiate withdrawal. Additionally, mildly elevated vital signs may occur; however, tachycardia and hypertension should always signal possible alcohol withdrawal. Pharmacologic management of withdrawal can include clonidine, a centrally acting alpha-2 agonist; buprenorphine, a mixed opiate agonist/antagonist; and methadone, a synthetic long-acting opiate. Lorazepam can be used to treat elevated vital signs.

674. **(B)** Your concern is greatest with sudden discontinuation of any sedative, hypnotic, or anxiolytic agent, which can cause seizures. Triazolam (Halcion) is a short-acting benzodiazepine. Thioridazine and fluphenazine are neuroleptics, and nortriptyline and imipramine are TCAs. Neither TCAs nor neuroleptics cause life-threatening withdrawal symptoms.

675. **(B)** As with the sudden discontinuation of alcohol, benzodiazepine or barbiturate withdrawal can be life-threatening. Withdrawal symptoms include tremors; anxiety; auditory, visual, and tactile hallucinations; autonomic hyperactivity; and seizures. The onset of symptoms depends on the half-life of the medication, the dose, and duration of use. The most concerning discontinuation side effect would be seizures.

676. **(A)** The best way to determine if the patient is withdrawing is to check the vital signs for autonomic instability. Of note, a phenobarbital challenge is performed to assess the amount of phenobarbital needed to keep a patient from withdrawing from barbiturates. Wada's test is the intracarotid administration of amytal, used to assess hemispheric language dominance.

677. **(D)** The patient is exhibiting typical signs of delirium, including impaired consciousness and difficulty with cognition, manifested as drowsiness and disorientation. Classically, these symptoms may fluctuate during the day. Patients who meet criteria for delirium may appear depressed with a decreased level of arousal or may appear overly active and energetic, with the depressed type occurring more commonly. Patients also show cognitive and memory impairments, which may be manifested as disorientation or decreased capacity to register, retain, and recall information. An MMSE during periods of delirium may be misleadingly low, suggesting a dementing or pseudodementing process. In this setting, it is important to gather information from the people who know the patient to evaluate for a possible coexisting depression

or dementia. Risk factors for delirium are extremes of age, prior history of delirium, alcohol dependence, sensory impairment (auditory or visual), and preexisting brain damage. There is a broad etiologic differential for delirium. In this case, causative factors may be infection, hypoxia, metabolic abnormalities, and current medications.

678. **(E)** Haloperidol is the drug of choice for managing the agitated or confused patient with delirium. Thioridazine, benztropine, and diphenhydramine all have anticholinergic properties that may exacerbate delirium. Lorazepam, especially in older patients, may have a paradoxical effect and exacerbate agitation and confusion. Haloperidol in low doses, such as 0.5 mg every 8 hours, will help manage the agitated patient. It has the advantage of intramuscular, intravenous, or oral administration.

679. **(A)** The most important next step is to perform a physical exam. Particular attention should be concentrated on the neurologic exam, looking for any evidence of focal deficit that would suggest an acute neurologic event that may have led to the sudden decline. The remainder of the test may be helpful in assessing the etiology of the deficit.

680. **(C)** A sudden decline in an otherwise slowly progressive course should alert the clinician to evaluate for an underlying cause. In this case, the patient is hypertensive, which increases the risk for stroke and therefore vascular dementia. Further workup for reversible causes of dementia should include a CBC with differential; electrolytes; BUN; creatinine; B_{12}; folate; VDRL; calcium, magnesium, and phosphorus; urinalysis; ESR; urine toxicology screen; thyroid studies; liver function tests; ECG; and chest x-ray. If focal neurologic deficits are found on the neurologic exam, a noncontrast head CT could be helpful in the assessment. The differential diagnosis of dementia includes pseudodementia (depression) and delirium. Depressed individuals may show evidence of cognitive impairment that can appear identical to dementia, which makes obtaining a history from those who know the patient crucial. Similarly, delirium may also present with cognitive deficits. In delirious states, these tend to fluctuate over time and may be associated with periods of agitation and confusion. Alzheimer's dementia is the most common form of dementia, followed by vascular dementia. Together, these account for between 70 and 80% of all dementias.

681. **(C)** This patient is exhibiting cognitive and memory difficulties consistent with a dementing process. Cognitive abnormalities seen in dementia include agnosia, aphasia, apraxia, and loss of executive function. This woman shows apraxic disturbances manifested as inability or diminished ability to carry out motor tasks, for example, dressing and eating. Loss of executive function is demonstrated by difficulties with paying bills. Finally, she also shows memory problems such as losing her purse and remembering recently learned information.

682. **(D)** This patient is exhibiting signs and symptoms consistent with MDD with psychotic features. For more than 2 weeks, the patient has displayed depressed mood, loss of interest in pleasurable activities, weight loss, inability to concentrate, poor sleep, and guilt about her current depressive state. She is also suffering delusional-type concerns about bodily functioning and possible infection. If the patient were complaining of contamination fears, and performing multiple compulsive tasks to rid herself of the pathogens, a diagnosis of OCD with comorbid depression could be considered. Somatization disorder would be characterized by more somatic complaints as well as at least one neurologic and pain symptom. Dysthymia would present with a chronic moderate level of depressive symptoms, but this patient is describing an episodic decompensation over the last month.

683. **(B)** Because of the delusional quality to her presentation, it is reasonable to treat this patient with a neuroleptic such as perphenazine for a few days prior to beginning a trial of an antidepressant. Antidepressants alone or with benzodiazepines would not help with the delusional aspects of her symptoms. Similarly, lithium and valproic acid would be used as mood stabilizers in bipolar depression or mania, but not commonly in the treatment of unipolar depression.

684. **(C)** The patient presents with classic symptoms and signs of schizophrenia, including delusions, hallucinations, and negative symptoms (flat affect and anhedonia). He has also had a marked change in his ability to care for himself and to attend school. Because these symptoms have been occurring for more than 1 month but less than 6 months, the appropriate diagnosis is schizophreniform disorder. Chronic schizophrenia would be the diagnosis if the symptoms had been occurring for more than 6 months.

685. **(C)** Brief psychotic disorder is diagnosed when symptoms have been persistent for more than 1 day but less than 1 month. Delusional disorder is a rare condition in which the primary symptoms are delusions that are usually nonbizarre; that is, they could occur. Delusional disorder is further classified into subtypes, including grandiose, jealous, persecutory, somatic, erotomanic, and unspecified. There are no symptoms of a mood disorder, and the other associated symptoms of schizophrenia are not present.

686. **(A)** The most helpful test would be a urine toxicology screen. Intoxication with a variety of substances including cocaine, PCP, or amphetamines may mimic the symptoms of schizophrenia, and thus it is necessary to rule out these intoxication syndromes. A CT scan would help rule out a mass lesion or a bleed, but in this age group and with a nonfocal neurologic exam, it is unlikely to contribute to the diagnosis and treatment. Because the patient does not present with signs or symptoms of a seizure disorder, an EEG is unlikely to provide information that will impact the diagnosis in this case. There is no diagnostic finding on CBC or electrolytes specific for any of the psychotic disorders.

687. **(D)** The treatment for any of the psychotic disorders should begin with a neuroleptic. In this case, haloperidol, a traditional neuroleptic, would be used rather than clozapine. Clozapine is an atypical antipsychotic that, because of its risk for agranulocytosis, is traditionally reserved for individuals whose disease processes are resistant to other medications or those who cannot tolerate other medications. Lithium is used traditionally for treatment of bipolar disorder. ECT had been used until as recently as the 1970s for schizophrenia but is not a first-line treatment. Psychotherapy may be helpful in the recovery phase but has limited utility in the acute phase of schizophrenia.

688. **(B)** Acute dystonic reactions are more common in young males and with high-potency antipsychotics such as haloperidol. Acute reactions may occur within a few hours after administration. The patient may describe difficulty swallowing or moving his tongue, or stiffness in the muscles around the head and neck. Laryngeal spasm may also occur and can be life-threatening. Treatment may be with either benztropine or diphenhydramine. More haloperidol would be contraindicated. Ketorolac is an injectable form of nonsteroidal anti-inflammatory medication that has no utility in the treatment of acute dystonic reactions. Demerol is also a pain reliever, but would have limited efficacy in this situation. Similarly, lorazepam would be sedating but would not be the most appropriate medication.

689. **(E)** Poor sleep, decreased concentration, thoughts of death, weight loss, feelings of guilt, and depressed mood are all symptoms consistent with a *Diagnostic and Statistical Manual of Mental Disorders*, 4th ed., Text Revision (DSM-IV-TR) diagnosis of MDD. For this patient, the symptoms have been occurring for more than 2 weeks and have caused difficulty with the patient's social and occupational functioning. While this illness seems to have occurred after the death of the patient's grandmother, the diagnosis of bereavement is usually made within 2 months of the death,

and the symptoms are usually not as severe in bereavement as with MDD. This episode could also represent the depressed phase of bipolar illness, but given the lack of personal or family mental illness history, it is less likely. Dysthymic disorder is not appropriate; although dysthymia has similar depressive symptoms, it usually occurs chronically over at least a 2-year period. Adjustment disorder usually occurs within 3 months of a stressor. The symptoms exhibited by this patient are in excess of what would be expected in this disorder.

690. **(B)** There are two choices for antidepressants in this group. Phenelzine, an MAOI, would not be the first choice of antidepressant because the SSRIs have a more favorable side effect profile, are safer in overdose, and have similar efficacy in the treatment of MDD. Fluoxetine, therefore, would be the best choice at this time. Triazolam is a benzodiazepine, flumazenil is an opioid antagonist, and fluphenazine is an antipsychotic.

691. **(A)** SSRIs have a number of side effects, including diarrhea, constipation, insomnia, nausea, headache, sexual dysfunction, and agitation. The side effect shared by the symptoms of depression is insomnia. Constipation and akathisia are also common side effects of antipsychotics.

692. **(B)** This patient is presenting with both depressive and manic symptoms, which is consistent with the diagnosis of a mixed episode of bipolar disorder. The manic symptoms are irritable mood, decreased sleep, flight of ideas, increase in pleasurable or goal-directed activity (e.g., a spending spree on stocks), and rapid speech. His depressive symptoms are decreased concentration, depressed mood, and suicidal ideation. A manic episode usually presents with elated or euphoric mood, rather than irritability, and there are usually no depressive symptoms. A hypomanic episode usually presents with similar symptoms as a manic episode, but the disturbance is not so great as to cause difficulty with everyday activities. Cyclothymia is a mood

disturbance occurring over at least a 2-year period with both hypomanic and depressive symptoms that are not severe enough to be considered a major depressive episode.

693. **(D)** It is essential to evaluate whether the behavioral disturbance is caused by an exogenous substance. The symptoms of bipolar illness can be mimicked by intoxication by a number of substances, including amphetamines and cocaine. A CT scan, VDRL, ESR, and electrolytes may all be appropriate to evaluate initially but are unlikely to change the diagnosis, and therefore will be of limited utility in making the diagnosis of bipolar illness.

694. **(D)** Given the severity of this patient's symptoms, it is likely that he will require the use of both lorazepam and valproic acid to control his illness. Valproic acid can be loaded rapidly to achieve therapeutic blood levels in 3 to 5 days. Prior to the onset of mood-stabilizing properties, a benzodiazepine such as lorazepam can be useful in keeping the patient calm.

695. **(A)** Valproic acid may cause a transient, asymptomatic elevation in the transaminases in approximately one third of patients. This usually occurs in the first few months of therapy. Prior to the induction of treatment, checking liver function tests is warranted to evaluate for the presence of hepatic disease and to establish a baseline. The drug should not affect kidney or heart function, so BUN, creatinine, and an ECG are not necessary.

696. **(E)** Adjustment disorder is characterized by the onset of emotional or behavioral disturbances within 3 months of a significant life event that may manifest as marked change in an individual's ability to function in school, work, or interpersonal relationships. The disturbances are not so severe, however, as to suggest the diagnosis of another disorder such as MDD. The differential diagnosis for adjustment disorder includes mood disorders such as MDD and anxiety disorders such as PTSD, GAD, and acute stress disorder. In this

case, the patient may be suffering from depressed mood but does not have other neurovegetative signs of depression. Acute stress disorder is usually diagnosed when an individual who has experienced an extreme stressor has dissociative experiences and anxiety after the stressful experience. This patient is not describing these symptoms. Similarly, PTSD usually requires exposure to or witnessing of a life-threatening event, with episodes of reexperiencing the event and making efforts to avoid settings that may remind the patient of that experience. In this case, the patient has experienced a significant stressor, but it is not a life-threatening event that is usually required for the diagnosis of acute stress response or PTSD. Bereavement is the normal response to the loss or death of an individual close to the patient.

697. **(C)** The diagnosis of adjustment disorder does not usually require pharmacotherapeutic intervention, but instead may respond to supportive individual or group psychotherapy. Risperidone is an atypical antipsychotic. Fluoxetine is an SSRI, while nortriptyline is a TCA and alprazolam is a benzodiazepine.

698. **(B)** This patient is describing symptoms associated with panic disorder. This disorder occurs in late adolescence or the early twenties and is more common in women than in men. People typically describe feelings of fear, dread, or intense discomfort associated with a variety of somatic symptoms, including tachycardia, chest pain, shortness of breath, tremulousness, diaphoresis, nausea, fears of dying, paresthesias, light-headedness, and hot or cold flashes. The diagnosis of agoraphobia is made when fears of having an attack or being unable to leave a place where they are having an attack force patients to remain in familiar places. The medical workup for panic disorder includes CBC, electrolytes, fasting glucose, calcium, liver function tests, BUN, creatinine, urinalysis, toxicology screen, ECG, and thyroid function studies. A careful substance abuse and caffeine intake history should also be taken. Social phobia or social anxiety disorder occurs

in the context of public appearances or performances. Individuals may experience anxiety and fear. These feelings cause great distress and may cause people to limit or avoid these settings. This disorder differs from panic disorder by having an identifiable trigger. Separation anxiety disorder is commonly diagnosed in young children when separated from their primary caregiver. GAD occurs in individuals experiencing continued anxiety and worry for periods greater than 6 months, occurring throughout the day. Unlike panic disorder, there do not seem to be discrete episodes.

699. **(A)** A variety of medications, including SSRIs (sertraline), TCAs, MAOIs (tranylcypromine), and benzodiazepines (alprazolam) have been used to treat panic disorder. While all have shown some efficacy in the treatment of panic, SSRIs are usually the first agent of choice because they are generally well tolerated, with fewer side effects than TCAs or MAOIs, and lack the dependency potential of benzodiazepines. Common side effects include sexual dysfunction, gastrointestinal disturbances, and insomnia. Lithium is used in the treatment of bipolar disorder, while propranolol is used for social phobia.

700. **(C)** The patient has OCD in which she suffers from recurrent, intrusive, unwanted thoughts or images (obsessions) and either repetitive behavior or mental acts (compulsions) that are performed in response to these obsessions. Patients realize that the obsessions and compulsions are intrusive, unreasonable, and unwanted and cause marked impairment in their lives. Many patients with OCD may hide their symptoms and may first come to the attention of other medical specialties. Somatization disorder presents with numerous somatic complaints that cannot be fully explained by the results of medical investigations. GAD is an appropriate diagnosis in people who have worries and concerns that are not limited to any particular aspect of their lives, with the anxiety significantly impairing their ability to function. Panic disorder occurs as recurrent, discrete episodes of

extreme anxiety and fear that occur unexpectedly and remit spontaneously.

701. **(A)** A common intervention for OCD is cognitive–behavioral therapy, during which the patient is exposed to the threat or fear (obsession) with the response (handwashing) prevented for progressively longer periods of time until the behavior is extinguished. SSRIs have been successful in treatment of OCD. Risperidone is an atypical neuroleptic that is used to treat psychotic disorders. Lithium is used in the treatment of bipolar disorder and has not been shown to be effective in the treatment of OCD. Psychodynamic psychotherapy is intensive, long-term therapy that may be helpful for people who wish to better understand the nature of their relationship with others.

702. **(A)** Symptoms of excessive worry and anxiety occurring for over 6 months without discrete episodes are best characterized by the diagnosis of GAD. Other symptoms of GAD include sleep difficulties, irritability, and difficulty concentrating. Patients with GAD may also suffer from muscle tension, fatigue, and restlessness. While this patient does admit to anxiety, it does not occur in episodic fashion or in response to public performances, as with panic disorder or social phobia. Similarly, while the symptoms of anxiety and worry are in excess of what would be expected, they do not reach the magnitude characteristic for OCD, nor are any compulsions elicited. There is no evidence of psychosis or a thought disorder in this patient.

703. **(C)** The diagnosis of conversion disorder is most likely, given that the primary symptoms are neurologic and exhaustive workup is negative for evidence of pathology that accounts for the deficits. Neurologic deficits in conversion disorder involve either motor or sensory modalities and are felt to be a result of psychological stressors. Had the symptoms been intentionally produced, the diagnosis of factitious disorder or malingering would be appropriate. If the primary incentive for the behavior was to assume the sick role, the diagnosis would be factitious disorder. If the symptoms are feigned or exaggerated for another reason, such as to gain monetary reimbursement, the diagnosis would be malingering. Somatization disorder is not appropriate in this case because the number and types of complaints do not extend past the neurologic complaints. An undiagnosed neurologic condition is a possibility, but given the extensive workup, it is less likely. It is important to note that as many as 50% of those diagnosed with conversion disorder are eventually diagnosed with a neurologic condition that could have produced the initial symptoms.

704. **(E)** Factitious disorder is an appropriate diagnosis when physical or psychological symptoms are intentionally produced in order to assume the sick role. It must be clear that these symptoms are not intentionally produced for other reasons, such as avoiding work, gaining monetary compensation, or avoiding legal issues. If any of these reasons are present, the diagnosis is malingering. Somatization disorder presents with complaints of pain, gastrointestinal symptoms, sexual dysfunction, and pseudoneurologic symptoms. The diagnosis of hypochondriasis is incorrect as this patient is not preoccupied with the idea of having a severe disease that is unrecognized despite repeated reassurances by medical personnel. Classically, people with factitious disorder are more likely to be male and to have experience in health care. Often, these patients will have numerous admissions to many different hospitals with a variety of symptoms. The psychological factors underlying this disorder are not well understood. No effective form of psychotherapy or pharmacotherapy has been identified for the treatment of factitious disorder.

705. **(B)** Obtaining height and weight is crucial for establishing the diagnosis of anorexia nervosa. Patients with anorexia nervosa are unable to achieve or maintain greater than 85% of expected body weight for height and frame structure. Additionally, they have continued concerns about thinness and body image despite being underweight. In contrast, most patients with bulimia nervosa are of normal height and weight or are slightly overweight. Some people with bulimia nervosa engage in recurrent binge eating with compensatory purging (e.g., via vomiting or laxatives) or other behaviors to control weight in the absence of binge eating. Both disorders occur more commonly in women than in men. Anorexia tends to begin in the teens to twenties, while bulimia's onset is somewhat later in the twenties. Patients with anorexia have a higher risk of comorbid disorders, including depression and anxiety.

706. **(E)** Patients with eating disorders may have a variety of medical complications including (1) amenorrhea secondary to starvation and alterations in hormonal regulation, (2) electrolyte abnormalities (low serum magnesium and potassium) due to purging, (3) elevated amylase, and (4) loss of cardiac muscle with resulting conduction abnormalities detected by ECG. Body dysmorphic disorder is a somatoform disorder with a preoccupation of physical imperfection. Anorexia and bulimia are considered eating disorders and not somatoform disorders.

707. **(C)** Given the patient's history of angry, aggressive outbursts around not understanding school work and difficulties with socialization and caring for himself, along with a family history of learning disabilities, you suspect the diagnosis of mental retardation. A diagnosis of mental retardation includes subnormal functioning with an intelligence quotient (IQ) of less than 70. Either the WISC or the Stanford–Binet Intelligence Scale is an adequate instrument for estimating IQ. The MMPI-2 is frequently used to assess personality structure, while the Goodenough Draw-a-Person Test and Kohs Block Test assess visual–motor coordination. The Peabody Vocabulary Test is used when patients suffer from a language barrier.

708. **(B)** Mental retardation is classified according to severity based on IQ scores: mild mental retardation, 50 to 70; moderate, 35 to 49; severe, 20 to 34; and profound, less than 20. Borderline intellectual functioning is a term no longer in use, but referred to IQ scores in the 71 to 84 range.

709. **(A)** Tourette's disorder is a syndrome of multiple motor and vocal tics that occur daily for at least 1 year, with the onset before age 18. Tourette's occurs more commonly in males than females and is associated with attention deficits and obsessive and compulsive behaviors. Currently, it is unclear whether obsessive–compulsive behaviors and ADD behaviors are separate entities from Tourette's or if these behaviors are always comorbid. This patient demonstrates none of the psychoses that characterize childhood schizophrenia.

710. **(A)** Haloperidol is the most commonly prescribed drug used to treat the tics of Tourette's disorder, but pimozide, another neuroleptic, is also effective. Clozapine is not appropriate. Stimulants such as methylphenidate, when used to treat hyperactivity and attention deficits, may worsen tics. Clonidine has also been effective in treatment of Tourette's. Comorbid obsessive–compulsive symptoms may respond to an SSRI. Lorazepam is a benzodiazepine anxiolytic and would not treat the underlying disorder.

711. **(E)** Prior to induction of therapy with pimozide, and while in active treatment, ECGs should be performed to evaluate the QT interval. Pimozide has been associated with QT prolongation and an increased risk of ventricular arrhythmias.

712. **(D)** Epilepsy is a complex set of disorders that may initially come to the attention of a psychiatrist because of unusual behaviors. Complex partial seizures, in particular, may be associated with a wide range of symptoms, including sensory auras and automatic behaviors. Prior to the seizure, the patient may notice a bad smell, an unusual taste, or gastrointestinal symptoms. During the event,

the patient may look dazed or frightened and may exhibit a number of automatisms such as lip smacking, eye blinking, and fumbling with his or her clothes. Additionally, there is impairment of consciousness. Complex partial seizures are usually associated with temporal lobe epilepsy but can also be derived from lesions elsewhere in the brain. In this case, another diagnosis to rule out is amphetamine intoxication. Amphetamines are commonly used to treat ADHD and may be drugs of abuse in this age group. Intoxication with amphetamines may present as seizures and can be easily ruled out by a urine toxicology screeen.

713. **(E)** Although syphilitic infections have been on the decline since World War I, they must still be considered in the differential for a wide variety of psychiatric disorders, especially when combined with neurologic abnormalities. In this case, two forms of neurosyphilis (tabes dorsalis and general paresis) are combined in one patient. The taboparetic form occurs in about 20% of patients with neurosyphilis. Patients demonstrate sensory ataxia with a wide-based gait, a positive Romberg sign, and a loss of vibratory and proprioceptive senses initially in the lower extremities. Deep tendon reflexes are decreased and pupil abnormalities are common, although the full Argyll–Robertson pupil is infrequent. General paresis is usually associated with a dementing process along with neurologic symptoms such as pupil abnormalities, tremors, dyscoordination, and spasticity in the lower extremities. Testing for neurosyphilis should include a blood test for VDRL and FTA-ABS (fluorescent treponemal antibody absorption test). Consideration should also be given to performing a lumbar puncture to test cerebrospinal fluid for evidence of treponemal infection. Although this patient has some symptoms of Wernicke's encephalopathy and Korsakoff's psychosis, neither diagnosis alone would account for this patient's constellation of neuropsychiatric symptoms. Finally, a diagnosis of NMS should not be entertained since the patient is currently not taking an antipsychotic medication.

714. **(C)** Pheochromocytoma is a tumor of the chromaffin cells, usually occurring in the adrenal medulla. Symptoms may differ according to the predominant catecholamine released. As norepinephrine-secreting tumors are the most common, baseline hypertension with paroxysmal exacerbations are frequent. Anxiety, fear, and palpitations may accompany exacerbations of hypertension. Because this may mimic symptoms of a panic attack or GAD, it is essential to consider this in the differential diagnosis when patients present with anxiety.

715. **(C)** Hepatic encephalophahy can present in many ways and may have a fluctuating course, making it difficult to diagnose without peripheral stigmata. Neurologically, the patient may exhibit asterixis, which, although characteristic for hepatic encephalopathy, is not specific for the disorder. Patients may suffer 6- to 9-Hz tremors, mildly increased deep tendon reflexes, and an altered sensorium. Typical psychiatric symptoms may include changes in personality, abrupt mood swings, and changes in cognitive ability. In an acute decompensation, depression, catatonia, psychosis, and delirium may develop. Physical stigmata reflecting changes in liver function can include ecchymosis, peripheral edema, ascites formation, palmar erythema, and spider angiomas.

716. **(B)** HIV may produce a spectrum of neuropsychiatric manifestations as a result of opportunistic infections, neoplasms, or direct invasion of the CNS by the virus. HIV-associated dementia is one of the most common manifestations of primary CNS invasion. It may present in a variety of ways, including motor abnormalities, cognitive decline, or behavioral changes. This case presentation describes typical behavioral change, apathy, and social withdrawal. HIV dementia may also have neurologic abnormalities such as weakness, imbalance, or ataxia. Occasionally,

patients present with irritability and apathy. Cognitively, this patient has been described as increasingly forgetful, and the results of the MMSE support the diagnosis of dementia. Criteria for dementia include the presence of multiple cognitive deficits, including aphasia, apraxia, agnosia, or disturbance in executive function.

717. **(H)** Hyperthyroidism may present with symptoms consistent with a variety of psychiatric disorders, including depression, anxiety, psychosis, mania, and, at an extreme, delirium. This case illustrates a more moderate presentation of hyperthyroidism with some depressive, hypomanic, and cognitive features. Hyperthyroidism may cause mild cognitive deficits in calculation and recent memory. Neurologically, patients may show a fine 8- to 12-Hz tremor, lid lag, brisk deep tendon reflexes, proximal myopathy with muscle wasting, and myalgias. Patients may report hot flashes and/or increased sensitivity to heat.

718. **(F)** Somatization disorder is characterized by a variety of somatic complaints that cannot be verified by laboratory and physical findings. The disorder has its onset before age 30 and is more common in women than in men. Diagnosis is based on the occurrence of four pain symptoms, two gastrointestinal symptoms, one sexual symptom, and one pseudoneurologic symptom. It is important to determine that these symptoms are not intentionally produced or feigned for other purposes. Similarly, it is important to ensure that the patient has received the appropriate medical workup since a number of disease processes may present with a constellation of symptoms.

719. **(A)** Neuropsychiatric complications occur in up to 60% of patients with SLE. While neuropsychiatric conditions may arise at any time during the course of the disease, they are most frequent during acute exacerbations or late in the disease process. Of the psychiatric manifestations, organic mental syndromes, including "lupus psychosis," schizophrenia-like syndromes, and affective disorders are the most common. Organic mental syndromes include psychotic symptoms, delirium, personality changes, anxiety, and emotional lability. Patients may also exhibit cognitive impairment on neuropsychological testing. Most of the reactions are short, lasting hours to days, and are associated with flares of the illness. Affective illnesses and schizophrenia-like syndromes are less common. Neurologically, patients can present with seizures, stroke, cranial nerve abnormalities, and headache.

720. **(G)** This patient is exhibiting signs and symptoms consistent with a delirium secondary to hypoglycemia. In this case, a psychiatric consultation was likely requested to evaluate the acute confusional state and to evaluate the refusal to provide blood. Signs of hypoglycemia manifested by this patient include tachycardia, tremor, hypertension, and, finally, seizure. Delirious states should receive immediate workup for an organic etiology, as delirium carries a high rate of morbidity and mortality. The standard workup consists of a CBC with differential, electrolytes, BUN, creatinine, VDRL, vitamin B_{12}, folate, urinalysis, TSH, calcium, magnesium, phosphorus, glucose, urine toxicology screen, liver function tests, peripheral oxygen saturation, chest x-ray, ECG, and mental status and physical exam.

721. **(H)** Alcohol intoxication and dependence are the most common substance abuse–related problems. This case exhibits some of the common signs of alcohol intoxication: impaired judgment, slurred speech, lack of coordination, unsteady gait, and impaired attention. Other signs can include nystagmus, stupor, and coma. This patient's vital signs are stable, and there is no mention in the case of diaphoresis or tremor. The presence of any of these would arouse suspicion for alcohol withdrawal.

722. **(B)** PCP intoxication can be quite striking in its similarities to schizophrenia, especially with regard to psychosis. In any case in which a substance-induced state may mimic psychiatric disorders, a toxicology screen should be obtained. This case highlights aspects of PCP intoxication, including nystagmus, hypertension, tachycardia, a decreased responsiveness to pain, and muscular rigidity. Violence or aggressive tendencies may be apparent with or without psychotic symptoms. No clear psychotic symptoms are occurring in this patient. Most patients recover in a few days from PCP-induced psychosis, but others may remain psychotic for periods up to 1 month.

723. **(A)** This case is typical for cocaine withdrawal or "crashing." After cessation or reduction of cocaine use, patients frequently report an intensely dysphoric mood, which may be associated with suicidal ideation. Additionally, patients are fatigued, with increased appetite, insomnia or hypersomnia, unpleasant dreams, and psychomotor agitation or retardation. The time frame for withdrawal can last hours to weeks depending on the pattern of use and the amount used.

724. **(C)** Although it is concerning that this patient has a family history of schizophrenia, the more likely cause of his failure at school is cannabis abuse. The findings of conjunctival injection, increased appetite, and dry mouth are consistent with this diagnosis. Mild tachycardia can also be associated with cannabis abuse. Behavioral abnormalities such as impaired coordination, poor judgment, social withdrawal, euphoria, or anxiety may also be present. At this point, there is no evidence of psychosis, but with a family history one would want to monitor closely for any prodromal symptoms of schizophrenia.

725. **(G)** This patient is exhibiting the classic signs of opiate withdrawal: piloerection, diaphoresis, abdominal cramps, yawning, lacrimation, and muscle aches. Other signs that may be suggestive of withdrawal include dysphoric mood, insomnia, fever, and nausea and/or vomiting. Shorter-acting opiates tend to produce withdrawal symptoms more quickly and more intensely than longer-acting agents.

726. **(E)** MDMA, or ecstasy, has stimulant properties, and its biologic effects include enhanced perception/sensation, increased heart rate, hypertension, dilated pupils, trismus (tightness of jaw muscles), bruxism (grinding of teeth), hyperthermia, and diaphoresis. Drug paraphernalia associated with MDMA use includes pacifiers, popsicle sticks, and candy necklaces to help alleviate MDMA-induced bruxism.

CHAPTER 9

Practice Test 1

Joseph R. Check, MD, and William Roman, MD

Questions

DIRECTIONS (Questions 1 through 110): Each of the numbered items or incomplete statements in this section is followed by answers or by completions of the statement. Select the ONE lettered answer or completion that is BEST in each case.

Questions 1 and 2

A 29-year-old man with a history of bipolar disorder presents to the psychiatric emergency department saying that he is the king of "Pumbar" and needs everyone's allegiance for the upcoming war with the Martians. In the past few days, he has slept a total of 3 hours but says that he is not tired. He has spent all of his money soliciting phone sex. Now, he is agitated, demanding, and threatening.

1. What is the best treatment for this patient in the acute setting?

    (A) hydroxyzine (Atarax)
    (B) lithium
    (C) valproic acid (Depakote)
    (D) haloperidol (Haldol)
    (E) carbamazepine (Tegretol)

2. After treating the patient acutely, a medication is needed to control his bipolar disorder. You find that he has a history of agranulocytosis. Which of the following would be the best choice for a mood stabilizer?

    (A) lithium
    (B) carbamazepine (Tegretol)
    (C) valproic acid (Depakote)

    (D) antipsychotic medication
    (E) lorazepam (Ativan)

Questions 3 through 5

A 44-year-old woman presents to her primary care doctor with multiple complaints, including weakness in her lower extremities, bloating, headaches, intermittent loss of appetite, and back pain. A careful review of symptoms reveals many other vague symptoms. Her complaints date back to adolescence, and she has seen many doctors. Thorough workups, including an exploratory laparotomy, have failed to uncover any clear, organic cause.

3. What is the most likely psychiatric diagnosis?

    (A) somatization disorder
    (B) conversion disorder
    (C) hypochondriasis
    (D) malingering
    (E) factitious disorder

4. What is the best approach to this patient?

    (A) Tell her any physical workup is unnecessary.
    (B) Tell her to come back in 1 month and, if the symptoms are still present, you will initiate a physical workup.
    (C) Tactfully ask her why she is inventing symptoms.
    (D) Assess her for other psychiatric illnesses.
    (E) Initiate a physical workup and arrange for follow-up in a year's time.

5. Which statement regarding this patient's diagnosis is correct?

(A) It has a good prognosis.
(B) It is most common in high socioeconomic groups.
(C) Women are overwhelmingly more likely to receive this diagnosis than are men.
(D) Conversion symptoms are uncommon.
(E) Regularly scheduled, frequent visits with a primary care doctor will exacerbate symptoms.

Questions 6 through 8

A 25-year-old man is a concern to his neighbors. He dresses in odd, outdated clothes; seems to utter his own language; and while he tends to keep to himself, he has told neighborhood children that witches who live down the road have it in for him.

6. This is most characteristic of which of the personality disorders?

(A) schizotypal
(B) schizoid
(C) avoidant
(D) dependent
(E) borderline

7. Which of the following statements about this personality disorder is true?

(A) Auditory hallucinations are common.
(B) Visual hallucinations are common.
(C) This diagnosis may be confused with schizophrenia in remission.
(D) This diagnosis is found overwhelmingly in men.
(E) Onset of symptoms is usually in the second or third decade of life.

8. The patient's brother brings him to a doctor after the death of their mother. Since then, the patient's paranoia has caused him to question his neighbors' activities. He moved into a hotel he couldn't afford to get away from the "spies" living next to him. What would be an appropriate intervention?

(A) no treatment
(B) psychoanalysis
(C) benzodiazepines
(D) a neuroleptic
(E) a selective serotonin reuptake inhibitor (SSRI)

Questions 9 through 14

A 25-year-old female college graduate is brought to her doctor by her mother. Described as "odd" since she lost her job a year ago, the patient has complained of hearing voices and believes that her body is a receiving antenna for a foreign spy operation. Her mother notes she has been isolating herself in her room. She is alert and oriented but suspicious and guarded on examination. Her affect is flat, and her speech reveals loose associations. A complete medical workup is negative.

9. What is the most likely diagnosis?

(A) major depressive disorder (MDD) with psychotic features
(B) bipolar disorder
(C) schizophrenia
(D) schizophreniform disorder
(E) brief psychotic disorder

10. Which of the following symptoms is considered a "negative symptom" with regard to her illness?

(A) auditory hallucinations
(B) delusions
(C) paranoia
(D) flat affect
(E) loose associations

11. What statement regarding this patient is true?

(A) Her negative and positive symptoms should respond about equally to medications.
(B) There is little evidence to suggest that she is at increased risk for drug and alcohol abuse or dependence.

(C) She has a good chance of being able to safely discontinue medications within the next 5 years.

(D) Lifetime prevalence is about 1% for her illness.

(E) She has a greater chance of having been born in the winter than the general population.

12. What is the most important consideration in choosing antipsychotic medications?

(A) renal function
(B) the presence of negative symptoms
(C) gender
(D) onset of action
(E) side effect profile

13. Which of the following pharmacologic interventions is most appropriate?

(A) haloperidol decanoate injection (Haldol LA)
(B) oral haloperidol
(C) lithium
(D) amitriptyline (Elavil)
(E) valproic acid (Depakote)

14. The patient is started on medication, and many of her symptoms improve. She begins a new job and does well. One year later, she is brought to her doctor floridly psychotic, actively hearing voices, and extremely paranoid. She thinks her boss is trying to kill her. She has an upper respiratory viral illness that she believes to be the work of a foreign government. She discontinued her medication 4 weeks ago because she felt too sedated. In the past year, her cigarette smoking habit has escalated to two packs per day. What is the most likely cause of her exacerbation?

(A) stress from work
(B) a reaction to the viral illness
(C) medication noncompliance
(D) medication side effects
(E) increased cigarette smoking

Questions 15 through 17

A 44-year-old man complains to his doctor that he is always tired and is having difficulty getting out of bed in the morning. Upon questioning, he reveals he has three or four drinks each night, and perhaps more on the weekends, but denies he has any problem with alcohol.

15. What would be the most important strategy in evaluating this patient for alcoholism?

(A) Quantify the average amount he drinks.
(B) Ascertain how often he drinks.
(C) Ask him how frequently he gets drunk.
(D) Ask him what his family and friends say about his drinking.
(E) Perform a complete laboratory investigation.

16. A diagnosis of alcohol dependence is made, and the patient comes to your office in acute alcohol withdrawal. He has a withdrawal seizure. What might be found on laboratory investigation?

(A) thrombocytosis
(B) elevated or depressed liver enzymes
(C) decreased prothrombin time
(D) hypermagnesemia
(E) a high blood alcohol level

17. Which of the following statements regarding this patient is true?

(A) Cerebellar degeneration is uncommon.
(B) He is at risk for developing a peripheral neuropathy.
(C) Alcoholic "fatty liver" is irreversible.
(D) He is at decreased or normal risk for heart disease.
(E) Immune function should remain relatively intact.

Questions 18 through 23

A 28-year-old woman is brought to the emergency department for active suicidal ideation, with a plan to overdose on acetaminophen. She has no history of a psychiatric illness but endorses many criteria for MDD, including poor sleep for the past 2 weeks. She recently lost her job and fears that she may not be able to pay her rent. You speak to a friend, who reports that the patient has been abusing alcohol. Attempts to obtain additional collateral information have been unsuccessful. You believe the patient requires inpatient evaluation but her health maintenance organization (HMO) denies authorization for inpatient care, alternatively authorizing eight outpatient visits with a psychiatrist. You speak to the weekend on-call MD reviewer and report that the patient remains unsafe and wishes to be discharged. Upon learning that the patient does not have a history of psychiatric illness, the reviewer fails to authorize inpatient care, despite your assessment.

18. The most appropriate intervention is to

(A) begin antidepressant therapy and arrange for outpatient follow-up the next day

(B) admit the patient on an emergency certificate to an inpatient facility on the basis of danger to self

(C) administer an antipsychotic medication and reevaluate the patient in 1 hour

(D) explain to the patient that her HMO did not authorize hospitalization and discharge her with follow-up care

(E) prescribe a medication to help her sleep, discharge her, and arrange for follow-up care

19. Which of the following disorders is most closely associated with suicide?

(A) alcohol dependence

(B) schizophrenia

(C) mood disorder

(D) multiple sclerosis

(E) cancer

20. Which of the following predictive factors is most associated with suicide risk?

(A) depression

(B) unemployment

(C) age 45 and older

(D) male gender

(E) divorce

21. Suicide rates

(A) are higher in Protestants and Jews than in Catholics

(B) are equal for men and women

(C) decrease with age

(D) are higher in nonwhites than in whites

(E) have not been stable over time

22. Suicide risk is

(A) decreased with higher social status

(B) greater for married individuals than for never-married individuals

(C) not associated with loss of physical health

(D) lowest in the first week of a psychiatric admission

(E) associated with a fall in social status

23. Which of the following individuals is least likely to attempt suicide?

(A) a white male

(B) an African-American male

(C) a white female

(D) an African-American female

(E) a Native American individual

Questions 24 and 25

A 29-year-old woman presents to the emergency department with her 3-year-old child, reporting that the child suffered a seizure while at home. Hospital records verify that this is the third emergency department visit in as many weeks for the same presentation. Neurologic workup for seizure disorder was negative. Initiation of an anticonvulsant has been ineffective.

24. Which of the following statements is likely to be true?

    (A) The child suffers from a conversion disorder.
    (B) The child is experiencing separation anxiety.
    (C) The child's history is falsified.
    (D) The child does not have a therapeutic level of anticonvulsant.
    (E) The child suffers from a seizure disorder.

25. The mother is most likely to suffer from

    (A) schizophrenia
    (B) bipolar disorder
    (C) depression
    (D) epilepsy
    (E) posttraumatic stress disorder (PTSD)

Questions 26 and 27

A 26-year-old man is being evaluated in the emergency department for sudden onset of chest pressure and dyspnea. This is his third emergency department visit for similar symptoms for which he reports "I feel like I'm going to die." An electrocardiogram (ECG) and stress test were normal. The patient denies risk factors for heart disease and does not have a family history of heart disease. Urine toxicology was negative.

26. Which of the following is the most likely diagnosis?

    (A) delirium
    (B) panic disorder
    (C) acute stress reaction
    (D) acute myocardial infarction
    (E) hypochondriasis

27. Which of the following medications would be most useful in the initial treatment of this disorder?

    (A) sertraline (Zoloft)
    (B) propranolol
    (C) clonidine (Catapres)
    (D) haloperidol (Haldol)
    (E) lithium

28. A woman being treated for major depression is brought to the emergency department after being found unconscious by a neighbor. The neighbor said that over the past few days the woman had been complaining of severe headaches. She also said the woman enjoys red wine. The woman's blood pressure is recorded as 220/110. This emergency is best managed by intravenous (IV) administration of

    (A) an alpha-blocking agent
    (B) a beta blocker
    (C) dantrolene sodium (Dantrium)
    (D) bromocriptine (Parlodel)
    (E) a calcium channel blocker

Questions 29 and 30

A 28-year-old man recently began taking clozapine (Clozaril) to treat symptoms of schizophrenia. He does not suffer from any medical illness.

29. Which of the following adverse effects is associated with this medication?

    (A) bradycardia
    (B) hypertension
    (C) weight loss
    (D) galactorrhea
    (E) seizures

30. Which of the following hematologic disorders associated with this medication can be life threatening?

    (A) a decreased granulocyte count
    (B) leukocytosis
    (C) thrombocytopenia
    (D) pancytopenia
    (E) microcytic anemia

31. A 35-year-old patient exhibits odd beliefs and thinking, paranoid behavior, and has no close friends. Which of the following diagnoses is the most appropriate to consider?

    (A) schizoid personality disorder
    (B) avoidant personality disorder
    (C) paranoid personality disorder
    (D) narcissistic personality disorder
    (E) schizotypal personality disorder

32. A 28-year-old woman demonstrates a pervasive pattern of unstable relationships, poor self-image, impulsiveness, and irritability. The most appropriate diagnosis to consider is

    (A) histrionic personality disorder
    (B) borderline personality disorder
    (C) antisocial personality disorder
    (D) dependent personality disorder
    (E) schizoid personality disorder

Questions 33 through 36

A 30-year-old woman is brought to the emergency department by the police after being arrested for breach of the peace. The woman was observed acting irrationally at a local business, where she demanded to speak with the president of the company, claiming that she had new ideas for product development. The patient reports that she has not slept for days and that her mood is "fabulous." Urine human chorionic gonadotropin (HCG) is positive. Illicit substances were not detected.

33. The most likely diagnosis is

    (A) delusional disorder
    (B) schizophreniform disorder
    (C) bipolar I disorder, manic episode
    (D) bipolar II disorder
    (E) schizoid personality disorder

34. Which of the following is most likely to be present on Mental Status Exam (MSE)?

    (A) racing thoughts
    (B) depressed mood
    (C) auditory hallucinations
    (D) daytime sleepiness
    (E) weight loss

35. Which of the following medical disorders can present with similar symptoms?

    (A) hyperglycemia
    (B) thyroid disorder
    (C) rheumatoid arthritis
    (D) diabetes mellitus
    (E) cirrhosis

36. Which of the following is the safest intervention to consider to treat her symptoms?

    (A) lithium carbonate
    (B) valproic acid (Depakote)
    (C) chlorpromazine (Thorazine)
    (D) electroconvulsive therapy (ECT)
    (E) diazepam (Valium)

Questions 37 through 39

A 24-year-old man with a history of seizure disorder and polysubstance abuse has been incarcerated for assaultive behavior. He is referred to you for an evaluation.

37. Which of the following classes of drugs is the most dangerous when abruptly withdrawn?

    (A) opiates
    (B) sedative–hypnotics
    (C) stimulants
    (D) psychedelics
    (E) cannabinoids

38. The patient is evaluated by a neurologist, who prescribes phenytoin (Dilantin). Which of the following conditions is associated with this medication?

    (A) leukocytosis
    (B) hypertension
    (C) gingival hyperplasia
    (D) hepatic failure
    (E) Ebstein's anomaly

39. The patient returns 1 month later for a follow-up examination and reports that he experienced a generalized seizure. Laboratory investigation reveals that the phenytoin level is 6.5 mg/dL (normal, 10–20). Which of the

following is the most appropriate intervention at this time?

(A) Increase the phenytoin dose to achieve a therapeutic level.

(B) Discontinue phenytoin and begin valproic acid (Depakote).

(C) Add a benzodiazepine as an adjunct medication.

(D) Ask the patient about compliance with medications.

(E) Add phenobarbital.

40. A 24-year-old woman with a history of schizophrenia tells you that she would like to become pregnant. What is the chance for familial transmission of schizophrenia?

(A) 0.1%

(B) 1%

(C) 2%

(D) 5%

(E) 10%

41. A 70-year-old man with a history of major depression is brought to the emergency department by his family, who is concerned because he was found wandering in the streets near his home. During the MSE, attention is best assessed by asking the patient to

(A) perform serial seven subtraction

(B) recite his Social Security number

(C) spell a five-letter word forward and backward

(D) perform digit recall

(E) repeat the examiner's first name

42. An 18-year-old patient experiences a sudden onset of euphoria, grandiose delusions, a decreased need for sleep, and paranoia. Which of the following conditions is most associated with these symptoms?

(A) schizophrenia, paranoid type

(B) cannabis intoxication

(C) MDD with psychotic features

(D) schizoaffective disorder

(E) cocaine intoxication

43. A Malayan man experiences a dissociative episode characterized by an outburst of homicidal behavior toward his friend, whom he believed was insulting his appearance. Which of the following conditions is most associated with this presentation?

(A) substance intoxication

(B) dissociative identity disorder

(C) Ganser syndrome

(D) factitious disorder

(E) culture-bound syndrome

Questions 44 through 47

A 26-year-old woman is diagnosed with schizophrenia. The psychiatrist decides to treat her symptoms with a high-potency antipsychotic medication.

44. Which of the following medications is an appropriate choice?

(A) thiothixene (Navane)

(B) chlorpromazine (Thorazine)

(C) trifluoperazine (Stelazine)

(D) thioperidol (Thiodol)

(E) daslaperizone (Daxplar)

45. The patient experiences abnormal involuntary movements associated with the use of the antipsychotic drug she has been prescribed. Realizing that side effects may affect further medication compliance, the psychiatrist should prescribe

(A) clozapine (Clozaril)

(B) risperidone (Risperdal)

(C) benztropine (Cogentin)

(D) methylphenidate (Ritalin)

(E) a cholinergic agonist

46. Despite the intervention, the patient abruptly stops taking her antipsychotic medication. Which of the following is commonly associated with the abrupt withdrawal of antipsychotic drugs?

    (A) persistent dyskinesia
    (B) seizures
    (C) dry mouth
    (D) constipation
    (E) blurred vision

47. The psychiatrist decides to change the patient's medication. Which of the following may be considered?

    (A) haloperidol (Haldol)
    (B) clozapine (Clozaril)
    (C) loxapine (Loxitane)
    (D) pimozide (Orap)
    (E) perphenazine (Trilafon)

Questions 48 and 49

A 30-year-old woman with a history of unstable interpersonal relationships, suicidal gestures, and marked impulsivity is referred to you for dialectical behavioral therapy (DBT).

48. Which of the following disorders is this patient likely to be suffering from?

    (A) avoidant personality disorder
    (B) bipolar disorder
    (C) passive–aggressive personality disorder
    (D) borderline personality disorder
    (E) schizoid personality disorder

49. The foundations of DBT include which of the following?

    (A) The patient is doing the best that she can.
    (B) The patient may fail in therapy.
    (C) At times the patient does not want to improve.
    (D) The patient should not learn new behaviors.
    (E) The patient is responsible for causing all of her own problems.

50. A 21-year-old man presents with a 4-week history of paranoid delusions and auditory hallucinations that comment on his appearance. After thorough evaluation, you diagnose him with schizophrenia, paranoid type, and prescribe haloperidol (Haldol) 5 mg bid. One week later, the patient returns for a follow-up examination and reports that, although his symptoms have improved, he now experiences muscle stiffness in his arms and neck. You prescribe benztropine (Cogentin) 1 mg bid and schedule a follow-up appointment in 2 weeks. One week later, the patient's mother calls you and reports that her son is more agitated and confused. Physical exam reveals tachycardia, dilated pupils, and flushed skin. The next appropriate measure would be to

    (A) discontinue benztropine and prescribe amantadine (Symmetrel)
    (B) increase haloperidol to 5 mg tid
    (C) increase benztropine to 2 mg bid
    (D) discontinue haloperidol and prescribe risperidone (Risperdal)
    (E) prescribe lorazepam (Ativan) 1 mg bid

51. A 28-year-old male medical student is found to have an enlarged testicle during a routine physical exam. The student reports that it has been gradually enlarging for several months. The physician asks why he didn't report these findings earlier. "I'm sure it's nothing," the student replies. This response is an example of

    (A) a mature defense
    (B) a neurotic defense
    (C) a narcissistic defense
    (D) an immature defense
    (E) confidence

52. A 45-year-old Asian-American woman is brought to the emergency department by her husband, who reports that for the past 3 days his wife has not been sleeping well, has been experiencing bad dreams, and appears "in a daze" with a sense of feeling "numb." The patient endorses feeling anxious but does not know why. She has been unable to perform

her usual activities of daily living. One week ago, the patient was discharged from the hospital after experiencing an anaphylactic reaction to intravenous contrast dye while undergoing an imaging procedure for sinusitis. Although she cannot recall specifics, her husband verifies the history, adding that the doctors "thought she was going to die." Upon returning to the hospital, she experiences intense fear about revisiting the same hospital from which she was recently discharged. The most appropriate diagnosis to consider is

(A) PTSD
(B) acute stress reaction
(C) generalized anxiety disorder (GAD)
(D) adjustment disorder
(E) depressive disorder

53. A 40-year-old woman without a past psychiatric history is admitted to the hospital for treatment of depression. During morning rounds, the patient appears unresponsive and does not respond to verbal stimuli. There are no signs of trauma or overdose. A review of her chart reveals that the patient was well the night before and went to sleep without incident. You determine that the patient's unresponsiveness is psychogenic. Which of the following findings is most likely to be apparent on exam?

(A) an abnormal electroencephalogram (EEG)
(B) nonsaccadic eye movements
(C) elevated temperature
(D) decreased respirations
(E) cold-caloric–induced nystagmus

54. A 24-year-old woman experiences fatigue, weight gain, and hyperphagia during the winter months. She reports a sad mood and "can't wait" until her vacation to Florida. The most likely diagnosis is

(A) dysthymia
(B) sundowning syndrome
(C) anxiety disorder
(D) stress disorder
(E) seasonal depression

55. A 27-year-old woman is brought to the emergency department by her parents, who report that their daughter is unable to recall her name. The emergency department physician reports that a complete neurologic workup is within normal limits. Collateral information reveals that the patient had episodes in which she would take unplanned trips, sometimes for days, without notice, and would return unable to recall the episode. A review of her medical chart notes a past history of possible sexual abuse as a child. Urine toxicology is negative, and she does not take any medications. Which of the following is the most likely diagnosis?

(A) partial complex seizure disorder
(B) delirium
(C) fugue state
(D) PTSD
(E) depressive disorder

56. A 26-year-old female graduate student reports to you a 4-week history of a depressed mood that has caused her significant difficulty in attending her classes. The patient reports difficulty falling asleep at night, weight loss, and passive suicidal ideation. A careful review of her history reveals that during the past year she also experienced brief and distinct periods of an elevated and expansive mood, a decreased need for sleep, and an increase in goal-directed activities. Which of the following is the most appropriate diagnosis to consider?

(A) MDD
(B) bipolar I disorder, current episode manic
(C) bipolar II disorder, current episode depressed
(D) cyclothymic disorder
(E) dysthymic disorder

57. You are asked to evaluate a 30-year-old male prisoner who reports a depressed mood and suicidal ideation. During your exam, you note that the prisoner responds to your questions with approximate answers. Which of the following is the most appropriate diagnosis to consider?

   (A) malingering
   (B) Ganser syndrome
   (C) Capgras syndrome
   (D) Munchausen syndrome
   (E) fugue state

58. A 75-year-old man is admitted to the hospital following a serious suicide attempt. The patient exhibits clinical features of depression and has a past history of suicide attempts. The medical chart reveals that he is prescribed levodopa/carbidopa, digoxin, aspirin, and a medication for cardiac arrhythmia. The most appropriate treatment at this time is to

   (A) prescribe risperidone (Risperdal)
   (B) administer supportive psychotherapy
   (C) prescribe nortriptyline (Pamelor)
   (D) prescribe diazepam (Valium)
   (E) administer ECT

59. A 38-year-old woman presents to your office with a 2-week history of symptoms of depression characterized by hypersomnolence and reaction sensitivity. She reports to you that she recently enrolled in graduate school and is having trouble with many of her classes. Which of the following diagnoses should be considered?

   (A) adjustment disorder
   (B) atypical depression
   (C) dysthymic disorder
   (D) melancholic depression
   (E) sleep disorder

60. A 33-year-old man changes his first name to honor a musician whom he idolizes. He recently bought the same guitar as the musician and formed a rock band to play his mu-

sic. During practice, the man dresses like his idol. This behavior is an example of

   (A) identification
   (B) regression
   (C) fixation
   (D) projection
   (E) idealization

61. A 60-year-old man with schizophrenia sits motionless in his chair. The patient is mute and reacts very little to his environment. His eyes appear fixated on a distant object. At times, he assumes bizarre postures and imitates the movements of others. The most likely explanation for his behavior is

   (A) partial complex seizure
   (B) absence seizure
   (C) catatonia
   (D) cataplexy
   (E) catalepsy

62. During an examination to evaluate muscle rigidity, a male patient is somewhat resistant to movement of his arms but maintains the arm in the position in which you place it. This is an example of

   (A) catalepsy
   (B) cataplexy
   (C) rigidity
   (D) dystonia
   (E) malingering

Questions 63 and 64

A 42-year-old healthy man is taking a medication to help him sleep at night. Unexpectedly, he experiences painful, persistent penile erection.

63. Which of the following medications is most likely to cause this condition?

   (A) fluoxetine (Prozac)
   (B) sertraline (Zoloft)
   (C) paroxetine (Paxil)
   (D) trazodone (Desyrel)
   (E) nortriptyline (Pamelor)

64. Which of the following statements regarding this condition is correct?

   (A) It is self-limiting.

   (B) It is dose-dependent.

   (C) It may require surgery.

   (D) It occurs after long-term therapy.

   (E) It is related to dopamine blockade.

Questions 65 through 67

A 60-year-old man reports a history of excessive worry about his daughter since she moved away to college 1 year ago. His wife of 40 years verifies his complaint, adding that "he worries about everything." Recently, his wife made plans to travel abroad to visit friends. The patient is unable to accompany his wife because of respiratory problems caused by years of heavy smoking, and is anxious about her leaving. He reports difficulty falling asleep, excessive daytime fatigue, and difficulty concentrating at work.

65. Which of the following is the most likely diagnosis?

   (A) panic disorder

   (B) GAD

   (C) MDD

   (D) separation anxiety

   (E) dependent personality disorder

66. Which of the following should be considered to treat his symptoms?

   (A) buspirone (BuSpar)

   (B) fluoxetine (Prozac)

   (C) alprazolam (Xanax)

   (D) diazepam (Valium)

   (E) lorazepam (Ativan)

67. Two weeks later, the patient reports that the medication you prescribed has helped everything but his difficulty falling asleep. He reports that during the past week he has slept only 4 hours per night. After careful consideration, you decide to prescribe a 1-week supply of medication to help him sleep. Which of the following medications is most appropriate to consider?

   (A) clorazepate (Tranxene)

   (B) zolpidem (Ambien)

   (C) oxazepam (Serax)

   (D) diphenhydramine (Benadryl)

   (E) temazepam (Restoril)

Questions 68 and 69

A 25-year-old woman is scheduled for a gynecologic procedure. Upon discharge from the hospital, she is likely to receive pain medication. For 1 year, you have been prescribing a monoamine oxidase inhibitor (MAOI) to treat a single episode of depression, with excellent results.

68. Which of the following medications may cause a fatal drug interaction in this patient?

   (A) codeine

   (B) acetaminophen

   (C) oxycodone

   (D) meperidine (Demerol)

   (E) ibuprofen

69. The patient tolerates the procedure well and 2 months later reports to you that she is pregnant. Which of the following interventions is most appropriate?

   (A) MAOIs are safe in pregnancy and should be continued.

   (B) Antidepressant therapy should be discontinued.

   (C) Discontinue the MAOI and initiate treatment with paroxetine (Paxil).

   (D) Discontinue the MAOI during the first trimester only.

   (E) Discontinue the MAOI and begin maintenance ECT.

70. A 62-year-old homeless man presents to the emergency department with impaired gait and nystagmus. His vital signs are stable, and an ophthalmologic exam is within normal limits. The patient is unable to recall the date and has difficulty sustaining attention without evidence of amnesia. The most appropriate initial intervention would be to

    (A) perform a breath analysis
    (B) obtain a head computed tomographic (CT) scan
    (C) perform a lumbar puncture
    (D) administer parenteral thiamine
    (E) administer IV dextrose

71. Which of the following language deficits is characteristic of Broca's aphasia but not of Wernicke's aphasia?

    (A) nonfluency
    (B) impaired repetition
    (C) impaired writing
    (D) impaired naming
    (E) impaired reading comprehension

72. A 34-year-old executive reports drinking up to six cups of caffeinated coffee per day. He boards a plane scheduled for an 18-hour flight on which only decaffeinated beverages are served. Which of the following symptoms is the executive most likely to experience?

    (A) depressed mood
    (B) muscle cramping
    (C) headache
    (D) irritability
    (E) nausea

Questions 73 through 75

A 25-year-old man with a history of medication-responsive schizophrenia presents to the emergency department with severe muscle stiffness and an elevated temperature. The patient appears confused, is diaphoretic, and vital signs are unstable. A urine toxicology screen is provisionally negative.

73. Which of the following is the most likely diagnosis?

    (A) tyramine-induced autonomic instability
    (B) neuroleptic malignant syndrome (NMS)
    (C) neuroleptic-induced dystonic reaction
    (D) serotonin syndrome
    (E) malignant hyperthermia

74. The most appropriate initial intervention would be to

    (A) administer IV dantrolene sodium (Dantrium)
    (B) apply cooling blankets
    (C) administer naloxone (Narcan)
    (D) administer bromocriptine (Parlodel)
    (E) discontinue medications

75. Which of the following laboratory abnormalities is most likely to be present?

    (A) anemia
    (B) leukopenia
    (C) elevated creatine phosphokinase (CPK)
    (D) decreased transaminases
    (E) elevated blood urea nitrogen (BUN)

76. An 18-year-old man presents to the emergency department after being involved in a motor vehicle accident. The medical chart reports a history of substance use. Which of the following tests can confirm your diagnosis of substance dependence?

    (A) serum liver function studies
    (B) breath analysis
    (C) urine toxicity screen
    (D) naloxone (Narcan) injection
    (E) elevated heart rate

77. A 72-year-old man without a prior psychiatric history presents to the outpatient clinic with a recent history of cognitive deficits. The patient has had a stable level of consciousness and denies any current or past substance abuse. The patient has not been prescribed any new medications. The medical chart reveals a history of megaloblastic anemia and a subtotal gastrectomy for severe peptic ulcer disease. Which of the following initial interventions is most appropriate?

(A) Order a magnetic resonance imaging (MRI) scan of the brain to confirm dementia, Alzheimer's type.

(B) Order a reversible workup for dementia.

(C) Discuss long-term extended-care facility admission.

(D) Obtain a forensic examination to evaluate competency.

(E) Obtain a neurologic consult.

78. A 37-year-old woman presents to the emergency department complaining of severe diarrhea and a coarse tremor. The medical chart notes a history of bipolar I disorder. The most appropriate intervention aimed at establishing a diagnosis is to

(A) obtain a serum medication level

(B) prescribe antidiarrheal medication

(C) obtain a urine toxicology screen

(D) obtain a urine pregnancy test

(E) obtain renal function studies

79. A young healthy man is diagnosed with bipolar I disorder and is prescribed lithium carbonate to treat his symptoms of mania. Which of the following lab tests should be obtained before initiating treatment with lithium?

(A) EEG

(B) creatinine clearance

(C) liver function studies

(D) 24-hour urine volume

(E) thyroid-stimulating hormone (TSH)

80. A 27-year-old woman has been prescribed fluoxetine (Prozac) for depression for the past year. She comes to you complaining of medication side effects and wishes to discontinue her antidepressant. As her physician, you discuss with her the appropriate risks and benefits, and you discontinue her treatment. Two weeks later, she returns complaining of depressive symptoms characterized by sleep and appetite changes, poor concentration, and a depressed mood for most of the day. You decide that she is experiencing a recurrent major depressive episode and decide to prescribe her a different class of medication to treat her symptoms. After discussing the appropriate precautions with her, you prescribe an MAOI. Within 1 week, she begins experiencing irritability, abdominal pain and diarrhea, and autonomic instability characterized by hypertension and tachycardia. Her temperature is 103.5°F. The patient also reports experiencing myoclonic-like jerking of her muscles and vivid visual hallucinations of colorful flowers spinning toward the sky. She states that she has followed your directions carefully while taking this medication. Which of the following can account for this presentation?

(A) NMS

(B) tyramine-induced hypertensive crisis

(C) malignant hyperthermia

(D) serotonin syndrome

(E) hallucinogen abuse

Questions 81 and 82

A 17-year-old girl is referred to the school nurse for frequent episodes of vomiting in the bathroom during lunch breaks. Her friends report that, despite a preoccupation with her body image, she eats "twice as much as anybody else." The parents are called to the school and recall that a recent bill from their charge account at the local pharmacy indicated a large number of laxative purchases. The girl reports that her mood is fine, and her records at school indicate that she is an above-average student.

81. Medical complications of this disorder are most often due to

    (A) chronic vomiting
    (B) weight loss
    (C) ritualistic fasting
    (D) suicide gestures
    (E) substance abuse

82. Which of the following medications is the most appropriate initial treatment for her symptoms?

    (A) antiemetics
    (B) antidepressants
    (C) antianxiety agents
    (D) appetite stimulants
    (E) hypnotic medications

Questions 83 through 85

A 16-year-old female high school student is referred by her parents for an evaluation. One year prior to the evaluation, the girl began restricting her food intake and started a rigorous exercise program in order to improve her appearance. Aspiring to be a model, the girl lost 25 pounds but remained preoccupied with her appearance despite weighing only 85 pounds. Her friends reported that she constantly referred to herself as being "fat" and did not seem interested in dating. The girl continued to lose weight and was reluctant to discuss her condition.

83. The girl is most likely to experience

    (A) normal breast development
    (B) three consecutive missed periods

    (C) the loss of feelings of hunger
    (D) body weight 85% of expected normal
    (E) sexual promiscuity

84. The mortality rate associated with this disorder may be as high as

    (A) 5%
    (B) 10%
    (C) 20%
    (D) 25%
    (E) 30%

85. Which of the following is common to both anorexia nervosa and bulimia nervosa?

    (A) normal sexual activity
    (B) amenorrhea
    (C) normal body weight
    (D) decreased triiodothyronine levels
    (E) normal appetite

Questions 86 and 87

A 50-year-old woman reports a depressed mood, poor appetite, and weight loss 1 month following the death of her husband. After his death, she began to feel that she would be "better off dead." At times, she believes that she can hear his voice calling to her. She denies any feelings of worthlessness but feels guilty about not being able to do the right things for him before he died. When talking with others, she believes that her feelings are normal.

86. Which of the following describes this condition?

    (A) uncomplicated bereavement
    (B) complicated bereavement
    (C) major depressive episode
    (D) adjustment disorder with depressed mood
    (E) dysthymic disorder

87. Which of the following is the most appropriate course of action?

    (A) no treatment
    (B) prescribing antidepressant medication
    (C) prescribing sedative–hypnotic medication

(D) admission to a hospital

(E) evaluating for a sleep disorder

88. A 25-year-old man reports a 5-year history of excessive hand washing and a preoccupation with feeling clean. The thought of contracting an infectious disease persists throughout the day even though he makes attempts to ignore it. His condition has progressively worsened and has caused significant impairment while at work and at home. Which of the following medications is the best initial choice to treat his symptoms?

(A) antipsychotics

(B) antianxiety agents

(C) antidepressants

(D) antiepileptic agents

(E) lithium

Questions 89 through 91

A 52-year-old obese man experiences excessive daytime sleepiness and a depressed mood. His wife reports that he snores loudly and is restless while sleeping. There is no evidence of substance abuse, and the patient does not have a prior psychiatric history.

89. Which of the following is the most likely cause of his symptoms?

(A) depression

(B) abnormal circadian rhythm

(C) periodic limb movements of sleep

(D) airway obstruction

(E) nocturnal myoclonus

90. Which of the following is the treatment of choice for his symptoms?

(A) breathing air under positive pressure

(B) nasal surgery

(C) benzodiazepine medication

(D) antidepressant medication

(E) uvulopalatoplasty

91. The most cost-effective intervention in treating his symptoms is

(A) air mattress pads

(B) weight loss

(C) curative surgery

(D) repositioning techniques

(E) benzodiazepine medications

Questions 92 and 93

A patient with chronic paranoid schizophrenia who has been stable for years on a low-potency antipsychotic agent begins experiencing parkinsonian-like side effects. His physician prescribes a drug to alleviate some of these side effects. One week later, the patient is seen in the emergency department with dilated pupils, dry mouth, warm skin, and tachycardia. He is experiencing visual hallucinations.

92. The most appropriate intervention would be to

(A) administer IV atropine

(B) administer an anticholinesterase medication

(C) administer IV dantrolene sodium (Dantrium)

(D) administer haloperidol (Haldol)

(E) administer a benzodiazepine

93. After the appropriate intervention, the patient experiences nausea and vomiting and has a seizure. Which of the following medications should be administered next?

(A) atropine

(B) lorazepam (Ativan)

(C) physostigmine

(D) epinephrine

(E) prochlorperazine (Compazine)

94. A 40-year-old woman suffers from depression and obsessive ritualistic behavior. The physician decides to prescribe an SSRI. Which of the following medications might the physician consider?

(A) buspirone (BuSpar)

(B) phenelzine (Nardil)

(C) clomipramine (Anafranil)

(D) doxepin (Sinequan)

(E) fluvoxamine (Luvox)

Questions 95 and 96

A 56-year-old man with a long history of alcohol abuse and liver disease is ordered by the court to enroll in an inpatient detoxification program for alcohol dependence. He begins to experience clinical signs and symptoms of withdrawal.

95. Which of the following medications is the most appropriate to prescribe during his treatment?

   (A) chlordiazepoxide (Librium)
   (B) phenobarbital
   (C) disulfiram (Antabuse)
   (D) lorazepam (Ativan)
   (E) alprazolam (Xanax)

96. Soon after his admission the man begins to report hallucinations and becomes agitated. Which of the following medications should be prescribed to treat these symptoms?

   (A) sertraline (Zoloft)
   (B) clonazepam (Klonopin)
   (C) haloperidol (Haldol)
   (D) lithium
   (E) diazepam (Valium)

97. A 48-year-old woman successfully completes an inpatient program for alcohol detoxification for which she was prescribed chlordiazepoxide (Librium). Upon discharge, the patient is prescribed a medication that disrupts alcohol metabolism. Soon after discharge, the patient attends an office party where she reports having a few drinks. She has been compliant with her prescribed medication and does not have any active medical problems. Which of the following symptoms is the patient likely to experience?

   (A) high blood pressure
   (B) euphoria
   (C) blurred vision
   (D) vomiting
   (E) urinary retention

98. A 22-year-old man with a history of bipolar disorder is prescribed lithium carbonate to

treat his symptoms. During a weekend rugby tournament, he hurts his knee and an orthopedic physician prescribes a medication to reduce his symptoms of pain and swelling. Although the patient reports relief from this medication, he begins to experience abdominal pain, diarrhea, and drowsiness. Which of the following medications may contribute to the production of these symptoms?

   (A) ibuprofen
   (B) acetaminophen
   (C) aspirin
   (D) codeine
   (E) meperidine (Demerol)

99. A patient experiences clinical signs and symptoms of depression. The physician decides to prescribe a medication whose mechanism includes significant blockade of serotonin reuptake. Which of the following antidepressants should be considered?

   (A) maprotiline (Ludiomil)
   (B) amitriptyline (Elavil)
   (C) bupropion (Wellbutrin)
   (D) desipramine (Norpramin)
   (E) clonazepam (Klonopin)

100. A patient who is HIV-positive reports a depressed mood, low energy, and hopelessness. Which of the following medications can the physician prescribe to achieve rapid relief of some of his symptoms?

   (A) methylphenidate (Ritalin)
   (B) fluoxetine (Prozac)
   (C) bupropion (Wellbutrin)
   (D) buspirone (BuSpar)
   (E) nefazodone (Serzone)

Questions 101 and 102

A college-aged man reports that he and his friends have been experimenting with the new drug craze on campus called "huffing." His roommate reports that he has been accumulating typewriter correction fluid, nail polish remover, and model airplane glue.

101. Which of the following findings is experienced by a person after "huffing"?

(A) staring into space
(B) tolerance
(C) depressed reflexes
(D) increased appetite
(E) diminished response to pain

102. Which of the following is the current treatment for this type of drug abuse?

(A) antidepressant agents
(B) dialectic behavioral therapy
(C) abstinence
(D) exposure and response prevention
(E) antipsychotic agents

103. A 30-year-old man with schizophrenia exhibits symptoms that have not been stable over time. Which of the predominant symptoms would support the diagnosis of the paranoid subtype?

(A) immobility
(B) inappropriate affect
(C) disorganized speech and behavior
(D) posturing
(E) prominent hallucinations or delusions

104. Hair loss is a reversible side effect of which of the following medications?

(A) valproic acid (Depakote)
(B) ziprasadone (Geodon)
(C) carbamazepine (Tegretol)
(D) clozapine (Clozaril)
(E) olanzapine (Zyprexa)

105. A young man experiences erectile dysfunction and is told that the medication he is prescribed is likely to be the cause. Which of the following medications is associated with erectile dysfunction?

(A) amantadine (Symmetrel)
(B) methylphenidate (Ritalin)
(C) SSRIs
(D) antihistamines
(E) cholinergic agents

Questions 106 through 108

A 21-year-old male college student without prior medical or psychiatric history is evaluated for poor work performance. The student reports to the dean that he finds it hard to follow through with assignments and is easily distracted by environmental stimuli. The dean comments to the student about how frequently he interrupts others during conversations and observes that it seems that the student is not paying attention to what he is saying. Overall, his grades are poor except in the class he considers "the most interesting class I have ever had." He often forgets required materials for classes, and his assignments are frequently late. The student's parents report that he was incompletely evaluated for similar difficulties while in public school. The student seemed to improve when the family moved out of the area and he attended private school.

106. Which of the following is the most likely diagnosis?

(A) attention deficit–hyperactivity disorder (ADHD)
(B) bipolar I disorder
(C) bipolar II disorder
(D) conduct disorder
(E) learning disability

107. Which of the following medications is the best initial choice to treat his symptoms?

(A) modafinil (Provigil)
(B) methylphenidate (Ritalin)
(C) fluoxetine (Prozac)
(D) lorazepam (Ativan)
(E) paroxetine (Paxil)

108. The patient is prescribed methylphenidate (Ritalin) for symptoms of inattention and hyperactivity. After an adequate trial and dose, the patient does not fully benefit from the medication. Which of the following actions is the most appropriate?

    (A) Add a low-dose amphetamine.
    (B) Add an anxiolytic medication.
    (C) Add an antidepressant.
    (D) Discontinue methylphenidate and prescribe a mixed amphetamine compound.
    (E) Discontinue methylphenidate and prescribe an antidepressant.

109. A 19-year-old man is brought to the emergency department by the police for an evaluation. The written police report states that the patient has been calling 911 for the past 4 weeks reporting that he is being spied on by aliens from a distant planet. The patient reports that he is receiving messages from the aliens through his radio and that he hears voices in his head commenting on his appearance. He has not been sleeping well at night because he has been "guarding his bedroom." You note that his affect is flat, and he appears tired during your examination. A urine toxicology screen is negative. Which of the following is the most likely diagnosis?

    (A) schizophrenia
    (B) bipolar I disorder with psychotic features
    (C) schizoaffective disorder
    (D) brief psychotic disorder
    (E) MDD with psychotic features

110. An 18-year-old woman with recently diagnosed schizophrenia is acutely psychotic and in labor with her first child. The obstetric service requests a psychiatric consultation for a safe medication to control the patient's psychosis while she is in labor. Which of the following would be relatively safe?

    (A) haloperidol (Haldol)
    (B) chlorpromazine (Thorazine)
    (C) thioridazine (Mellaril)
    (D) droperidol (Inapsine)
    (E) trihexphenidyl (Artane)

DIRECTIONS (Questions 111 through 120): Each set of items in this section consists of a list of lettered headings followed by several numbered words or phrases. For each numbered word or phrase, select the ONE lettered option that is most closely associated with it. Each lettered option may be selected once, more than once, or not at all.

Questions 111 through 113

Match the appropriate test to assess for intelligence in each age group.

    (A) Wechsler Preschool and Primary Scale of Intelligence (WPPSI)
    (B) Wechsler Adult Intelligence Scale–Revised (WAIS-R)
    (C) Wechsler Memory Scale (WMS)
    (D) Wechsler Intelligence Scale for Children (WISC)

111. A 4-year-old girl whose parents wish to have her evaluated for entrance into an "elite" kindergarten

112. A 65-year-old female physician who is now concerned about memory difficulties

113. An 8-year-old boy whom the school system wants evaluated for possible special needs in the classroom

Questions 114 through 116

Match the clinical presentation with the appropriate neuropsychological test.

- (A) Minnesota Multiphasic Personality Inventory-2 (MMPI-2)
- (B) WISC
- (C) Rey–Osterreith Test
- (D) Beck Depression Inventory
- (E) Blessed Rating Scale
- (F) WAIS-R
- (G) Boston Diagnostic Aphasia Examination
- (H) Rorschach Test
- (I) Mini-Mental Status Exam (MMSE)
- (J) Bender–Gestalt Test
- (K) Wisconsin Card Sorting Test (WCST)
- (L) Wada's Test

114. A 35-year-old woman with a protein S deficiency shows evidence of left side hemineglect.

115. A 7-year-old boy with difficulty in school needs further evaluation of academic potential.

116. You would like to address the deficits of a 69-year-old man with nonfluent speech and formulate a specific treatment plan.

Questions 117 through 120

Select the drug most likely to cause the associated symptoms.

- (A) lysergic acid diethylamine (LSD)
- (B) phencyclidine (PCP)
- (C) cocaine
- (D) marijuana
- (E) opiates
- (F) nicotine

117. An 18-year-old high school student with conjunctival redness, increased appetite, dry mouth, tachycardia, and a sensation of slowed time

118. A 31-year-old man with miosis, bradycardia, hypotension, hypothermia, and constipation

119. An assaultive 26-year-old man with vertical nystagmus, echolalia, paranoid ideation, and hallucinations

120. A 16-year-old girl with abdominal cramps, confusion, palpitations, and muscle twitching

Answers and Explanations

1. **(D)** Antipsychotics are indicated for acute treatment of agitation and violence sometimes seen in manic patients. Haloperidol works quickly (20–30 minutes). Doses of 2 to 5 mg PO or IM are usual initial doses. It may be given IV as well, especially in the intensive care unit (ICU) setting. Hydroxyzine is an antihistamine; it is not effective in mania. Lithium, valproic acid, and carbamazepine have all been shown to control mood fluctuations in manic patients. However, these agents take days to work and are not effective in the acute management of this patient.

2. **(A)** Lithium is not associated with significant blood dyscrasias, although it can cause a modest benign increase in the white blood cell (WBC) count. Carbamazepine is commonly associated with reduced WBC count, but the incidence of agranulocytosis is approximately 1 in 10,000. Agranulocytosis is a rare complication with valproic acid; a bit more common is benign thrombocytopenia. Antipsychotic medication is occasionally associated with a decrease in leukopoiesis, but the WBC count usually returns to normal with continued treatment. Agranulocytosis can also occur in the setting of antipsychotic medication use in approximately 1 in 10,000 cases (clozapine has a higher incidence). Lorazepam is not associated with WBC abnormalities.

3. **(A)** Somatization disorder is characterized by multiple physical complaints that cannot be explained by any objective physical findings. As in this case, patients' symptoms frequently date back many years and have prompted multiple doctor visits, even hospitalizations. Conversion disorder is a loss or deficit of motor or sensory function that is inconsistent with any known physiologic basis; paralysis of both hands would be an example. Conversion disorders typically follow an identifiable stressor. Hypochondriasis is a fear of serious disease; it results from a hypervigilance and misinterpretation of normal bodily sensations. Malingering is the confabulation of symptoms with the conscious goal of personal gain; for example, using a doctor's diagnosis to get one out of work. Factitious disorder is the purposeful production of signs or symptoms for the express purpose of becoming a patient (and assuming the sick role).

4. **(D)** Somatization disorder often coexists with other psychiatric illnesses, such as anxiety, depressive, and personality disorders. The suspected presence of a somatization disorder should prompt a search for other, treatable illnesses. In managing patients with somatization disorder, it is important to accept that symptoms are not consciously produced and to let patients know that you realize their symptoms are a source of great consternation. Regardless of history, any patient presenting to a physician with physical complaints deserves a reasonable physical investigation; patients with somatization disorder are as likely, if not more likely, to develop identifiable medical conditions. However, rather than repeat tests, it may be necessary to contact previous treaters. Sending this patient away for a year would not be helpful; rather, regular, frequent checkups and foster-

ing a therapeutic alliance and support are in order.

5. **(C)** Women are as much as 20 times more likely to receive the diagnosis of somatization disorder than are men. Rarely will any therapy or intervention "cure" the patient of somatization disorder; at best, patients will learn to minimize the impact somatization has on their lives. Somatization disorder is found more commonly in lower socioeconomic groups. Conversion symptoms are common in somatization disorder and are included in the diagnostic criteria. Patients with this disorder benefit from regular, scheduled visits that allow them to forge a trusting therapeutic alliance.

6. **(A)** People with schizotypal personality disorder are actively odd. They expose peculiar thoughts, may speak in an idiosyncratic language, and exhibit eccentric behaviors. Someone with schizoid personality disorder, while cool and aloof, would not endorse the mild delusion that witches live down the road. Unlike the schizotypal patient, the avoidant patient longs for relationships, yet is morbidly shy and fears them. The patient in this question displays no trace of an overwrought dependence on others, as would be seen in dependent personality disorder. Nor does this patient appear to be involved in the chaotic, intensely troublesome relationships in which the borderline patient finds himself.

7. **(C)** Schizotypal personality disorder, with its attendant social isolation and subtle distortions of reality, may indeed resemble schizophrenia in remission; the diagnosis can be sorted out by a thorough history. Frank hallucinations of any type are uncommon; only subtle distortion of environmental cues is seen. While men may be slightly more at risk for being diagnosed with schizotypal personality disorder, the disparity is not stark. As with any personality disorder, schizotypal personality disorder represents a lifelong maladaptive approach to life and does not suddenly express itself well into adulthood.

8. **(D)** In schizotypal personality disorder, the subtle disconnection from reality, which may be exacerbated in times of stress as in this case, can be treated with low doses of neuroleptics. These patients lack the capability, stable sense of self, and trust to be able to engage in, or benefit from, psychoanalysis. Antidepressant medication of any type, including tricylics and SSRIs, would be helpful in the schizotypal patient who displays significant affective (mood) symptoms, which is not seen in this case. There is no evidence of anxiety that would make benzodiazepines useful.

9. **(C)** Schizophrenia, schizophreniform disorder, and brief psychotic disorder include similar signs and symptoms and are differentiated largely on the basis of time course. Episodes of 1 day to 1 month, 1 to 6 months, and more than 6 months are associated with a diagnosis of brief psychotic disorder, schizophreniform disorder, and schizophrenia, respectively. As symptoms persist, the diagnosis changes. With her delusions, hallucinations, disorganized speech, social dysfunction, and negative symptoms, this patient meets criteria for one of these psychotic illnesses; because these symptoms have lasted for longer than 6 months, the most likely diagnosis is schizophrenia. MDD and bipolar disorder are both remote possibilities, but the bizarreness of her delusion and lack of report of a significant mood component make these diagnoses less likely.

10. **(D)** Symptoms of schizophrenia are commonly divided into positive and negative symptoms. Flat affect, a negative symptom, represents an absence, in this case, of a normally reactive and variable affect. Auditory hallucinations, delusions (including paranoid delusions), and loose associations are all positive symptoms.

11. **(D)** The lifetime prevalence rate for schizophrenia is about 1%. The remaining statements are false. Positive symptoms tend to respond more readily than negative symptoms to medication; there is some hope that the

newer atypical antipsychotics target negative symptoms better than the older typical antipsychotics, but this is the subject of considerable study. Patients with schizophrenia experience significantly higher rates of drug and alcohol abuse and dependence. Most patients diagnosed with schizophrenia will need to be on medications indefinitely; remission in 5 years is the exception. It has been repeatedly shown that persons diagnosed with schizophrenia are born more frequently in winter months than the general population. The meaning of this is unknown.

12. **(E)** When starting a patient on antipsychotic medication (neuroleptics), the most important consideration is the side effects the patient will experience. Compliance with medication is usually a major issue, and there is a general tendency to want to "get off on the right foot." Renal function is less important with neuroleptics, because they are cleared principally by the liver. The presence of negative symptoms may steer a clinician toward the atypical antipsychotics, but today these are often chosen because of their superior side effect profile. Gender and onset of action do not typically guide the choice of neuroleptic.

13. **(B)** Of the choices presented, oral haloperidol is most appropriate. This patient needs an antipsychotic drug. Haloperidol decanoate, a long-acting (usually dosed monthly) intramuscular preparation, is reserved for patients known to respond well to, and tolerate, oral haloperidol. It would not be used first line, for legal and medical reasons. Untoward side effects, if experienced, would persist as there is no easy way to increase the metabolism or elimination of a decanoate prep. Lithium and valproic acid (mood stabilizers) and amitriptyline (a tricyclic antidepressant [TCA]) may be used in schizophrenia if there is a significant affective component, but that is not seen here.

14. **(C)** The exacerbation seen is most likely precipitated by medication noncompliance. Stress from work or a viral illness may in-deed contribute to a relapse, but they are less strongly predictive of a reemergence of psychotic symptoms than medication noncompliance. Nicotine has been shown to lower neuroleptic levels—which has been offered as a reason cigarette smoking is rampant among patients with schizophrenia—but not to the extent that it would incite an exacerbation of symptoms.

15. **(D)** Because the defense mechanism of denial is active in alcoholism, the best approach in evaluating a patient would be to explore how alcohol affects his life, rather than direct questions about drinking behavior. Hearing about his drinking from his friends and family may provide a more accurate description of a patient's alcoholism than the alcoholic would provide of himself. While lab work might provide clues to the presence of alcoholism, it cannot be relied on to make the diagnosis.

16. **(B)** Classically, patients with hepatitis secondary to alcohol abuse or dependence will have elevated liver enzymes (such as gamma-glutamyl transpeptidase, aspartate transaminase, or alanine transaminase). However, in advanced alcoholism, the liver may be "burnt out," and liver function tests may reveal low or normal levels of these enzymes. As a result of liver damage, prothrombin time is typically increased. Hypomagnesemia, not hypermagnesemia, is more likely to be found in alcoholism, usually as a result of dietary deficiency. In the patient having a withdrawal seizure, the problem is absence, not presence, of alcohol. His blood alcohol is expected to be zero. The alcoholic is more likely to have thrombocytopenia than thrombocytosis.

17. **(B)** As a result of vitamin deficiencies and the direct insult alcohol exacts on the nerve function, peripheral neuropathy can be seen in 10% of heavy drinkers. Another important nervous system effect of alcohol and its metabolites is cerebellar degeneration, which can be suggested by an unsteady gait and nystagmus. Alcoholic "fatty liver"—a swollen

liver resulting from the deposition of fats and proteins in the hepatocytes—will reverse with abstinence from alcohol. While there is some evidence that a glass of wine each day may impart some protective cardiac effects, heavy drinking is certainly destructive to the cardio-vascular system. It raises the blood pressure and raises levels of triglycerides, thus increasing the risk of myocardial infarction. Heavy drinking also lowers WBC count and interferes with many specific aspects of the immune system; for example, it compromises T-cell function.

18. **(B)** The patient does not have a history of mental illness, which gives you information about past behaviors, especially suicidality. She is unable to contract for safety, and attempts to contact collaterals have been unsuccessful. Collateral information is essential to validate the present history as well as to provide data about baseline mental status. In the absence of collateral input, from both family and health care professionals, and the important fact that she remains suicidal, the patient should not be discharged from the emergency department. The patient does not exhibit psychotic behavior and is not a management problem. The administration of an antipsychotic medication can cause side effects and may affect future compliance with psychotropic medications. A thorough history, physical, and MSE, in conjunction with sound judgment based on the available facts, supplants judgment based on a telephone presentation or decisions by managed care organizations.

19. **(C)** The psychiatric disorder that carries the greatest risk for suicide in both males and females is a mood disorder. Although up to 15% of all alcohol-dependent persons commit suicide and up to 10% of schizophrenic patients commit suicide, the age-adjusted suicide rates for patients with mood disorders is estimated at 400 per 100,000 males and 180 per 100,000 females. Multiple sclerosis and cancer are distractors.

20. **(C)** Suicidal ideation is a serious manifestation of myriad disease processes. High-risk characteristics of suicidal persons have been studied extensively, and predictive variables exist to assist the physician when called to assess suicidal ideation. Age 45 or greater is the most predictive factor. Alcohol dependence, rage or violence, prior suicidal behavior, and male gender follow, in that order.

21. **(A)** Men successfully complete suicide attempts more than three times as often as women do, and suicide rates increase with age. However, the frequency of suicide attempts is roughly equal among men and women. The rate of suicide among whites is almost twice that of nonwhites, and the rates have been stable over time. Historically, suicide rates among Catholics have been lower than the rates among Protestants and Jews.

22. **(E)** The higher the individual's social status, the greater the risk of suicide. A fall in social status also increases the risk. The rate for never-married individuals is almost double the rate for married individuals. Physical illness has been shown to be a significant contributing factor in suicide risk, and the risk of suicide in both sexes is highest during the first week of a psychiatric admission.

23. **(D)** The rate of suicide is greater for whites than for nonwhites. White females are more likely to attempt suicide than African-American females, and two thirds of all suicides are white males. Native American groups exceed the national rate. Suicide is higher in the immigrant population.

24. **(C)** This scenario represents a case of Munchausen syndrome by proxy, in which one person feigns illness in another to vicariously gain medical attention. Commonly, the victim is a child and the perpetrator is the child's mother. Apparent bleeding, seizures, and central nervous system (CNS) depression are typical presentations. The disorder is underdiagnosed and typically will take more than a year to diagnose, due both to the elusive and crafty planning of the perpetrator and the un-

willingness of health care providers to accuse the ostensibly caring parent. Conversion disorder is a disorder characterized by the presence of one or more neurologic symptoms that are left unexplained by a known medical or neurologic disorder. It is associated with such comorbid psychiatric disorders as MDD, anxiety disorder, or schizophrenia, and adolescents and young adults suffer from this disorder most commonly. Paralysis, blindness, and mutism are the most common conversion disorder symptoms. The diagnosis requires the association of psychological factors to the initiation and exacerbation of conversion symptoms. In this case, there are no data to support this diagnosis.

25. **(C)** The mental status of the mother has been described as depressed, anxious, and suicidal. Borderline and histrionic personality disorders are the most common Axis II diagnoses associated with Munchausen by proxy, and most sufferers demonstrate a dissociation of affect. Schizophrenia has been reported in only a few cases. Of the choices listed, depression is the most likely, as bipolar disorder and PTSD have not been clearly described in the literature. Epilepsy is not associated with the disorder to any significant extent.

26. **(B)** Panic disorder is characterized by the sudden unexpected occurrence of panic attacks and periods of intense anxiety or fear accompanied by somatic symptoms, commonly causing the misdiagnosis of a medical illness such as myocardial infarction. The frequency of panic attacks varies widely from many per day to a few per year. Panic disorder is often associated with agoraphobia, the fear of being alone in public places. The lifetime prevalence is up to 3%. Concerns of death from cardiac or respiratory disorders occur frequently. Delirium is characterized by the sudden onset of a disturbance of consciousness with cognitive changes caused by a general medical condition. Acute stress disorder is diagnosed in individuals who have experienced a traumatic event and subsequently develop symptoms within 4 weeks of

the event that remit after 1 month. The traumatic event must be reexperienced by the patient, and this causes the patient to avoid stimuli that arouse recollections of the trauma. Other criteria necessary for the diagnosis are the presence of dissociative symptoms and marked anxiety or increased arousal not better accounted for by other medical or psychiatric illnesses.

27. **(A)** Tricyclic and tetracyclic medications, MAOIs, SSRIs, and the benzodiazepines are effective in the treatment of panic disorder. Beta-adrenergic drugs like propranolol are not effective for the treatment of panic disorder. Haloperidol, an antipsychotic agent; lithium, a mood stabilizer; and clonidine, an alpha-2 adrenergic agonist, are ineffective. Of the choices listed, sertraline, an SSRI, is most effective.

28. **(A)** Hypertensive crisis is a potentially life-threatening complication that occurs when patients taking an MAOI eat tyramine-containing foods such as wine, beer, pickled foods, and aged cheese. Clinical features include hypertension, severe occipital headache, stiff neck, nausea, vomiting, and sweating. Phentolamine, an alpha-adrenergic receptor-blocking drug, is given intravenously to control hypertension. It has been shown to be more effective than beta blockers or calcium channel blockers. Admission to an ICU and supportive measures are indicated. Although muscle rigidity can occur, the use of dantrolene, a muscle relaxant, is not indicated.

29. **(E)** Clozapine is an effective antipsychotic medication that has been associated with fewer extrapyramidal side effects than the conventional antispychotics (which primarily act by blocking dopamine type 2 receptors). About 5% of patients taking more than 600 mg per day of clozapine will experience clozapine-associated seizures. Tachycardia, hypotension, sedation, fatigue, and weight gain have all been associated with clozapine treatment. Clozapine, unlike the conventional antipsychotic agents, does not affect

prolactin secretion and thus does not cause galactorrhea.

30. **(A)** Agranulocytosis is a potentially life-threatening side effect of clozapine treatment. It is defined as a decrease in the number of WBCs, with a specific decrease in the number of neutrophil granulocytes. It occurs in 1 to 2% of all patients treated with clozapine. The other choices are bone marrow disorders that are not associated with clozapine.

31. **(E)** Schizotypal personality disorder is characterized by a pervasive pattern of social and interpersonal deficits. Individuals demonstrate a reduced capacity to establish any close relationships, and eccentric behavior is present. The presence of odd beliefs or magical thinking separates schizotypal personality disorder from schizoid personality disorder. Paranoid ideation is common in both schizotypal and paranoid personality disorders but not in the others. Schizoid personality disorder represents a pervasive pattern of detachment from social relationships and a restricted range of expressed emotions. Avoidant personality disorder represents a pervasive pattern of behavior characterized by social inhibition, feelings of inadequacy, and hypersensitivity to negative evaluation. Narcissistic personality disorder represents a pervasive pattern of grandiosity, lack of empathy, and a need for admiration.

32. **(B)** Borderline personality disorder is a pervasive pattern of instability of interpersonal relationships, self-image, affect, and marked impulsivity. Antisocial personality disorder describes individuals with long histories of disregard for the rights of others and often dishonesty used in attempts to gain something for themselves. Patients with histrionic personality disorder, like those with borderline personality disorder, may display excessive emotionality and attention-seeking behavior, but their core symptoms center around superficial seductiveness and theatricality. Those with dependent personality disorder require an excessive amount of advice, reassurance, and approval from others.

Schizoid personality disorder represents a pervasive pattern of detachment from social relationships and a restricted range of expressed emotions.

33. **(C)** Bipolar I disorder is characterized by the presence of major depressive and manic episodes. A manic episode describes a period of an abnormally elevated mood with associated symptoms of grandiose behavior, a decreased need for sleep, pressured speech, racing thoughts, distractibility, an increase in goal-directed activity or an increase in energy, and excessive involvement in potentially dangerous activities. Bipolar II disorder shares the expansive mood and associated symptoms as bipolar I disorder, but symptoms are less severe and referred to as hypomania. Delusional disorder requires the presence of nonbizarre delusions that occur in real life, and evidence of mania should not be present. Schizophreniform disorder describes individuals who meet criteria for schizophrenia but whose symptoms have not been present for 6 months.

34. **(A)** Racing thoughts, pressured speech, expansive mood, a decreased need for sleep, and an increase in goal-directed activity are all common manifestations of mania. The patient is usually energized during the day even after only a few hours of sleep. Weight loss and depressed mood are characteristic of a depressive disorder. Auditory hallucinations may be present in severe cases of mania but are usually a symptom of a psychotic disorder such as schizophrenia.

35. **(B)** Many disorders can mimic symptoms of mania. A complete history, physical exam, and routine laboratory tests can sufficiently rule out most medical causes of mania. They include endocrine disorders such as thyrotoxicosis and Cushing's disease, hypoglycemia, electrolyte disorders, substance abuse and withdrawal, medications such as steroids and anticholinergic agents, nutritional deficiencies, and CNS insults.

36. **(D)** Lithium and valproic acid are indicated as first-line agents for the treatment of bipolar manic episodes. Antipsychotic agents like chlorpromazine are important for the treatment of psychosis, sometimes associated with mania, but are not considered effective as single agents. Fluoxetine is an antidepressant that may actually activate patients with bipolar disorder and precipitate a manic episode. Ideally, all medications should be discontinued during pregnancy, but in many instances they are necessary. Considering the risk–benefit ratio is important. Low-potency antipsychotics (chlorpromazine), lithium, and valproic acid are all associated with an increased risk of congenital abnormalities, especially when taken during the first trimester. The benzodiazepines are associated with an increased risk for oral clefts after first-trimester exposure. However, this remains controversial. ECT has been used in pregnancy for more than 50 years, and its safety and efficacy is well-documented.

37. **(B)** Cessation or a reduction in sedative, hypnotic, or anxiolytic medications that have been used heavily or for a prolonged period of time may result in a withdrawal syndrome characterized by symptoms that develop within hours to a few days after cessation or reduction. Autonomic hyperactivity, orthostatic hypotension, muscle weakness, tremor, insomnia, nausea, vomiting, auditory/visual/tactile hallucinations, agitation, or anxiety may occur. By far, the most serious sequelae are grand mal seizures or delirium. As many as 75% of patients may experience grand mal seizures on the second or third day of withdrawal and two thirds of these patients will have more than one seizure. Delirium may develop between the third and eighth day of withdrawal. Minor symptoms may persist for up to 2 weeks.

38. **(C)** Gingival hyperplasia is associated with administration of phenytoin. Other, dose-related symptoms include nystagmus, dizziness, slurred speech, ataxia, mental confusion, and decreased coordination. Hepatic failure is associated with valproic acid, and

Ebstein's anomaly is associated with lithium therapy.

39. **(D)** Before any pharmacologic changes are considered, the physician must assess compliance with medications. The subtherapeutic phenytoin level may be due to patient noncompliance, especially if side effects are being experienced.

40. **(E)** The risk of schizophrenia among first-degree relatives of patients with the disease may be as high as 10%, compared with a 1% risk in the general population.

41. **(D)** Attention is defined as the ability to focus one's perception on an outside or inside stimulus. A simple test of attention is digit recall. Most people can recall a seven-digit number forward and five to seven digits in reverse. Concentration refers to sustained attention to an internal thought process. The serial seven examination, in which the examiner asks the patient to subtract 7 from 100 and continue the subtraction process for as many calculations as possible, is a good test of concentration. Another test of concentration is to have the patient spell a five-letter word forward and backward. Asking the patient to recall the examiner's name is an example of recent memory, and asking him to recall his Social Security number is a test of remote memory.

42. **(E)** Cocaine intoxication can appear like a manic episode associated with bipolar I disorder, with an increase in energy, euphoria, grandiosity, and impaired judgment. The acute onset of symptoms makes the diagnosis of major depression unlikely. A diagnosis of schizophrenia requires the presence of symptoms during a significant portion of the previous month, which is not evident. In this case, the patient experiences a sudden onset of euphoria that is not characteristic of schizophrenia. Negative symptoms (e.g., flattened affect, avolition, alogia) are more common in schizophrenia. The diagnosis of schizoaffective disorder requires that during the period of illness there are symptoms that suggest a

diagnosis of both schizophrenia and a mood disorder (major depressive episode, manic episode, or a mixed episode). Cannabis intoxication can present with euphoria, paranoia, and impaired judgment in association with physical symptoms of conjunctival injection, increased appetite, dry mouth, and tachycardia. A decreased need for sleep does not suggest cannabis intoxication.

43. **(E)** Culture-bound syndromes denote recurrent, locality-specific patterns of behavior. The syndrome of amok is a culture-bound syndrome of Malayan origin that refers to a violent or furious outburst with homicidal intent. Four defining characteristics are prodromal brooding, a homicidal outburst, persistence in reckless killing without an apparent motive, and a claim of amnesia. The attack typically will result in multiple casualties and is most common in young men whose self-esteem has been injured. Ganser syndrome is characterized by a patient who responds to questions by giving approximate or outright ridiculous answers. Additional features include altered consciousness, hallucinations, conversion phenomenon, and amnesia for the episode. Dissociative identity disorder is a chronic state in which two or more separate ongoing identities or personalities alternate in consciousness. It usually occurs in patients who experienced severe and repeated abuse as young children.

44. **(A)** High-potency antipsychotics such as thiothixene and haloperidol block dopamine receptors more potently than the low-potency antipsychotics such as chlorpromazine. Thioperidol and daslaperizone are nonsense names of drugs that do not exist.

45. **(C)** Neuroleptic-induced extrapyramidal side effects, due to the blockade of dopamine, are common in the treatment of psychosis. The higher-potency neuroleptic drugs are more likely to cause extrapyramidal side effects than the lower-potency neuroleptics. Extrapyramidal side effects are diminished by agents such as benztropine, antihistamines, benzodiazepines, and dopamine agonists.

There are four types of extrapyramidal side effects: acute dystonic reactions, akathisia (restlessness), pseudoparkinsonism, and tardive dyskinesia or tardive dystonia. In this case, the treatment of the involuntary movements involves evaluation of dose and type of neuroleptic. Reducing the dose, substituting with a higher-potency agent, or adding an antiparkinsonian drug are all feasible therapeutic interventions.

46. **(A)** Antipsychotic agents lower the seizure threshold and do not precipitate seizures on withdrawal. Dry mouth, constipation, and blurred vision are all anticholinergic side effects and not associated with medication discontinuation. Movement disorders such as dyskinesia often persist despite the discontinuation of the antipsychotic medication likely to have caused them.

47. **(B)** Atypical antipsychotic agents are thought to act on various subpopulations of dopamine neurons as well as on various dopamine receptor subtypes and other neurotransmitter systems. They are considered atypical agents because they are associated with a lower risk of extrapyramidal symptoms. Clozapine, introduced to the United States in 1989, is the first antipsychotic to be labeled atypical. The other choices are all considered typical antipsychotics.

48. **(D)** Borderline personality disorder is a pattern of instability in interpersonal relationships, self-image, affect, and marked impulsivity. Dialectical behavioral therapy, a manualized treatment for chronically parasuicidal patients that incorporates elements of cognitive, behavioral, and supportive therapies, is a form of cognitive–behavioral treatment for borderline personality disorder. Avoidant personality disorder represents a pervasive pattern of behavior characterized by social inhibition, feelings of inadequacy, and hypersensitivity to negative evaluation. Schizoid personality disorder represents a pervasive pattern of detachment from social relationships and a restricted range of expressed emotions. Bipolar disorder is an affec-

tive illness characterized by alternating periods of mania and major depression. Passive–aggressive personality disorder describes a pervasive pattern of negativistic attitudes and passive resistance to demands for adequate performance.

49. **(A)** General principles of DBT include believing that the patient wants to improve and is doing the best he can. The patient is encouraged to take responsibility and solve his own problems. Patients may not have caused all of their problems, but they are encouraged to solve them anyway. Patients learn new behaviors in a relative context and believe that they cannot fail in therapy.

50. **(A)** The patient is experiencing anticholinergic toxicity as evidenced by dilated pupils, dry or flushed skin, agitation, confusion, and tachycardia. Additional manifestations include disorientation and urinary retention. More severe toxicity may result in hyperthermia or coma. In this case, the patient reported benefit from haloperidol but experienced extrapyramidal side effects, common to the high-potency antipsychotic medications. Benztropine, an anticholinergic medication, is prescribed to alleviate extrapyramidal side effects, but in this patient it caused anticholinergic side effects. Amantadine is an antiviral medication that is used to help alleviate extrapyramidal side effects and should be instituted to replace benztropine.

51. **(C)** Denial, a narcissistic defense, is a common unconscious emotional defense mechanism used to avoid becoming aware of a painful aspect of reality. Denial can be used in both normal and pathologic states. As a defense mechanism it serves to keep internal or external reality out of the conscious in order to avert stress and anxiety. Regression, an immature defense, is an emotional and physical retreat from adult standards of behavior toward an infantile level of passivity and dependence. At times, regression represents a retreat from the arduous task of recovery. Rationalization is a neurotic defense mechanism in which unacceptable behavior, feelings, or

thoughts are logically justified by elaborate and reassuring answers. Suppression, a mature defense, is a conscious act of controlling and inhibiting unacceptable impulses, emotions, or ideas.

52. **(B)** The essential feature of acute stress disorder is the development of anxiety and dissociative symptoms within 1 month of exposure to an extremely traumatic stressor. The diagnosis should be considered if the symptoms persist at least 2 days and cause significant distress or impairment. While experiencing the stressor, the individual must experience three of these five symptoms: a subjective sense of numbing, detachment, or absence of emotional responsiveness; a reduction in awareness of surroundings; derealization; depersonalization; or dissociative amnesia. In addition, the person must reexperience the event in some way (e.g., bad dreams), must experience anxiety or increased arousal, and must experience a marked avoidance of the stimuli that arouse recollections of the traumatic event. The diagnosis of PTSD requires more than 1 month of symptoms. Adjustment disorder can be considered for those individuals who do not meet criteria for acute stress disorder but develop similar symptoms in excess of what is to be expected given the nature of the stressor. GAD is characterized by excessive anxiety and worry that occur for at least 6 months. MDD can exist in the context of an acute stress reaction. However, in this case, the symptoms are not suggestive of a depressive illness.

53. **(E)** Psychogenic unresponsiveness can be delineated from coma by obtaining an EEG, which will be normal in a psychogenic state. On physical examination, deep tendon reflexes may be suppressed. In patients who are awake, cold water introduced into the ear produces nystagmus, with the fast component away from the ear. In coma, the eyes either do not react or they may slowly and smoothly deviate toward the ear in which the cold water was introduced. Voluntary eye movements, called saccades, are rapid and smooth. Saccadic eye movements are elicited

in patients by asking them to stare at an object at one side of the visual field and then ask them to shift their gaze to the opposite visual field. Typically, eye movements in coma or persistent vegetative states are spontaneous and random.

54. **(E)** Seasonal affective disorder describes a seasonal pattern of symptoms associated with major depressive episodes in MDD, bipolar I disorder, and bipolar II disorder. The essential feature is the onset of depressive symptoms at characteristic times of the year. More common in females, most episodes begin in the fall or winter and remit in the spring. Major depressive episodes that occur in a seasonal pattern are typically characterized by anergy, hypersomnia, overeating, weight gain, and carbohydrate craving. Age is a strong predictor, with young persons at higher risk.

55. **(C)** The essential features of dissociative fugue are sudden and unexpected travel away from home or one's usual place of daily activities, with a subsequent inability to recall the episode, accompanied by confusion about personal identity or the assumption of a new identity. The disorder is more common in women and is often associated with a childhood history of sexual abuse. Partial complex seizures tend to be brief and do not last as long as the clinical picture presents. Delirium is characterized by a disturbance of consciousness and a change in cognition that develops over a short period of time.

56. **(C)** Bipolar II disorder is characterized by the occurrence of one or more major depressive episodes accompanied by at least one episode of hypomania (a distinct period of a persistently elevated, expansive, or irritable mood that lasts at least 4 days). It differs from bipolar I disorder in that, although the manic and hypomanic episodes of these two disorders have identical list criteria, bipolar II disorder is not severe enough to cause marked impairment in social or occupational functioning or to cause hospitalization. Cy-

clothymic disorder and dysthymic disorder require a 2-year history of symptoms.

57. **(B)** The hallmark of Ganser syndrome is that the patient responds to questions by giving approximate or ridiculous answers. Often confused with malingering, Ganser syndrome is primarily described in the prison population. It involves the production of answers to questions that are relative but not quite correct (e.g., $4 \times 5 = 19$). It is classified in the *Diagnostic and Statistical Manual of Mental Disorders*, 4th edition, Text Revision (DSM-IV-TR), as a dissociative disorder not otherwise specified. Munchausen syndrome is a factitious disorder with physical symptoms. Capgras syndrome describes a content-specific delusion in which the patient believes that a significant other, usually a family member, has been replaced by an identical imposter.

58. **(E)** ECT provides safe and effective treatment of MDD in the elderly, especially in a patient with a high risk of suicide or medical contraindications (e.g., heart disease) to the use of psychotropic medications. Nortriptyline, a TCA, is lethal in overdose and should not be prescribed in an acutely suicidal patient. Cardiac arrhythmia is also a contraindication to TCA use.

59. **(B)** The specifiers of melancholic features and atypical features can be applied to a current or recent major depressive episode that occurs in the course of MDD and to a major depressive episode in bipolar I or bipolar II disorder. The atypical features specifier can also be applied to dysthymic disorder. The essential features of the atypical specifier are mood reactivity and two of the following four features: increased appetite or weight gain, hypersomnia, leaden paralysis, and rejection sensitivity. The essential feature of a major depressive episode with melancholic features is a loss of interest or pleasure in all or almost all activities or a lack of reactivity to usually pleasurable stimuli.

60. **(A)** Identification is an unconscious defense mechanism in which the person incorporates

the characteristics and qualities of another person or object into his or her own ego system. The defense serves to strengthen the ego. Regression, an immature defense, is an emotional and physical retreat from adult standards of behavior toward an infantile level of passivity and dependence. Projection is the false attribution of one's own unacceptable feelings to another. Fixation refers to an overactive attachment to a person or object, while idealization is the attribution of near-perfect, unrealistic attributes to that person or object.

61. **(C)** The essential feature of the catatonia observed in patients with schizophrenia is a marked psychomotor disturbance involving motor immobility, excessive motor activity, mutism, negativism, peculiar voluntary movements, echolalia (parrotlike senseless repetition of words or phrases), or echopraxia (imitation of movements of another person). Catalepsy, classically associated with schizophrenia, is a general term for an immobile position that is constantly maintained. It can also occur in dementia or in the twilight states of disturbed consciousness, and represents one symptom of catatonia. Cataplexy is a sudden and brief loss of muscle tone involving either a few muscle groups or most of the antigravity muscles of the body. The fact that the patient occasionally mimics the movements of others makes seizure activity unlikely.

62. **(A)** Catalepsy is a general term for the assumption of an immobile position that is constantly maintained, especially after an examination. Cataplexy is a sudden and brief loss of muscle tone involving either a few muscle groups or most of the antigravity muscles of the body. Dystonia is a stiffening of muscle groups sometimes seen after administration of typical neuroleptics. The patient does not seem to have a secondary gain for his symptoms, making malingering unlikely.

63. **(D)** Priapism can occur with a number of antidepressant or antipsychotic agents but occurs most often with the use of trazodone (1

in 1,000 to 1 in 10,000 incidence). The three SSRIs (fluoxetine, sertraline, and paroxetine) listed can cause impotence, but are unlikely to cause priapism. Nortriptyline is a TCA not associated with priapism.

64. **(C)** The condition usually occurs within the first 4 weeks of treatment but can happen as late as 18 months into treatment. The condition is independent of dose. Priapism is a medical emergency and may require surgery. The condition may respond to intracavernosal injection of an alpha-adrenergic agonist to promote detumescence and constriction of veins.

65. **(B)** GAD is defined by excessive anxiety or worry occurring for at least 6 months. Associated symptoms include feeling restless, fatigued, or irritable; muscle tension; difficulty with concentration; and sleep disturbance. Patients with panic disorder are usually more disabled by their symptoms and seek help much earlier than patients with GAD. Although depression and dysthymia share some symptoms with GAD, the depressive symptoms are more severe in the mood disorders than with the anxiety disorders. The onset of anxiety with panic disorder is more sudden and more intense, with the fear of choking or dying more common. Separation anxiety requires the onset of symptoms before the age of 18, and dependent personality disorder represents a pervasive need to be taken care of, leading to submissive, clinging behavior that begins in early childhood.

66. **(A)** Treatment of GAD includes antidepressants, benzodiazepines, buspirone, and cognitive–behavioral therapies. However, benzodiazepines should be avoided in patients with respiratory compromise, because these medications can exacerbate breathing-related disorders. Alprazolam, diazepam, and lorazepam are all benzodiazepines. Buspirone, a nonbenzodiazepine anxiolytic, is a logical alternative and has been demonstrated to be effective in the treatment of GAD. Beta-blocking agents such as propranolol are effective but should not be first-line therapy in patients with

chronic obstructive pulmonary disease or other respiratory disorders.

67. **(B)** The long-term use of benzodiazepines (temazepam, oxazepam, and clorazepate) for sleep is controversial, especially in patients with substance abuse or breathing-related disorders. Zolpidem is not a member of the benzodiazepine class but does produce its effects at the gamma-aminobutyric acid (GABA)–benzodiazepine (BZ) receptor and as a result has a much lower risk of dependence. Zaleplon (Sonata) is a newer nonbenzodiazepine hypnotic that interacts with the GABA–BZ receptor complex. It has an ultrashort half-life of 1 hour. A nonbenzodiazepine medication is a logical alternative in cases in which respiratory function is compromised. Benadryl should be avoided in the elderly because of its anticholingeric effects.

68. **(D)** Hypertensive crisis is a life-threatening emergency that may result from the combination of meperidine and an MAOI. The combined use of these medications is absolutely contraindicated. The treatment of hypertensive crisis is with intravenous alpha-adrenergic blocking agents and ICU admission and support. All of the other medications are safe in combination with MAOIs.

69. **(B)** The use of any medications in pregnancy requires examining the risks and benefits of treatment. The use of MAOIs is contraindicated in pregnancy, partly because they can exacerbate pregnancy-induced hypertension. Although ECT is safe in pregnancy, maintenance ECT is indicated after an initial course is completed. The safety of newer antidepressants such as paroxetine in pregnancy has not yet been completely established, although limited studies of fluoxetine suggest that it is relatively safe. Specific recommendations regarding the course of treatment for a single episode of MDD do not exist. Many physicians find that the treatment of a single episode requires 9 to 12 months of pharmacotherapy. The return of symptoms suggests a recurrent MDD that requires longer-term pharmacotherapy.

70. **(D)** The patient presents with clinical symptoms of Wernicke's encephalopathy, a medical emergency, characterized by ophthalmoplegia, ataxia, and delirium and caused by thiamine deficiency. If the thiamine deficiency is not corrected, Wernicke–Korsakoff syndrome emerges, characterized by amnesia, ataxia, and nystagmus. The syndrome results from chronic thiamine deficiency, with resultant pathology in the mamillary bodies and the thalamus. A history of alcohol abuse is common but other causes of thiamine deficiency, such as starvation, prolonged vomiting, and gastric carcinoma, can cause this syndrome. The use of intravenous dextrose prior to the administration of thiamine may aggravate Wernicke's encephalopathy. The other interventions may be appropriate if thiamine does not resolve the symptoms.

71. **(A)** Aphasia is characterized by the loss of language abilities produced by brain dysfunction. Cardiovascular disorders, brain tumors, infection, trauma, and degenerative diseases are the most common causes. Broca's aphasia is characterized by short, nonfluent output with intact comprehension. Reading comprehension is preserved. Wernicke's aphasia presents as fluent speech output with poor reading comprehension. Repetition, naming, writing, and reading aloud are impaired in both disorders. Wernicke's aphasia results from lesions of the posterior superior left temporal gyrus (Wernicke's area). Broca's aphasia results from a lesion of the middle third of the left inferior frontal gyrus (Broca's area).

72. **(C)** Caffeine withdrawal occurs after the abrupt cessation or a marked reduction in the use of caffeinated products. Studies estimate that up to 75% of caffeine users will experience symptoms of withdrawal at some point. Caffeine withdrawal symptoms have their onset 12 to 24 hours after the last dose, and symptoms peak in 24 to 48 hours. Symptoms typically remit in 1 week. Although all the possible choices are associated with caffeine withdrawal, up to 50% of sufferers will experience headache, the most common symptom.

73. **(B)** NMS is a rare, life-threatening complication that can occur at any time during treatment with antipsychotic medications. The pathophysiologic mechanism is unclear, but patients suffer from severe muscle rigidity, elevated temperature, autonomic dysfunction (increase or decrease in blood pressure and heart rate), and an altered level of consciousness, ranging from disorientation to coma. Associated findings include diaphoresis, dysphagia, incontinence, mutism, and tremor. There is no evidence that this patient is taking MAOIs that might induce a tyramine crisis. Similarly, there is no evidence that he is taking SSRIs that might induce serotonin syndrome, characterized by flushing, diarrhea, and diaphoresis. Malignant hyperthermia can be a symptom of NMS, as can dystonias.

74. **(E)** Death, reported in up to 30% of cases, usually results from the failure to recognize the syndrome or from delayed treatment. Discontinuation of the offending agent and supportive treatment in an ICU setting is imperative. Cooling measures reduce hyperthermia. Intravenous dantrolene sodium and oral bromocriptine have been used, but their benefits are unclear. The exact frequency remains unknown, with some studies suggesting up to 1.9% of all patients treated with antipsychotics experience this syndrome. NMS may be more frequent in men and younger patients. Naloxone does not have a place in the treatment of NMS.

75. **(C)** An elevated serum CPK demonstrates muscle injury. Leukocytosis is also seen. Elevated BUN may be seen in dehydration resulting from NMS, but is not as common as CPK elevation.

76. **(D)** Physical dependence emphasizes the presence of tolerance or withdrawal. Naloxone injection can precipitate opiate withdrawal in dependent persons. Positive urine toxicology or breath analysis can identify only substance abuse, not dependence. Elevated liver function studies can be present in individuals who abuse alcohol but can also be present in other non–substance-related disorders. Elevated heart rate can be present in many withdrawal syndromes or medical disorders and is not specific for any substance.

77. **(B)** Dementia is an organic and global decline of functioning without impaired consciousness. (This differentiates it from delirium, characterized by a waxing and waning consciousness.) The most common type of dementia (50 to 60%) is the Alzheimer's type. Vascular dementia is the second most common type of dementia, occurring in 10 to 20% of cases. Other degenerative processes that cause dementia are Parkinson's disease, Huntington's disease, and Pick's disease. Infectious, metabolic, endocrine, neoplastic, and toxic processes can also cause dementia. In this case, the history of cognitive decline without impaired consciousness suggests a diagnosis of dementia. The history reveals a megaloblastic anemia, the cause of which may be a vitamin B_{12} deficiency possibly secondary to a subtotal gastrectomy. Folate deficiency can also cause megaloblastic anemia. Vitamin deficiencies such as B_{12} and folate can cause clinical signs of dementia but represent one of a few possible reversible causes of this process. A complete reversible workup for dementia should also include thyroid function studies and an RPR (rapid plasma reagin) to test for syphilis. Alzheimer's disease is confirmed only by autopsy.

78. **(A)** Lithium, commonly used to treat bipolar disorder, can be dangerous in intoxication, which is a neurotoxic event and can lead to death or permanent damage to the nervous system, particularly the cerebellum. Cardiovascular and renal manifestations may also be present. Lithium has a low therapeutic index with a therapeutic range of 0.5 to 1.5 mEq/L. Plasma concentrations above the therapeutic range, especially greater than 2.0 mEq/L, will precipitate severe CNS and renal impairment. Early clinical signs of intoxication include dysarthria, coarse tremor, and ataxia. Impaired consciousness, fasciculations or myoclonus, seizures, and coma are omi-

nous manifestations. The goal of treatment is removal of lithium from the body. Gastric lavage, rehydration, and hemodialysis are possible interventions. Given the danger of lithium intoxication, a serum drug level should be obtained before any of the other interventions.

79. **(E)** Baseline medical tests should be obtained and documented before starting many psychotropic medications, including the mood stabilizers lithium, carbamazepine, and valproate. Assessment of thyroid function, complete blood count, electrolytes, ECG, and renal function studies (BUN, creatinine, urinalysis) are important before the initiation of lithium. Older patients require additional tests, including EEG, thyrotropin-releasing hormone test, 24-hour urine volume determination, and creatinine clearance. Lithium-induced polyuria results from the inhibition of the effect of antidiuretic hormone. Reversible T-wave changes on the ECG are common.

80. **(D)** The serotonin syndrome occurs when an SSRI is combined with another drug that can potentiate serotonin, such as the monoamine oxidase–inhibiting drugs, pentazocine, L-tryptophan, lithium, and carbamazepine. Symptoms of the syndrome include abdominal pain, diarrhea, diaphoresis, hyperpyrexia, tachycardia, hypertension, myoclonus, irritability, agitation, seizures, and delirium. Coma, cardiovascular collapse, and death have been reported. In this case, the serotonergic effects of fluoxetine are potentiated by the MAOI. Fluoxetine has a prolonged half-life with active metabolites that require up to 6 weeks' clearance time. Treatment with the MAOI was initiated before adequate washout of the fluoxetine and resulted in the serotonin syndrome. Management involves discontinuation of the offending agent and supportive care. There is no evidence that the patient is continuing to take her MAOI and eat a tyramine-heavy diet, that she has been abusing hallucinogens, or that she is taking antipsychotics that might induce any of the remaining choices.

81. **(A)** Bulimia nervosa, more common than anorexia nervosa, consists of repeated episodes of binge eating of large amounts of food associated with the feeling of being out of control. The patient usually purges by self-induced vomiting or repeated laxative or diuretic use and engages in excessive amounts of exercise to prevent weight gain. Unlike individuals with anorexia nervosa, individuals with bulimia nervosa usually maintain a normal body weight. Medical complications of bulimia nervosa are usually secondary to either chronic vomiting or laxative abuse. Fluid and electrolyte imbalances (alkalosis, hypokalemia, hypochloremia, dehydration); dental caries and enamel loss; gastrointestinal disturbances such as esophagitis, Mallory–Weiss tears, and constipation; and sore throat are also common.

82. **(B)** Antidepressant medications reduce binge eating and purging independent of the presence of a mood disorder. Imipramine, desipramine, MAOIs, and fluoxetine have been effective in controlled studies. The other choices treat symptoms of the illness without treating the underlying disorder.

83. **(B)** Anorexia nervosa is clinically characterized by a deliberate self-imposed starvation in the pursuit of being thin, driven by a fear of being fat. The patient refuses to maintain accepted normal body weight appropriate for age and height. Failure to achieve 85% of expected body weight, the intense fear of being fat, a disturbed perception of the body weight or shape (or denial of the seriousness of the current low body weight) and amenorrhea in postmenarchal females are diagnostic criteria. Underdeveloped breasts, abnormal insulin secretion, endocrine disorders, and poor sexual development with a marked decreased interest in sexual activity, are also associated with this disorder. For anorexia nervosa to be diagnosed, a postmenarchal female must have missed at least three consecutive periods. Patients do not lose their feelings of hunger despite their refusal to eat properly.

84. **(C)** The mortality rate for anorexia nervosa ranges from 5 to 20%.

85. **(E)** Bulimia nervosa differs from anorexia nervosa in that patients with bulimia nervosa maintain a normal body weight and have a normal interest in sexual activity. Patients with bulimia nervosa do not experience amenorrhea and have normal triiodothyronine levels. In both disorders, appetite is normal.

86. **(A)** Bereavement refers to the reaction to the death of a loved one. Some individuals develop symptoms of a major depressive episode. For example, 50% of all widows and widowers meet criteria for major depression within the first year. The bereaved usually refers to feeling depressed as being normal. If the symptoms of a major depressive episode begin within 2 months of the loss and do not persist beyond the 2-month period, they are considered the result of bereavement unless associated with marked impairment of any of the following: thoughts of death other than feelings that they would be better off dead or should have died with the deceased person, expressing guilt other than about the actions taken or not taken by the survivor at the time of the death, a morbid preoccupation with worthlessness, marked psychomotor retardation, or hallucinations other than that he or she hears the voice of (or sees the image of) the deceased individual. Complicated bereavement is chronic and unremitting distress. Chronic grief may occur if the relationship between the bereaved and the deceased was close or ambivalent, if they were dependent on one another, or if few other support systems are available. Bereavement reactions are very intense after sudden or unexpected deaths. Prolonged denial, anger, or guilt complicates the course of bereavement. Adjustment disorder requires the development of symptoms within 3 months of an identifiable stressor, with marked distress in excess of what would be expected from experiencing the stressor: In this case, the symptoms are considered acceptable reactions to the death of a spouse. Dysthymic dis-order requires 2 years of symptoms marked by a depressed mood.

87. **(A)** Most bereaved do fine without treatment. Support and reassurance usually come from family, friends, or clergy. When the bereaved feel unable to move beyond the grief, psychotherapeutic measures are appropriate. The treatment of anxiety or insomnia with medications remains controversial, and no controlled studies have established clear efficacy. However, medications may be warranted if cognitive or other higher functions of daily living are substantially affected.

88. **(C)** The treatment of patients with obsessive–compulsive disorder (OCD) requires integrating multiple treatment modalities, including medications, psychotherapy, and collateral support systems. The best-studied medication to treat obsessions is clomipramine (Anafranil), a TCA. SSRIs have also been effective in treating symptoms of OCD, but at doses higher than those used to treat depression. MAOIs are helpful for those who suffer from comorbid anxiety. Lithium has not been proven to be helpful in the treatment of OCD. Antipsychotic agents are used in conjunction with antidepressants but are not usually indicated as individual agents. Anxiolytic agents are of little use in treating obsessions. Antiepileptics are not indicated for the treatment of OCD.

89. **(D)** Sleep apnea is defined as the cessation of respirations lasting at least 10 seconds. The presence of more than five episodes of apnea per hour of sleep is diagnostic. Sleep apnea is classified as obstructive, central, or a mixed picture of both types. Classified as a breathing-related sleep disorder, sleep apnea leads to excessive sleepiness or insomnia. Characterized by upper airway obstruction, obstructive sleep apnea is associated with snoring, morning headache, excessive movements at night, and mental dullness. The typical patient is a middle-aged obese man.

90. **(A)** Nasal continuous positive airway pressure (CPAP) is the treatment of choice for ob-

structive sleep apnea. No medications are consistently effective in normalizing sleep in these patients. The use of nasal CPAP appears to prevent long-term morbidity and mortality and provides restorative sleep. Surgical procedures are reserved for CPAP treatment failures.

91. **(B)** Weight loss measures and the avoidance of alcohol and sedatives are important and the most cost-effective measures in the treatment of this disorder. Surgical procedures introduce the element of risk–benefit ratios and may not be curative in many cases.

92. **(B)** Anticholinergic toxicity can be caused by many psychotropic medications. The low-potency agents chlorpromazine and thioridazine and the TCAs amitriptyline and imipramine are particularly anticholinergic. The syndrome often results when an anticholinergic medication is coadministered with an antipsychotic medication to prevent or treat extrapyramidal side effects such as parkinsonism and dystonia. Clinical features include decreased secretions, agitation, dry skin, flushing of the skin, hyperthermia, tachycardia, dilated pupils, urinary retention, constipation, and hypotension. Seizures, hallucinations, and coma may result from severe intoxication. Drugs that inhibit the enzyme that breaks down acetylcholine (anticholinesterase medications such as physostigmine) reverse the syndrome and are usually administered intravenously with appropriate monitoring. Atropine would further increase the heart rate; haloperidol would likely worsen anticholinergic symptoms, and benzodiazepines are reserved for use in agitation and anxiety.

93. **(A)** Anticholinesterase toxicity, manifesting as nausea, vomiting, bradycardia, and seizures, result from excessive action of acetylcholine at specific receptors. Atropine, an antimuscarinic agent, can reverse the symptoms. Physostigmine would worsen the toxicity; while prochlorperazine would combat vomiting, it would not treat the underlying condition and might worsen the anticholinergic

toxicity. Similarly, epinephrine would treat the bradycardia without treating the underlying condition.

94. **(E)** SSRI medications are used to treat a variety of medical and psychiatric disorders. Fluvoxamine is an SSRI particularly indicated for both depression and OCD. Doxepin and clomipramine are TCAs, and phenelzine is an MAOI. Buspirone is a nonbenzodiazepine medication used to treat anxiety disorders.

95. **(D)** Because they act at the same GABA receptors as alcohol, the benzodiazepines are the preferred medications used in detoxification from alcohol. For uncomplicated detoxification, the long-acting benzodiazepines, such as chlordiazepoxide and diazepam, are appropriate because they are essentially self-tapering. The shorter-acting benzodiazepines such as lorazepam or oxazepam are used in patients with impaired liver function, because they are not oxidized to long-acting metabolites and do not accumulate. Patients with unstable medical problems, cognitive impairment, or old age are also candidates for the shorter-acting medications. Phenobarbital was formerly used for detoxification and has been replaced by benzodiazepines. Disulfiram, which interferes with the metabolism of alcohol, is reserved for long-term behavioral therapy of alcohol dependence.

96. **(C)** The patient is experiencing hallucinations due to alcohol withdrawal. In addition to benzodiazepines (e.g., clonazepam and diazepam) for the underlying withdrawal, hallucinations can be treated with an antipsychotic agent. The patient shows no evidence of a mood disorder that would be best treated with sertraline, an SSRI, or lithium, a mood stabilizer.

97. **(D)** Ethanol is metabolized in the liver to acetaldehyde, which is enzymatically converted to acetate by the enzyme alcohol dehydrogenase. Disulfiram is a medication that irreversibly inhibits the action of alcohol dehydrogenase. Acetaldehyde accumulates and

accounts for the aversive effects associated with the disulfiram–ethanol reaction. Flushing, sweating, dyspnea, hyperventilation, tachydardia, hypotension, nausea, and vomiting are common symptoms. Extreme reactions can result in respiratory depression, cardiovascular collapse, myocardial infarction, seizures, and death. Blurred vision and urinary retention are anticholinergic effects associated with antispychotic, antidepressant, and antiparkinsonian medications. Hypertension is associated with but not characteristic of the disulfiram–ethanol reaction. Disulfiram is not recommended for patients with moderate to severe liver disease, renal failure, severe cardiac disease, pregnancy, or peripheral neuropathy. In this case, the patient was prescribed chlordiazepoxide and presumably had preserved liver function.

98. **(A)** Many nonsteroidal anti-inflammatory drugs (NSAIDs) can decrease the clearance of lithium and produce significant increases in serum levels. Ibuprofen, indomethacin, ketoprofen, diclofenac, phenylbutazone, naproxen, and piroxicam have all been reported to produce such potential dangerous interactions. The symptoms of abdominal pain, diarrhea, and drowsiness indicate mild to moderate (1.5 to 2.0 mEq/L) lithium toxicity. Acetaminophen, aspirin, and the opiates do not interfere with lithium clearance. Meperidine, however, can cause dangerous interactions with MAOIs.

99. **(B)** Clinically effective antidepressant medications potentiate the actions of serotonin, norepinephrine, and dopamine in the brain. The antidepressant action of amitriptyline, a TCA, is to significantly block the reuptake of serotonin and to a lesser degree norepinephrine. Bupropion is a weak inhibitor of dopamine reuptake with modest effects on norepinephrine. It does not have any effect on serotonin. Lorazepam is an anxiolytic medication whose actions are mediated by GABA receptors. Maprotiline is a TCA with modest effects on norepinephrine and no effect on serotonin. Desipramine, a TCA, has potent effects on norepinephrine reuptake

and has weak effects on the serotonergic system.

100. **(A)** Medically ill patients with depressive disorders may respond to psychostimulants, an excellent choice if the patient is unable to tolerate TCAs. The rapid onset of action and rapid clearance are beneficial. Nefazodone, fluoxetine, and bupropion are effective antidepressants but may take 4 to 6 weeks to accomplish beneficial results. Buspirone is a nonbenzodiazepine anxiolytic medication not indicated in the treatment of depression.

101. **(C)** Inhalant abuse is commonly a social activity undertaken in groups. Volatile or toxic solvents such as toluene (found in glues and adhesives), trichloroethane (found in correction fluid), or hydrocarbons (gasoline) are placed in a bag and the fumes are inhaled. The practice is known as huffing, sniffing, or bagging. Effects are almost immediate because the substances are rapidly absorbed. Signs and symptoms of intoxication include visual disturbances, dyscoordination (a drunken appearance), depressed reflexes, euphoria, and nystagmus. An increased appetite suggests marijuana use, and staring into space and euphoria are associated with phencyclidine use.

102. **(C)** Abstinence is the only treatment for inhalant abuse. Antipsychotic agents are of no use and may aggravate organic presentations of inhalant abuse. Agitation can be managed by benzodiazepine medications such as lorazepam.

103. **(E)** The five subtypes of schizophrenia (paranoid, catatonic, residual, disorganized, and undifferentiated) are based on the presence or absence of predominant symptoms. The paranoid type is marked by prominent hallucinations or delusions; the disorganized type is marked by disorganized speech and behavior and inappropriate affect; the catatonic type is marked by waxy flexibility or motoric immobility, excess motor activity, negativism, bizarre posturing, and echolalia or echopraxia. The residual type is marked by the

absence of predominant hallucinations or delusions, disorganized speech, or catatonic behavior. The undifferentiated type is reserved for patients who meet criteria for schizophrenia but do not meet criteria for the other four types.

104. **(A)** Valproic acid, indicated for the treatment of simple or complex absence seizures or as an adjunct medication in the treatment of partial seizures, can cause sometimes significant hair loss that is usually reversible. Common side effects associated with valproic acid are nausea, vomiting, and indigestion. Sedation and mildly elevated serum transaminase levels are also seen. Hepatic failure resulting in fatalities has occurred, usually during the first 6 months of treatment. Valproic acid is also used in the treatment of migraine headache and as a mood stabilizer. Hair loss is not associated with the other medications, although these too have side effects. Carbamazepine, clozapine, olanzapine, and ziprasidone (the newest antipsychotic on the market) are not known to cause significant hair loss.

105. **(C)** Sexual dysfunction has become an increasingly common side effect associated with many antidepressant medications. It may be underreported for many reasons. Decreased libido, erectile dysfunction, ejaculatory dysfunction, and anorgasmia have been reported. None of the other choices are associated with sexual dysfunction to the same degree as the SSRIs, and some of the choices may be used to reverse the dysfunction. Various pharmacological strategies aimed at treating these side effects include the alpha-2 antagonist yohimbine; the dopamine agonists methylphenidate and amantadine; bupropion; cyproheptadine (an antihistamine with serotonin antagonist properties); and bethanacol, a cholinergic agonist.

106. **(A)** ADHD is a disorder of unclear etiology. As many as 9% of children suffer from this disorder, and up to 60% of those diagnosed will carry the diagnosis into adulthood. The disorder is characterized by symptoms of inattention, hyperactivity, and impulsivity that are inappropriate for age. Although the DSM-IV-TR criteria suggest that symptoms must have been present before the age of 7 years, many cases are not diagnosed until adolescence or adulthood. In these cases, a retrospective history from both the patient and the family often support the presence of early-life symptoms. Although some symptoms are reminiscent of the manic component of bipolar disorder, these disorders represent two separate entities. A careful history by astute physicians will secure the proper diagnosis. Depressive, anxiety, and substance-abuse disorders are common comorbid conditions that often make the diagnosis of ADHD more difficult. The absence of prominent mood symptoms and the relative degree of impairment help distinguish ADHD from other disorders.

107. **(B)** The psychostimulant medications are the treatment of choice for ADHD. Methylphenidate (Ritalin) is the best-studied medication, with well-established efficacy in treating the core symptoms of this disorder. Appropriate doses and dosing intervals are often arrived at by trial and error as each individual case is unique. Modafinil is indicated only to treat narcolepsy. In adults, antidepressants are used to treat comorbid depressive symptoms rather than the core symptoms of ADHD. However, in children, TCAs demonstrate some efficacy and are used for treatment of ADHD.

108. **(D)** The approach to the treatment of the core symptoms of ADHD has been the initiation of a trial of a psychostimulant medication. Often, if one stimulant fails to treat symptoms, another stimulant is prescribed. Many patients benefit from one stimulant and not another. The appropriate choice in this case would be to try a second type of stimulant before alternative strategies are implemented.

109. **(A)** The median age of onset for the first psychotic episode of schizophrenia is in the early to mid-twenties for men and the late twenties

for women. The onset can be abrupt or insidious. Estimates of prevalence have ranged from 0.2 to 2.0%. Schizophrenia is characterized by a 1-month period of two of the following symptoms: delusions, hallucinations, disorganized speech, disorganized behavior, and negative symptoms such as affect flattening, alogia, or avolition. Continuous signs of the disturbance should be present for 6 months, with a decline in functioning in at least two areas (work, school, interpersonal, or self-care). A prodrome often precedes the acute phase of the disorder. Distinguishing schizophrenia from mood disorders with psychotic symptoms (e.g., bipolar I disorder with psychotic features) and schizoaffective disorder can often be difficult in that a mood disturbance is common during the prodromal and active phases of schizophrenia. If psychotic symptoms occur exclusively without the presence of mood symptoms, then schizophrenia is more likely. Schizoaffective disorder describes the presence of a major depressive episode, a manic episode, or a mixed episode concurrent with symptoms that are characteristic of schizophrenia: delusions, hallucinations, disorganized speech or behavior, or negative symptoms. A brief psychotic disorder is defined by the presence of delusions, hallucinations, disorganized speech or behavior, or catatonic behavior lasting for at least 1 day but less than 1 month.

110. (A) In the context of labor, high-potency typical antipsychotics are considered relatively safe to use to control psychosis. For a mother suffering psychosis during delivery, the benefit of using high-potency antipsychotics outweighs the risk because strictly speaking during delivery, it is unclear if there is any risk in using these medications. Thorazine and droperidol could lower blood pressure significantly. A related issue is postpartum psychosis, characterized by an agitated, highly changeable psychosis that usually develops between the 3rd and 14th day postpartum and can lead to the fatal complication of infanticide. The incidence of postpartum psychosis in primiparous women is about 1 in 500. For those affected after the first pregnancy, subsequent pregnancies carry a risk of about 1 in 3.

111–113. (111-A, 112-B, 113-D) Wechsler developed a variety of scales each to be used depending on the age of the examinee. WPPSI is designed for children ages 4 to 6.5, the WISC is for children ages 5 to 15, and the WAIS-R is for people age 15 and older. The WMS was designed to evaluate a variety of memory deficits in adults.

114. (C) The Rey–Osterreith figure is sensitive to deficits in copying and lack of attention to detail in people with right-sided parietal lobe lesions. It appears that this young woman may have had a stroke in this area resulting from her protein S deficiency, hypercoagulable state.

115. (B) The appropriate test to evaluate IQ would be the WISC.

116. (G) The Boston Diagnostic Aphasia Examination is a series of tests given by an experienced clinician to evaluate and make treatment recommendations for individuals with aphasia. The Beck Depression Inventory is a 21-item test, with three responses per item, that is an easily used screening tool to evaluate for depression. As it would be unusual for an individual so young to have a dementing illness and because many of the answers reflect a lack of interest, the Beck Depression Inventory in conjunction with the MMSE may help distinguish depression from dementia. The Wisconsin Card Sorting Test assesses executive functions of the brain such as mental flexibility and the ability to abstract and reason. These capacities are believed to be located in the frontal lobes. Damage to the frontal lobes can lead to abnormalities on this test. The Blessed Rating Scale is a tool that asks friends or families of the patient to assess the ability of the patient to function in his usual environment. The WAIS-R is used in this instance, as the patient is older than 15, to provide an assessment of IQ, which may help to explain behavioral difficulties as

well as to help the school provide adequate aids for this student. The Rorschach Test is a projective test used to assess personality structure. The patient has characteristics of schizoid personality disorder that may be better elucidated with further skilled assessment in the context of the clinical history. The MMSE is a quick, easily administered test that allows for immediate assessment of dementia. Scores of less than 24 are suggestive of a dementing process. The MMPI-2 is an objective test, interpreted by skilled evaluators, used in personality assessment. It is the most widely used and highly standardized test of personality structure. Wada's Test is used to evaluate hemispheric language dominance prior to surgical amelioration of seizure focus. While most right-handed individuals show left hemispheric dominance for language, left-handed individuals may either be right- or left-dominant. The test consists of injecting sodium amytal into the carotid artery and observing the transient effects on speech. Injection into the left carotid artery will anesthetize the left side of the brain; those with left hemispheric language dominance will show interrupted speech. The Bender–Gestalt Test involves copying figures, which helps determine if organic brain disease is present.

117. **(D)** Cannabis (marijuana) is the most commonly abused illicit drug in the United States. The onset of action after smoking is immediate, and symptoms include conjunctival injection, mild sedation, dose-dependent hypothermia, dry mouth, increased appetite, tachycardia, and euphoria. A sensation of slowed time and paranoid ideation can also occur.

118. **(E)** The onset of action for opiates can be almost immediate when smoked, about 5 minutes when injected, and longer if taken orally. Symptoms include miosis, bradycardia, hypotension, hypothermia, and euphoria. Intoxication can lead to fatal respiratory depression.

119. **(B)** PCP is a hallucinogen that produces a dissociative anesthesia. It can cause unpredictable behavior, assaultiveness, and belligerence. Agitation, nystagmus (vertical or horizontal), tachycardia, a numbed response to pain, muscle rigidity, hyperacusis, hypertension, echolalia, and anticholinergic effects are associated symptoms.

120. **(F)** Nicotine found in tobacco smoke produces symptoms of excitement. Intoxication may produce symptoms of confusion, muscle twitching, weakness, abdominal cramps, depression, palpitations, coma, and respiratory failure.

Use of hallucinogens (e.g., LSD, MDMA [3,4-methylenedioxy-N-methylamphetamine, or "Ecstasy"]) causes symptoms that usually begin 1 hour after ingestion and generally last 8 to 12 hours. Most hallucinogenic drugs have stimulant-type effects and produce elevated vital signs and increased activity. Hallucinations and a heightened sense of perception of objects and colors are typical.

CHAPTER 10

Practice Test 2

Vladimir Coric, MD, and Chung-Che Charles Wang, MD

Questions

DIRECTIONS (Questions 1 through 114): Each of the numbered items or incomplete statements in this section is followed by answers or by completions of the statement. Select the ONE lettered answer or completion that is BEST in each case.

Questions 1 through 3

A 86-year-old widow is brought to your office by her son after she is found wandering the streets of her neighborhood. The son reports that over the last 8 months his mother has been acting unusual. She has become more forgetful and often misplaces various items including her keys and purse. The patient has also had several episodes during which she would drive to the store and not remember how to return home. She intermittently does not remember the names of her neighbors who have lived in the neighborhood for several years. On examination, the patient is unable to correctly state the date or place, but otherwise appears to be in good health.

1. You suspect a diagnosis of dementia. Which of the following is the most common cause of dementia?

    (A) vascular disease
    (B) Alzheimer's-type dementia
    (C) Pick's disease
    (D) head trauma
    (E) Parkinson's disease

2. Which of the following laboratory tests should be performed as part of your initial evaluation?

    (A) serum rapid plasma reagin (RPR)
    (B) thyroid function tests
    (C) vitamin B$_{12}$ level
    (D) folate level
    (E) all of the above

3. Which of the following treatments for dementia is associated with a high incidence of hepatotoxicity and requires regular monitoring of liver function tests?

    (A) donepezil (Aricept)
    (B) methyldopa (Aldomet)
    (C) levothyroxine (Synthroid)
    (D) tacrine (Cognex)
    (E) none of the above

4. An 18-year-old woman recently diagnosed with a first episode of schizophrenia agrees to take a neuroleptic medication to help decrease her hallucinations, but she is adamantly opposed to taking any medication that may cause her to gain excessive weight. Which of the following atypical neuroleptic medications is not associated with significant weight gain?

    (A) quetiapine (Seroquel)
    (B) olanzapine (Zyprexa)
    (C) risperidone (Risperdal)
    (D) ziprasidone (Geodon)
    (E) clozapine (Clozaril)

5. A 38-year-old man that you started on a neuroleptic medication 2 days earlier for a psychotic disorder presents to your office complaining of restlessness. Which of the following is an effective treatment for neuroleptic-induced akathisia?

   (A) propranolol
   (B) benztropine
   (C) benzodiazepines
   (D) decreasing the dose of neuroleptic
   (E) all of the above

6. A 72-year-old woman complains to her physician that she has been seeing "little people" walking around her house over the past few days; moreover, she saw one while waiting in the doctor's office. Exam proves her to be alert and oriented. What term best describes this phenomenon?

   (A) illusion
   (B) hallucination
   (C) flashback
   (D) formication
   (E) hallucinosis

7. You decide to start a patient with bipolar disorder on lithium. Which of the following is a potential adverse effect of lithium?

   (A) impairment of thyroid function
   (B) tremor
   (C) diarrhea
   (D) weight gain
   (E) all of the above

Questions 8 and 9

A 25-year-old patient presents to her primary care doctor complaining of a sudden onset of intense fear and a feeling that she was going to die while stuck in traffic earlier in the week. She was short of breath, diaphoretic, and tremulous, and she could feel her heart pounding. Her initial impulse was to drive to an emergency department, but her distress subsided on its own in about 20 minutes.

8. An appropriate course of action for the primary care doctor would be to

   (A) prescribe a short-acting benzodiazepine for the next such episode
   (B) refer the patient to a psychiatrist
   (C) reassure the patient that her symptoms are most likely benign and not a cause for concern
   (D) prescribe a selective serotonin reuptake inhibitor (SSRI) and ask to see the patient back in 1 week
   (E) conduct a thorough medical screening for heart and lung disease

9. After appropriate intervention, a diagnosis of panic disorder is made. Which statement regarding panic disorder is true?

   (A) The time course of onset and resolution of panic attacks is rarely helpful in making the diagnosis.
   (B) Panic attacks usually do not require medical investigation.
   (C) Panic disorder is essentially refractory to behavioral therapy.
   (D) Left untreated, panic disorder tends to run a chronic, unremitting course.
   (E) Panic disorder affects men more often than women.

10. On Mental Status Examination (MSE), a patient speaks coherently and articulately, but makes no sense because many of the words he uses are of his own invention. This patient demonstrates

    (A) word salad
    (B) negative symptoms
    (C) dysarthria
    (D) neologisms
    (E) clang associations

11. A 34-year-old female is diagnosed with dysthymic disorder. Which of the following statements regarding this patient is likely true?

    (A) She has had a feeling of depression, for most of the day, for at least the past 6 months.

(B) At some point in her illness, she may have experienced mood-congruent delusions.

(C) Her presenting complaint was suicidality.

(D) She has a comorbid diagnosis of alcohol dependence.

(E) Her presenting complaint was of poor appetite, insomnia, fatigue, poor concentration, and a feeling of hopelessness.

12. A man brings his wife to the doctor because she believes that her husband is actually an imposter who looks exactly like her husband. The term for this delusion is

(A) koro
(B) amok
(C) Capgras syndrome
(D) pseudocyesis
(E) couvade syndrome

13. A 49-year-old woman with diabetes presents to her primary care physician. She says that as a result of divorcing her husband 1 month ago, she has been sleepless, agitated, and depressed. In her twenties, she drank alcohol abusively, but she has not had any alcoholic drinks in many years. In terms of the classification of psychiatric disease within the *Diagnostic and Statistical Manual of Mental Disorders*, 4th edition, Text Revision (DSM-IV-TR) multiaxis system, which of the following statements is true?

(A) Her Axis II diagnosis is adjustment disorder.
(B) Alcohol abuse, in remission, should be placed on Axis I.
(C) Diabetes should be included on Axis IV.
(D) Recent divorce should be included on Axis V.
(E) Her Global Assessment of Functioning (GAF) should be included on Axis III.

Questions 14 and 15

You are asked to evaluate a 12-year-old boy who has a history of Tourette's disorder and complex vocal and motor tics. On evaluation, you note the patient intermittently making obscene gestures and repeating your phrases.

14. In your report, you should describe the motor tics as

(A) blepharospasm
(B) bruxism
(C) copropraxia
(D) echopraxia
(E) torticollis

15. When noting the vocal tics that were observed, the term best used is

(A) coprolalia
(B) echolalia
(C) palilalia
(D) parapraxis
(E) dysarthria

Questions 16 and 17

A wealthy middle-aged woman presents to you after being arrested for shoplifting. The patient says she has been stealing for years, although she would have no difficulty affording the objects stolen. She states that she steals "on the spur of the moment" and that these impulses seem foreign and distressing.

16. This form of impulse control disorder is called

(A) pyromania
(B) trichotillomania
(C) intermittent explosive disorder
(D) kleptomania
(E) pathologic gambling

17. The fact that these impulses are distressing to her indicate that they are

(A) ego-syntonic
(B) ego-dystonic
(C) mood-congruent
(D) mood-incongruent
(E) delusional

18. A 49-year-old man comes to you complaining of headaches, memory loss, disorientation, and occasional paralysis that affects his arms and lasts several hours. During the MSE, you notice that the patient is giving approximate answers to many questions (e.g., there are 6 toes on the foot, and 2 + 2 = 5). You also notice that the patient is talking past the point. Feeling that this is a dissociative-type disorder, you could label it

    (A) amok
    (B) Ganser syndrome
    (C) piblokto
    (D) malingering
    (E) fugue state

Questions 19 and 20

A 19-year-old woman presents with complaints of fear, apprehension, and trembling without predisposing situations noted. On exam, you note brown skin, smoky brown rings on the outer cornea, and occasional rapid, seemingly purposeless movements. After completing your workup, your diagnosis is Wilson's disease.

19. In preparing your report, the ocular findings are best termed

    (A) Kayser–Fleischer rings
    (B) arcus senilis
    (C) xanthelasma
    (D) Brushfield spots
    (E) subconjunctival hemorrhage

20. The rapid, jerky movements that worsen with voluntary movement are best termed

    (A) choreiform
    (B) athetoid
    (C) hemiballismus
    (D) myoclonus
    (E) myotonia

Questions 21 and 22

A 21-year-old woman is brought to the psychiatric emergency department after calling the police to turn herself in. She claims that she was responsible for the loss of her neighbor's pregnancy. She believes her negative thoughts toward the woman caused her miscarriage. On further questioning, she tells you that she felt threatened by her neighbor because she believed her thoughts could be heard through the walls. She feels that this is an invasion of her privacy.

21. The delusion that the patient's thoughts toward the neighbor were the responsible factors for the lost pregnancy is best termed

    (A) magical thinking
    (B) ideas of reference
    (C) displacement
    (D) projection
    (E) reaction formation

22. The patient's fear that her thoughts could be overheard is best termed

    (A) thought broadcasting
    (B) thought insertion
    (C) thought control
    (D) transference
    (E) echolalia

Questions 23 through 26

A 25-year-old man who is hospitalized for bipolar disorder tells you that he has his doctorates in six fields and currently is the richest person in the world. He states that he speaks 28 languages, one of which is an angelic language. He tells you that he is concerned, however, because a well-known supermodel is infatuated with him, and she will not leave him alone. He wishes to leave the hospital in order to spend some time with her.

23. The patient's belief that a famous supermodel is in love with him is best termed

    (A) erotomania
    (B) satyriasis
    (C) nymphomania
    (D) thought broadcasting
    (E) alexia

24. The patient's incorrect perception of his wealth and education is most likely a form of

    (A) micropsia
    (B) macropsia

(C) palinopsia

(D) delusion of grandeur

(E) delusion of infidelity

25. What term would best describe the patient's affect?

(A) euphoric

(B) euthymic

(C) anhedonic

(D) alexithymic

(E) apathetic

26. The outward expression of the patient's internal state is termed

(A) affect

(B) mood

(C) insight

(D) perception

(E) ego-dystonic

Questions 27 and 28

A devout husband finds that his wife is having an affair with his best friend. One week later, he finds that he cannot walk. A thorough neurologic workup fails to reveal a cause to his sudden paraplegia. His neurologic exam is not consistent with upper or lower motor neuron findings. Despite this dramatic disability, he seems quite unaffected by it emotionally.

27. The sudden neurologic symptom without evidence of etiology is best labeled as

(A) projection

(B) conversion

(C) sublimation

(D) dissociation

(E) rationalization

28. This patient's disregard for the severity of his symptoms is called

(A) déjà entendu

(B) jamais vu

(C) déjà vu

(D) la belle indifference

(E) folie à deux

29. A 67-year-old woman with pulmonary carcinoma and secondary brain metastases recently drafted a will in the presence of her family attorney. She has a history of major depressive disorder (MDD) that is now in remission. She decides that her children, who are well established in their careers, do not need any inheritance and that her estate would best serve charity. In order to secure the validity of the will, the patient asks her psychiatrist to submit a letter to her attorney regarding her competency. Which of the following is most important in determining a person's testamentary capacity?

(A) knowledge of natural heirs to the estate

(B) the presence of a conservator of person

(C) history of mental illness

(D) actus reus

(E) presence of a judge to witness the signing of the will

30. Which of the following is an exception to informed consent?

(A) nonemergent situations

(B) patient waiver of informed consent

(C) inability to read or write

(D) presence of a language barrier

(E) a living will

31. A deputy sheriff serves you a subpoena for the records of one of your patients who is the defendant in a civil liability lawsuit. The most appropriate course of action is to

(A) release the patient's records to the plaintiff since the subpoena overrides patient consent

(B) hand over only information that is relevant to the case

(C) contact the patient and ask if she would like the information released

(D) release the patient's records directly to the court

(E) refuse to tell the sheriff if you are the patient's physician in order to maintain confidentiality

32. A 23-year-old graduate student you have been seeing in long-term psychotherapy has stopped paying his bills despite being reimbursed by his insurance company. The next appropriate course of action is to

(A) notify a collection agency to obtain reimbursement

(B) contact the patient's insurance company and demand that they issue you another payment

(C) inquire with family members whether the patient has financial problems

(D) directly address this issue with the patient at the next scheduled appointment

(E) send the patient a letter of termination and instruct him to no longer call your office

Questions 33 through 35

You are asked to perform a "competency to stand trial" evaluation of an 18-year-old man who was arrested for violently assaulting his girlfriend. The patient has no past psychiatric history, and friends report that he has never demonstrated any violent tendencies. The patient reports that his relationship with his girlfriend "went downhill" shortly after they graduated high school and his girlfriend stopped calling him. On MSE, his affect is constricted and his mood is reported as "crazy." Thought processes are goal directed, and he denies any hallucinations or delusions. The patient is unable to correctly perform simple calculations. Each time he is asked to multiply, subtract, or add a pair of numbers, his answers are wrong by 1 or 2 digits. For example, he responds "22" when asked to multiply 7 by 3.

33. Which of the following is most consistent with the patient's tendency to give approximate answers?

(A) "first-break" psychosis

(B) amok

(C) Ganser syndrome

(D) irresistible impulse

(E) koro

34. Intentionally feigning symptoms to avoid prosecution is consistent with which of the following disorders?

(A) factitious disorder

(B) malingering

(C) Munchausen syndrome

(D) conversion disorder

(E) Munchausen by proxy

35. Which of the following statements best distinguishes malingering from conversion disorder?

(A) Malingerers seek primary-gain incentives, whereas individuals with conversion disorder seek secondary-gain incentives.

(B) Malingerers are usually friendly and cooperative, whereas individuals with conversion disorder are uncooperative.

(C) Malingering and conversion disorder can be distinguished based on the absence of an underlying neurologic problem.

(D) Malingering represents an unconscious process, whereas conversion disorder results from conscious feigning of symptoms.

(E) Malingerers avoid evaluation/treatment, whereas patients with conversion disorder are usually eager for evaluation/treatment.

36. A 7-year-old girl is brought to the emergency department for evaluation of a sore throat and fever. Her parents took her to the pediatrician's office about 1 week ago, and he recommended fluids and bed rest. Within the last 2 days, the patient developed dysphagia and severe abdominal pain. History from the parents indicates the patient has been anxious and impulsive over the last month. There has also been a marked decline in school performance, and she has not been interested in playing with her friends. Physical exam is remarkable for significant erythema over the posterior pharynx with gray exudate. There are abrasions in the region of the patient's labia. Complete blood count (CBC) shows a white blood cell (WBC) count of 14,000 with a left shift. The next appropriate step is to

(A) detain the parents while you notify the police

(B) arrange for a family meeting to determine a safe disposition

(C) refer the patient to the family's pediatrician

(D) notify the probate court to have the patient legally removed from the alleged perpetrator

(E) contact the state's child protective services while keeping the patient safe

Questions 37 and 38

A 30-year-old man with a history of paranoid schizophrenia is arrested after opening fire with a shotgun in a crowded public square. He is taken into custody and awaits trial.

37. Which of the following statements best characterizes the defendant's use of the insanity defense?

(A) Insanity defenses are infrequently used.

(B) When asserted, the insanity defense is generally successful.

(C) Insanity defenses often lead to less time incarcerated compared to individuals found guilty.

(D) The insanity defense is typically used to establish competency to stand trial.

(E) Agreement by both prosecution and defendant is required to assert an insanity plea.

38. A forensic psychiatrist is asked by the defendant's attorney to evaluate this individual. Which of the following best characterizes the role of an expert witness?

(A) provides only factual information in court

(B) offers an opinion in court based on his or her knowledge

(C) presents a written report to the judge but does not testify in court

(D) works with the jury in establishing a verdict

(E) establishes pretrial parameters for the individual's likelihood of guilt

Questions 39 and 40

A 26-year-old man with a history of paranoid schizophrenia is seen in your office for monthly medication evaluation. After talking with him, you uncover that he believes his girlfriend is poisoning his food and he plans to "do something about it." You are concerned because the patient has a history of intense paranoid delusions during which he has become violent. As you explore his intentions toward the girlfriend, he confides that he must "kill her before she gets me." You tell the patient that he has to increase his medications and is likely to be hospitalized. He becomes outraged and storms out of your office.

39. The next appropriate step is to

(A) allow for a "cooling-down" period and attempt to contact the patient at home

(B) notify your staff that the patient is dangerous and to call the police if he returns

(C) anonymously call the girlfriend and tell her to "watch out"

(D) call the police and make them aware of the threats to his girlfriend

(E) call the patient's family and ask them to monitor the patient closely.

40. *Tarasoff II v. Regents of University of California* (1976) is the landmark legal precedent establishing

(A) physician–patient confidentiality

(B) duty to warn

(C) police power

(D) duty to protect

(E) fiduciary protection

41. Which of the following statements is most accurate regarding suicide statistics?

    (A) Suicide is the second leading cause of death among individuals aged 15 to 24.
    (B) Suicide is common in children under the age of 13.
    (C) Women are more likely to commit suicide than men.
    (D) Men are more likely to attempt suicide than women.
    (E) Risk of suicide decreases with increasing age.

42. According to the American Medical Association's (AMA's) Code of Medical Ethics, physician-assisted suicide is

    (A) justifiable if a patient's suffering becomes intolerable despite adequate pain control
    (B) unethical
    (C) defined as euthanasia
    (D) a matter on which the AMA has no official position
    (E) not an ethical issue and must be left to state legislatures

43. A 16-year-old girl is brought to your office by her parents to get a pregnancy test. She consents for the evaluation but requests that you keep the results confidential. Beta-human chorionic gonadotropin (HCG) is positive. The patient's parents demand to know the results. You should

    (A) notify the parents of the results since they pay her medical bills
    (B) encourage the patient to discuss the results with her parents
    (C) report the results to child protective services
    (D) invoke testimonial privilege
    (E) disclose the results in a meeting with the patient and her parents

Questions 44 through 45

After you ask her how many siblings she has, a patient launches into a long discussion first on her sister Sally, then one of Sally's old boyfriends Mark,

who is now an accountant, she says, which in turn leads her to a monologue on accountants and bankers, whom she says are all "in cahoots with the IRS and CIA—you can't trust 'em!" You note that she never comes back to answering the question fully until prompted to do so by you. She further tells you that she believes "the government has experimentally planted alien eggs in my ovaries, you know. I know they've told you. They think I don't know."

44. The above patient's thought processes when asked about her siblings are an example of

    (A) trichotillomania
    (B) flight of ideas
    (C) tangentiality
    (D) circumstantiality
    (E) isolation of affect

45. Delusions as in the above patient's case are an example of

    (A) a perceptual disturbance
    (B) a disturbance in thought content
    (C) disorganized thought processes
    (D) a cognitive deficit
    (E) impaired judgment

46. Which type of schizophrenia is most consistent with the above patient's presentation?

    (A) residual
    (B) catatonic
    (C) disorganized
    (D) undifferentiated
    (E) paranoid

47. If, instead of the prominent delusions above, the patient exhibited milder, merely "eccentric" delusions at most, did not show grossly disordered behavior or speech, but clearly evinced multiple negative symptoms and mild, nonbothersome auditory hallucinations, the most appropriate type of schizophrenia would be

    (A) residual
    (B) catatonic
    (C) disorganized

(D) undifferentiated

(E) paranoid

Questions 48 through 52

A 60-year-old patient has suffered from bipolar illness for decades, developing along the way severe reactions to each of the mood stabilizers you have tried him on. He is currently in the midst of a severe manic episode. His family is "at wit's end," according to a daughter. You suggest electroconvulsive therapy (ECT), to which the patient agrees. His daughter, however, says she has heard of "depressed and psychotic people who had it done to them, with little or no benefit. And it seems so barbaric."

48. You respond by saying your advice is to still consider ECT. One factor you base this on is the fact that

(A) bipolar illness, especially in a manic episode, has an extremely high rate of response to ECT, perhaps higher than either of the other two disorders the daughter mentioned

(B) ECT is proven to be safer in bipolar illness than in any other of the disorders for which ECT is used

(C) ECT is proven to have more lasting results in bipolar disorder than in the other two

(D) bipolar illness is shown to respond best in late life to ECT

(E) ECT is shown to have more lasting effects than medications

49. Treating bipolar illness is believed to

(A) have no change on the likelihood of further episodes

(B) have no effect on future episodes

(C) decrease the likelihood of further episodes, as well as the severity of them

(D) increase the patient's response to medications or ECT in the future

(E) decrease the patient's response to medications or ECT in the future

50. Something that could also be considered in this patient to benefit him (and his family) would be to

(A) commit him to a long-term mental institution

(B) consider antipsychotic medication

(C) consider antidementia medication

(D) consider psychosurgery

(E) consider antiepileptic medication

51. Known medical causes of mania include

(A) thyroid and rheumatologic disorders

(B) uremia and central nervous system (CNS) infections

(C) phenytoin administration and dermatologic crises

(D) menopause and gout

(E) blood cell dyscrasias and cerebellar degeneration

52. Of the following, the drug of abuse most likely to be associated with mania-like symptoms is

(A) phencyclidine (PCP)

(B) marijuana

(C) heroin

(D) meperidine (Demerol)

(E) methaqualone (Quaalude)

Questions 53 through 57

A 60-year-old widow is brought to your clinic by her daughter, who reports that her mother said to her this afternoon that she "wanted to end it all." She reports thoughts of overdosing on her pills, which she has stockpiled. This woman has no prior history of suicide attempts but has had thoughts of suicide on multiple prior occasions over the course of her near-lifelong history of depression. She lost her husband to a sudden heart attack 1 year ago, but her daughter says that she still has many very supportive friends whom she spends significant amounts of time with. She still carries on her avid hobby of gardening, although "at a slower pace" because of her worsening arthritis. She expresses worries over a recent "big drop" in the value of retirement stocks she has.

53. Of the following, the factor that causes you to worry most about this woman's risk for suicide is her

    (A) age
    (B) gender
    (C) race
    (D) financial situation
    (E) stockpile of medications

54. The most significant factor mitigating her risk for suicide is

    (A) her social supports
    (B) her gardening hobby
    (C) her race
    (D) her slower movements secondary to arthritis
    (E) the fact that she has not attempted suicide before, despite her long history of depression

55. If this woman did eventually commit suicide, you would expect to find low levels of which of the following in her cerebrospinal fluid (CSF)?

    (A) cortisol
    (B) norepinephrine
    (C) gamma-aminobutyric acid (GABA)
    (D) opiates
    (E) serotonin

56. Which of the following would most likely be abnormal in this depressed woman?

    (A) ventricular size on computed tomographic (CT) scan
    (B) CSF albumin level on lumbar puncture
    (C) thalamic activity on magnetic resonance spectroscopy
    (D) liver function tests
    (E) dexamethasone suppression test

57. Important medical causes of depression to rule out in this and any depressed patient include

    (A) vitamin B_{12} and tryptophan deficiency
    (B) thyroid illness and malignancy

    (C) adrenal illness and basement membrane disorders
    (D) vascular disease and phospholipid metabolism disorders
    (E) infectious illness and lipid disorders

Questions 58 through 60

A 20-year-old college sophomore is brought to the emergency department after being found passed out in her bathroom. She had been vomiting, which she admits now was self-induced. History is significant for a breakup 4 months ago with her boyfriend of 2 years. Her weight is in the 82nd percentile for her height. She is amenorrheic. There is no history of binge eating.

58. You would most expect her examination to show

    (A) dental decay
    (B) pitting fingernails
    (C) pectus excavatum
    (D) palpable spleen
    (E) café au lait spots

59. Her diagnosis is most likely

    (A) bulimia nervosa
    (B) anorexia nervosa
    (C) MDD
    (D) obsessive–compulsive disorder (OCD)
    (E) adjustment disorder

60. Additional social history would be most likely to reveal that she is

    (A) a gymnast
    (B) a victim of rape
    (C) an identical twin
    (D) a genius
    (E) a "type A" personality

61. A 14-month-old girl presents with her parents, who report that she has become less responsive to them and less interactive with her 6-year-old brother. In addition, her gait has become clumsy, and most recently she has been noted to habitually rub her knuckles together. The parents also bring the chart

from their daughter's pediatrician with a note indicating that although her head circumference was normally sized at birth, it has now fallen into the 10th percentile for her age. The girl most closely fulfills criteria for

(A) autistic disorder

(B) childhood disintegrative disorder

(C) Rett syndrome

(D) Asperger syndrome

(E) childhood-onset schizophrenia

Questions 62 through 64

A 16-year-old boy began having repetitive eye blinking at the age of 6. By age 12, he began blurting stereotyped phrases such as "Balls!" and "Shitty!" as well as making kissing noises. Concomitant with this, he had increasing difficulty with paying attention in school and occasionally displayed wild, disinhibited behavior.

62. This adolescent is most appropriately diagnosed with

(A) chronic vocal tic disorder

(B) Tourette's disorder

(C) transient tic disorder

(D) tic disorder not otherwise specified

(E) pervasive developmental disorder not otherwise specified

63. The comorbid condition least likely to be diagnosed here is

(A) attention deficit–hyperactivity disorder (ADHD)

(B) MDD

(C) OCD

(D) conduct disorder

(E) childhood-onset schizophrenia

64. The treatment of choice for the primary condition evident in this case is

(A) pimozide (Orap)

(B) methylphenidate (Ritalin)

(C) fluoxetine (Prozac)

(D) topiramate (Topamax)

(E) clonidine (Catapres)

65. A 12-year-old boy has recently been arrested for setting fire to a neighbor's barn. He has been in trouble before for playing with fireworks in the neighborhood, and when he was 10 years old he was suspended for lighting matches at his school. The most frequently diagnosed DSM-IV-TR diagnosis associated with fire setting in children is

(A) a pervasive developmental disorder

(B) mental retardation

(C) conduct disorder

(D) a tic disorder

(E) destructive personality disorder of childhood

Questions 66 and 67

A 9-year-old boy with a history of normal developmental milestones has been wetting his bed for the last 6 months. His parents report that the bedwetting initially occurred sporadically, but for the last 2 months it has been happening about every other night.

66. The most accurate description of this boy's problem is

(A) primary diurnal enuresis

(B) primary nocturnal enuresis

(C) secondary diurnal enuresis

(D) secondary nocturnal enuresis

(E) primary diurnal encopresis

67. Once medical causes have been ruled out, the pharmacologic treatment of choice for this condition is

(A) clonidine (Catapres)

(B) haloperidol (Haldol)

(C) carbamazepine (Tegretol)

(D) diphenhydramine (Benadryl)

(E) imipramine (Tofranil)

Questions 68 through 70

An 11-year-old boy was adopted at age 6 months. His biological mother suffered from severe alcohol dependence. He has been in a special education school due to his global learning difficulties, and his intelligence quotient (IQ) has recently been measured at 50.

68. According to his IQ measurement, the patient would be diagnosed as having

   (A) borderline intellectual functioning
   (B) mild mental retardation
   (C) moderate mental retardation
   (D) severe mental retardation
   (E) mental retardation, severity unspecified

69. Given the history of prenatal alcohol exposure in this patient, we may expect

   (A) microcephaly
   (B) cleft palate
   (C) chromosome 13 translocation
   (D) congenital blindness
   (E) prominent jaw

70. The causes of mental retardation that are attributed to prenatal causes account for roughly

   (A) 10% of cases
   (B) 30% of cases
   (C) 50% of cases
   (D) 75% of cases
   (E) 95% of cases

71. Which of the following statements is least accurate with regard to psychopharmacologic treatments in children?

   (A) Most groups of psychiatric drugs, including neuroleptics, antidepressants, anticonvulsants, psychostimulants, and lithium, have shorter half-lives in children compared to adults.
   (B) Neuroleptics are known to have greater potency in children compared to similar weight-adjusted doses in adults.

   (C) Low-potency neuroleptics should be used cautiously in children due to cognitive dulling.
   (D) Fluoxetine (Prozac) should be used as a last resort in children due to risk of worsening violent behavior and provoking suicide.
   (E) Tricyclic antidepressants (TCAs) have not proven themselves to be effective after double-blind placebo-controlled trials for MDD in children and adolescents.

72. A 5-year-old girl has come under the care of state child protection services. Her mother was known to be using crack cocaine and intravenous heroin, and supporting her habit with prostitution. The girl's temporary foster parents reported to state workers that she was indiscriminately social with adults and unusually clingy. In her social interactions with other 5-year-old children at her preschool, she was described as being inappropriately aggressive with them. This case most closely illustrates a diagnosis of

   (A) mixed receptive–expressive language disorder
   (B) reactive attachment disorder of infancy and early childhood
   (C) childhood disintegrative disorder
   (D) ADHD
   (E) conduct disorder

Questions 73 through 75

A 12-year-old girl has recently come under psychiatric care for her depression and treatment of alcohol abuse. During the course of her evaluation, she revealed that she had a 3-year-long sexual relationship with her stepfather beginning when she was 8 years old.

73. Which of the following generalizations related to this case is most accurate?

   (A) Sexual activity between daughter and father (or stepfather) is the most common form of incest.

(B) The patient is at decreased risk of future sexual abuse or rape due to her heightened defense mechanisms around sexual issues.

(C) The patient has increased risk of developing borderline personality disorder.

(D) The patient has increased risk of developing schizophrenia after adolescence.

(E) The patient's history of alcohol abuse makes her a less reliable historian and her story about the sexual abuse less likely to be true.

74. The patient's stepfather has a decreased likelihood, compared to the general population, of having

(A) other paraphilias
(B) alcohol dependence
(C) a history of violence
(D) a sexually gratifying relationship with spouse
(E) a personal history of childhood sexual abuse

75. The fraction of child victims of sexual abuse reporting repeated incidents rather than single instances of the abuse is closest to

(A) 10%
(B) 30%
(C) 50%
(D) 70%
(E) 90%

76. A 27-year-old law student presents to you as a referral for treatment of depression diagnosed by his primary care physician. On MSE, you find that the patient's speech is pressured and that he quickly jumps from one topic to another. He says that his mood has improved greatly since he last saw his primary care doctor: "In fact, I'm on top of the world." The patient relates that now he doesn't get much sleep. He reports 3 to 4 hours a night for the last week, "not that I need that much sleep anyway." The most appropriate single pharmacotherapy strategy for this patient would be

(A) lorazepam (Ativan)
(B) imipramine (Tofranil)
(C) fluoxetine (Prozac)
(D) valproic acid (Depakote)
(E) citalopram (Celexa)

Questions 77 and 78

A 36-year-old woman presents with depressed mood, a sense of hopelessness, and thoughts of suicide for the last month. She also reports increased appetite. She also has been sleeping up to 16 hours a day. On MSE, her mood is sad most of the time, but she laughs in response to humorous statements. The patient did say that last week her mood brightened a bit when she won $150 from playing the lottery.

77. Additional history that would suggest a diagnosis of an atypical major depression versus a melancholic depression would be

(A) severe concentration difficulty and cognitive impairment
(B) a normal dexamethasone suppression test
(C) rejection hypersensitivity
(D) the presence of psychotic symptoms
(E) a history of manic symptoms after antidepressant treatment

78. A psychiatric drug class specifically associated with good treatment response for atypical major depression as in this case is

(A) anticonvulsants
(B) monoamine oxidase inhibitors (MAOIs)
(C) SSRIs
(D) TCAs
(E) typical neuroleptics

Questions 79 and 80

You have been treating a 34-year-old man for depression with an SSRI for the last 2 months. He had been on fluoxetine (Prozac) 20 mg once a day for the first month, and then you raised the dose to 40 mg PO qd for the last month. His depressive symptoms have remained refractory despite the increase in dosage. You have decided to change the medication to phenelzine (Nardil), an MAOI, in hopes of eliciting a better antidepressant response.

79. In making the transition from the SSRI to the MAOI, the best strategy is to

    (A) begin tapering down the dose of the SSRI, and start tapering up on the dose of the MAOI simultaneously

    (B) stop the SSRI abruptly, and immediately begin tapering up on the MAOI

    (C) taper off SSRI, and then 5 weeks after the last dose, begin tapering up on the MAOI

    (D) stop the SSRI abruptly, and begin with the MAOI at an equipotent dose the next day

    (E) start the MAOI until therapeutic levels have been reached, then taper off the SSRI

80. With regard to taking the MAOI, it is very important that the patient be aware that

    (A) he may experience stiffness and tremor

    (B) he should take the medications with bland food

    (C) he should avoid foods rich in tryptophan

    (D) he should avoid foods rich in tyramine

    (E) he may feel overly sedated

81. A 42-year-old accountant presents for long-term psychotherapy treatment. In the first session, you find that he has been divorced three times. The poor quality of his romantic and other relationships are the focus of his concerns. Over the course of months, you find out that he is a perfectionist and inflexible within relationships. He typically idealizes his partner, then devalues her, before ending the relationship suddenly. At times,

he loses "a sense of self" in relationships, not knowing who he is or what he wants. During this time he relies on others to advise him on what he should do. However, if he takes this advice and his plans fail, he uses this to devalue his advising friend. The patient makes it very clear that he sought your treatment as a psychotherapist "because I'll only accept the best in the city." The patient also reports to you that he has some unique abilities of perception that allow him to detect what or who will provide the best possible outcome for him. For example, he picked you as a therapist not only because of your reputation, but also because of your office phone number, which has digits in ascending value order. The most appropriate Axis II DSM-IV-TR diagnosis for this patient is

    (A) borderline personality disorder

    (B) narcissistic personality disorder

    (C) obsessive personality disorder

    (D) personality disorder not otherwise specified

    (E) schizotypal personality disorder

82. A 43-year-old woman is hospitalized during a psychotic episode in which she had the delusion that she was being shot with invisible laser beams from satellites in Earth orbit. According to her family, she had stopped taking her regimen of haloperidol (Haldol) and lithium 4 weeks prior to her admission to the hospital, and she had been telling her family about her concerns regarding the laser beams for the last 2 weeks. Her MSE on presentation to the hospital revealed primarily thought disorder and delusional symptoms without a prominent mood component. The patient's past psychiatric history is significant for three prior hospitalizations over the last 20 years. At the time of her first admission, she presented with a 3-week history of manic symptoms and psychosis. During her second hospitalization, she was suicidal and noted to be depressed without psychosis. During her third admission, she was again depressed with prominently disorganized behavior. The most appropriate diagnosis for this patient is

(A) bipolar disorder

(B) MDD

(C) psychotic disorder not otherwise specified

(D) schizoaffective disorder

(E) schizophrenia

Questions 83 and 84

The medical team on an inpatient service calls you to help them with a 72-year-old female patient. They report that at night she becomes confused, thinking that she is in a hotel. She makes demands of the nursing staff that they feel are unreasonable, and she has become disruptive of their other work. She has the most trouble from 10 P.M. until about 2 A.M., when she usually falls asleep. In the morning, she is much better oriented and cooperative. A review of her medications reveals that she is taking cimetidine 400 mg PO bid, furosemide 40 mg PO qd, atenolol 50 mg PO qd, digoxin 0.125 mg PO qd, and diphenhydramine 50 mg PO qhs and 25 mg PO qhs (second dose 3 hours post first dose for insomnia).

83. The medication most likely to cause this patient's nighttime confusion is

(A) atenolol

(B) cimetidine

(C) digoxin

(D) diphenhydramine

(E) furosemide

84. The neurotransmitter system most directly implicated in the etiology of this medication-induced confusion is

(A) acetylcholine

(B) dopamine

(C) GABA

(D) serotonin

(E) norepinephrine

85. A clinical research psychiatrist at university A has been running a double-blind placebo-controlled trial of a new antidepressant. The psychiatrist concludes after a statistical analysis of the data that there is no better effect of the drug compared to placebo. The psychiatrist's colleagues at 5 separate institutions (universities B, C, D, E, and F) have run identical studies and determine that there is a treatment effect of the drug compared to placebo. Given this information, one may conclude that the research trial at university A resulted in a

(A) high variance

(B) low predictive value

(C) standard error

(D) type I error

(E) type II error

Questions 86 through 88

A 56-year-old man with a long history of paranoid schizophrenia has been taking his chlorpromazine regularly for 27 years. About 5 years ago, he developed writhing movements of his wrists and fingers that disappear when he goes to sleep.

86. Which of the following extrapyramidal syndromes is most consistent with this case?

(A) akathisia

(B) dystonia

(C) neuroleptic malignant syndrome (NMS)

(D) parkinsonism

(E) tardive dyskinesia

87. The anatomic structure in the brain most likely implicated in the etiology of this movement disorder is the

(A) basal ganglia

(B) cerebellum

(C) frontal cortex

(D) midbrain

(E) motor cortex

88. The annual risk of developing the form of movement disorder illustrated in this case, while taking typical neuroleptics chronically, is closest to

(A) 1% per year on the medication

(B) 5% per year on the medication

(C) 10% per year on the medication

(D) 15% per year on the medication

(E) 20% per year on the medication

89. A poor prognostic indicator for a diagnosis of posttraumatic stress disorder (PTSD) is

(A) existence of premorbid personality disorder

(B) exposure to trauma in middle adulthood

(C) rapid onset of symptoms

(D) short duration of symptoms

(E) strong social supports

90. A 29-year-old man presents to your outpatient psychiatric clinic complaining of anxiety and depression. His social history reveals that he is a junior faculty member of a local university, working about 90 hours per week. He reports stress arising from his marital relationship that is exacerbated by his occupational demands. You identify a central conflict in this patient of issues of intimacy versus self-absorption borrowing from the theoretical work of

(A) Carl Jung

(B) Karen Horney

(C) Erik Erikson

(D) Jean Piaget

(E) Sigmund Freud

Questions 91 and 92

A 46-year-old man with a history of complex partial epilepsy is referred to your psychiatric clinic by his neurologist for onset of delusional thinking.

91. You may inform the patient's family that the prevalence of psychotic episodes in patients with complex partial epilepsy is closest to

(A) 1%

(B) 5%

(C) 10%

(D) 20%

(E) 50%

92. An investigation into the history of this patient's personality traits may reveal classic signs of complex partial epilepsy–associated personality including increased or decreased sexuality, hypergraphia, heightened experience of emotions, and

(A) depression

(B) hyperreligiosity

(C) urinary incontinence

(D) obsessive–compulsive behaviors

(E) sleep disorders

93. After being called to the emergency department to evaluate a young woman who overdosed on barbiturates, you find her in bed with her eyes closed. She opens her eyes briefly in response to pain and demonstrates flexion from pain, but makes no sounds. Her Glasgow Coma Scale score is

(A) 7

(B) 6

(C) 5

(D) 4

(E) 3

94. A 46-year-old man with a history of schizophrenia had been maintained on thioridazine (Mellaril) 700 mg qd since he was diagnosed at the age of 20. Over the last 8 months, he has been complaining of hearing derogatory voices, and his dose has been increased to 800 mg qd. He has no signs of tardive dyskinesia. What is the most harmful side effect associated with 1,000 mg or more of thioridazine?

(A) constipation

(B) dry eyes

(C) urinary retention

(D) pigmentary retinopathy

(E) nephrogenic diabetes insipidus

95. A 24-year-old man is admitted to the psychiatric ward with new-onset command suicidal auditory hallucinations. He is given haloperidol (Haldol) 10 mg IM. Fifteen hours later, he develops torticollis. What is the best treatment for this occurrence?

(A) acetaminophen

(B) labetalol (Normodyne)

(C) benztropine (Cogentin)

(D) a lower-potency neuroleptic

(E) penicillamine

96. A 28-year-old woman with a history of bipolar disorder is admitted to the medical service because of weakness, mental status changes, and a serum sodium of 154 mmol/L. Over the last 2 weeks, she has had polyuria, excessive thirst, and polydipsia. What drug is most likely associated with this medical condition?

    (A) lithium carbonate
    (B) haloperidol (Haldol)
    (C) diazepam (Valium)
    (D) valproic acid (Depakote)
    (E) buspirone (BuSpar)

Questions 97 and 98

A 47-year-old man who is addicted to heroin has been admitted to the inpatient psychiatric ward for detoxification.

97. What is the most effective treatment of autonomic dysregulation during detoxification?

    (A) haloperidol (Haldol)
    (B) thioridazine (Mellaril)
    (C) amantadine (Symmetrel)
    (D) clonidine (Catapres)
    (E) pimozide (Orap)

98. If the patient did not want detoxification but did want to stop using heroin, which of the following medications would be most appropriate for maintenance?

    (A) lorazepam (Ativan)
    (B) alprazolam (Xanax)
    (C) methadone
    (D) sertraline (Zoloft)
    (E) lithium

Questions 99 through 101

A 75-year-old man with Alzheimer's disease presents to your clinic complaining of depression. He has a past medical history including diabetes mellitus, two myocardial infarctions, atrial fibrillation, and one coronary artery bypass graft.

99. Assuming this patient is suffering from depression, which antidepressant class would you most want to avoid?

    (A) SSRIs
    (B) TCAs
    (C) butyrophenones
    (D) dibenzodiazepines
    (E) benzodiazepines

100. Blockade of which neurotransmitter system would most likely result in a cognitive decline in this patient?

    (A) histamine
    (B) serotonin
    (C) dopamine
    (D) acetylcholine
    (E) norepinephrine

101. Which of the following drugs would cause the most blockade of the neurotransmitter system most associated with cognitive function?

    (A) haloperidol (Haldol)
    (B) imipramine (Tofranil)
    (C) clonidine (Catapres)
    (D) fluoxetine (Prozac)
    (E) amantadine (Symmetrel)

102. A 35-year-old woman presents to the emergency department after taking an overdose of lithium. Which of the following signs is most associated with lithium toxicity?

    (A) acute dystonia
    (B) abdominal pain
    (C) paresthesias
    (D) paranoid delusions
    (E) leg pain

Questions 103 through 105

A 67-year-old woman presents to your office with a long history of depression. She has tried a number of different antidepressant medications in the past but has not had a remission with any of them. Currently, she is on lithium, venlafaxine (Effexor), nortriptyline (Pamelor), lorazepam (Ativan), risperidone (Risperdal), and benztropine (Cogentin). She is starting to believe that her next-door neighbors are out to harm her. You want to offer her ECT.

103. Which of her medications would be most acceptable to continue?

    (A) lithium
    (B) venlafaxine (Effexor)
    (C) haloperidol (Haldol)
    (D) lorazepam (Ativan)
    (E) clozapine (Clozaril)

104. Which of the following are relative contraindications to ECT?

    (A) a space-occupying lesion of the brain
    (B) a history of seizures
    (C) diabetes mellitus
    (D) a small-bowel obstruction
    (E) catatonia

105. Which of the following are absolute contraindications to ECT?

    (A) fractured femur
    (B) recent myocardial infarction
    (C) space-occupying lesion of the brain
    (D) severe coronary artery disease
    (E) there are no absolute contraindications to ECT

Questions 106 and 107

A 26-year-old man presents to the psychiatric emergency department with paranoia, visual hallucinations, feelings of unreality, depersonalization, and extreme agitation. A urine toxicology screen is positive for PCP.

106. What is the best treatment for extreme agitation in this patient?

    (A) a phenothiazine antipsychotic
    (B) a butyrophenone antipsychotic
    (C) trihexphenidyl (Artane)
    (D) trazodone (Desyrel)
    (E) fluoxetine (Prozac)

107. If this patient were not extremely agitated, what would be the best treatment?

    (A) vitamin B_{12}
    (B) IV haloperidol (Haldol)
    (C) supportive care
    (D) vitamin E
    (E) cheese

Questions 108 and 109

A 58-year-old man arrives in your office complaining of impotence. He suffers from hypertension but does not have cardiac disease, renal disease, glaucoma, or a history of peptic or duodenal ulcers.

108. Which of the following drugs is best for the treatment of impotence?

    (A) paroxetine (Paxil)
    (B) citalopram (Celexa)
    (C) molindone (Moban)
    (D) diphenhydramine (Benadryl)
    (E) yohimbine

109. If the patient is taking clonidine for hypertension, which of the following drugs would directly inhibit clonidine's mechanism of action?

(A) paroxetine (Paxil)

(B) citalopram (Celexa)

(C) molindone (Moban)

(D) diphenhydramine (Benadryl)

(E) yohimbine

110. A 45-year-old woman is admitted to the psychiatric inpatient ward. She is severely depressed, believes that her neighbors are conspiring to murder her, and occasionally can hear a man's voice that says she should die. After talking with the neighbors, you find out that they are the ones who brought the patient to the hospital. They have been good friends for 20 years and have noticed the patient has not been leaving the house much, has taken to looking out of her windows with suspicious glances, and has not cleaned her house in the last 2 months. Which of the following medication combinations would be proper treatment for this patient?

(A) sertraline (Zoloft) and lithium

(B) paroxetine (Paxil) and thyroid augmentation

(C) fluoxetine (Prozac) and risperidone (Risperdal)

(D) sertraline and lorazepam (Ativan)

(E) lorazepam and clozapine (Clozaril)

111. A 45-year-old woman who travels often to Europe from the United States presents to your office complaining of not being able to fall asleep at night after she arrives in Germany. What is the first line of treatment for insomnia?

(A) diphenhydramine (Benadryl)

(B) trazodone (Desyrel)

(C) clozapine (Clozaril)

(D) benzodiazepines

(E) amitriptyline (Elavil)

Questions 112 and 113

A 60-year-old man presents to your office complaining of the sudden onset of palpitations, sweating, shaking, shortness of breath, choking, and feeling that he is "going crazy." He has been seen by his cardiologist, who has ruled out a cardiac etiology. The patient fears future attacks.

112. Which of the following is the safest drug with which to treat panic disorder?

(A) fluvoxamine (Luvox)

(B) imipramine (Tofranil)

(C) phenelzine (Nardil)

(D) bupropion (Wellbutrin)

(E) deprenyl (Selegiline)

113. If the patient's symptoms were due to a cardiac etiology, and he subsequently became depressed, which antidepressant would be the most dangerous?

(A) amitriptyline (Elavil)

(B) sertraline (Zoloft)

(C) amphetamines

(D) bupropion (Wellbutrin)

(E) venlafaxine (Effexor)

114. A 33-year-old woman with a diagnosis of chronic paranoid schizophrenia has been maintained on haloperidol (Haldol) since she was diagnosed at age 24. In your office, she says she has not had her period in several months, has diminished sex drive, has been unable to conceive, has been discharging milk from her breasts, and has suffered pain on sexual intercourse. Assuming that these complaints are caused by her antipsychotic medication, which of the following is most likely to explain her symptoms?

(A) increased adrenocorticotropic hormone (ACTH) levels

(B) decreased prolactin levels

(C) increased prolactin levels

(D) increased serotonin levels

(E) increased dopamine levels

DIRECTIONS (Questions 115 through 120): Each set of items in this section consists of a list of lettered headings followed by several numbered words or phrases. For each numbered word or phrase, select the ONE lettered option that is most closely associated with it. Each lettered option may be selected once, more than once, or not at all.

Questions 115 through 118

Match the clinical vignette with the most likely substance-induced disorder.

(A) cannabis intoxication
(B) cocaine intoxication
(C) cocaine withdrawal
(D) alcohol intoxication
(E) alcohol withdrawal
(F) heroin intoxication
(G) heroin withdrawal
(H) MDMA (ecstasy) intoxication
(I) phencyclidine (PCP) intoxication
(J) methamphetamine intoxication
(K) inhalant intoxication
(L) nicotine intoxication
(M) nitrous oxide intoxication
(N) psilocybin withdrawal

115. A 23-year-old man is brought to the emergency department by the police. He shows agitation, vertical nystagmus, and analgesia.

116. A 62-year-old homeless man admitted to a psychiatric unit begins having visual hallucinations, tremor, and seizures.

117. A 43-year-old woman presents in the psychiatric emergency department complaining of paranoia and hearing voices. She is observed to have fatigue, depression, and irritability.

118. A 30-year-old musician presents in the outpatient clinic. He complains of fever, constipation, and myoclonus of extremities for the last 24 hours.

Questions 119 and 120

Choose the medication most likely associated with side effects in the following scenarios.

(A) benztropine (Cogentin)
(B) clozapine (Clozaril)
(C) desipramine (Norpramin)
(D) fluoxetine (Prozac)
(E) haloperidol (Haldol)
(F) lorazepam (Ativan)
(G) lithium
(H) nefazodone (Serzone)
(I) olanzapine (Zyprexa)
(J) phenelzine (Nardil)
(K) valproic acid (Depakote)
(L) venlafaxine (Effexor)

119. A 34-year-old man with schizophrenia presents with fever and chills. He is found to be bacteremic and has a WBC count of 900.

120. A 41-year-old woman on medications for her affective disorder presents with fatigue, weight gain, cold intolerance, constipation, and decreased concentration.

Answers and Explanations

1. **(B)** Alzheimer's-type dementia and vascular dementia account for over 70% of all cases of dementia. Alzheimer's dementia is the most common form of dementia and is characterized by a slow but progressive cognitive decline, memory impairment, aphasia, apraxia, agnosia, and/or impairment in executive functioning. These deficits must cause a significant impairment in social or occupational functioning, and there must not be any other medical causes of cognitive and memory deterioration.

2. **(E)** Before diagnosing Alzheimer's dementia, reversible causes of dementia should be considered. Therefore, it is important to perform a complete history and physical examination. Reversible causes of dementia such as vitamin B_{12} and folate deficiencies, hypothyroidism, neurosyphilis, hypercalcemia, and HIV should be considered in the differential diagnosis. Other causes such as vascular dementia, normal pressure hydrocephalus, a subdural hematoma, Parkinson's disease, and brain tumors should also be ruled out.

3. **(D)** Donepezil (Aricept) and tacrine (Cognex) are used in the treatment of Alzheimer's dementia. These medications can slow the progression of the dementia somewhat, but they generally cannot reverse the memory and cognitive impairments that have taken place. Tacrine is no longer prescribed as much due to its higher incidence of hepatotoxicity and need for frequent monitoring of liver function tests (every 2 weeks for 4 months and then every 3 months thereafter). Methyl-dopa is used for Parkinson's disease, and levothyroxine is used for hypothyroidism.

4. **(D)** Quetiapine, olanzapine, clozapine, and risperidone have all been shown to cause weight gain as a side effect. The only atypical antipsychotic to date that has not been shown to cause significant weight gain is ziprasidone (Geodon).

5. **(E)** All of the listed medications can be helpful in the treatment of akathisia, including decreasing the dose of the neuroleptic or switching to another antipsychotic medication.

6. **(E)** While this woman is having hallucinations—perceptions created without any corresponding sensory stimuli—her experience is best characterized as hallucinosis. Hallucinosis is a hallucination occurring in a patient who is completely alert and oriented, and most commonly occurs in alcohol withdrawal or chronic alcohol abuse. An illusion is a misinterpretation of something that is already there (e.g., a floor lamp being seen as a standing person). A flashback is a sensory re-experience of a past, emotionally intense event (e.g., a war veteran's having a flashback of the sights and sounds of a battle). Formication is the tactile experience of bugs crawling over, or within, one's body.

7. **(E)** Hypothyroidism, tremor, gastrointestinal side effects such as diarrhea, weight gain, and renal impairment (such as inhibiting the effects of antidiuretic hormone causing the

induction of diabetes insipidus) are all potential side effects of lithium. Lithium levels, thyroid function tests, and renal function should be carefully monitored.

8. **(E)** This patient has described a panic attack. Panic attacks are characterized by a sudden onset of intense fear, dread, or anxiety, and accompanied by a variety of physical symptoms. While virtually any organ system can seem to be the source of distress in panic disorder, common symptoms include diaphoresis, palpitations, shortness of breath, tremulousness, flushing, chest pain, and dizziness. Regardless of the clinical setting or psychiatric history, patients presenting with symptoms suggestive of panic disorder must be thoroughly worked up to rule out physiologic pathology as the source of the symptoms. Untreated, panic disorder tends to run a chronic course and can cause severe disability.

9. **(D)** The time course of a panic attack is important diagnostically. Such attacks tend to come on acutely and resolve in less than 30 minutes. Panic disorder is typically treated pharmacologically (with antidepressants or anxiolytics), with cognitive–behavioral therapies, and frequently with some combination of the two. Women are affected by panic disorder up to twice as often as men.

10. **(D)** Neologistic speech, a positive symptom of schizophrenia, consists of words made up by the patient, having meaning only to him. Word salad is an illogical, incoherent collection of words or phrases. Clang associations are words or phrases strung together because of the sound they make, not because of the meaning they convey. Dysarthria is a problem with pronunciation and articulation of words; it does not imply an inherent inability to understand and use language; for example, a dysarthric person could conceivably write a coherent and meaningful sentence.

11. **(E)** Dysthymia is a low-grade, chronic, intermittent depression. The symptoms must be present in adults for at least 2 years. Like depression, other than a subjective feeling of depressed mood, or "the blues," the key features of dysthymia are alterations in appetite and sleep, feelings of hopelessness, difficulty concentrating, and low energy or fatigue. While dysthymia and MDD share a number of features, it is generally the severity and duration of symptoms that distinguish the two disorders. In the presence of alcohol dependence, it would be difficult to convince any clinician that the mood disturbance is not due to the effects of the drug, and would exclude a diagnosis of dysthymia.

12. **(C)** Patients with Capgras syndrome suffer from the delusion that someone familiar is an identical-appearing replacement. Koro is a traumatic fear that the penis is shrinking into the body cavity. Amok is a violent fit, followed by amnesia. Pseudocyesis is the physiologic signs and symptoms of pregnancy developing in the absence of pregnancy. Couvade syndrome occurs when the husband of a pregnant woman goes into a sort of labor. Koro, amok, and couvade syndrome are culture-bound, that is, they describe unusual, recurrent patterns of behavior that resist placement in any Western diagnostic category (i.e., the DSM).

13. **(B)** The multiaxis system of diagnosis in criteria uses the signs and symptoms of psychiatric illness to assign diagnosis and to provide a snapshot picture of a particular patient. It was originally intended to lend objectivity to psychiatric diagnoses, principally in the service of research; today, it is widely used clinically. Axis I includes psychiatric illnesses that appear in a defined period or periods, and result in some diminished function as compared to previous functioning. Common Axis I diagnoses are schizophrenia, generalized anxiety disorder (GAD), and drug-related illnesses, such as alcohol abuse. Axis II represents long-standing pervasive problems in mental life such as personality disorders and mental retardation. Axis III is for all medical conditions, which may or may not relate directly to the psychiatric diagnosis. Axis IV is for psychosocial stressors. Axis V, the GAF, is a numerical value, from 1 (lowest) to 100 (highest), characterizing the over-

all level of impairment resulting from the conditions described on Axis I through Axis IV. The multiaxis representation of this patient would appear as:

Axis I: Adjustment disorder, alcohol abuse, in remission
Axis II: Deferred
Axis III: Diabetes
Axis IV: Psychosocial stressor (recent divorce)
Axis V: GAF: 70

14. **(C)** Both *copropraxia* and *echopraxia* are terms used in relation to movements and are specifically used in reference to obscene gestures and repeating another's movements, respectively. Bruxism is the grinding of the teeth. Blepharospasm is the spasm of the periorbital muscles causing sustained or exaggerated blinking. Torticollis is a spasm of the neck muscles such as the sternocleidomastoid on one or both sides. This usually brings the neck to one side or another but can also pull forward or backward.

15. **(B)** *Coprolalia* and *echolalia* are terms used in relation to language or speech and are specifically used in reference to obscene speech and repeating another's words, respectively. Palilalia is also a repetition of words but is the repetition of one's own words as the person appears to get stuck on the same word or phrase. Parapraxis is a slip of the tongue, and dysarthria refers to a problem of word articulation, usually secondary to cerebellar or motor control abnormalities.

16. **(D)** All of the terms listed are impulse control disorders of various forms. The content of each is listed below:
   • *Pyromania:* Fire setting that is deliberate, more than once
   • *Trichotillomania:* Hair pulling with appreciable hair loss
   • *Kleptomania:* Stealing objects not out of need or monetary value
   • *Pathologic gambling:* Maladaptive gambling behavior
   • *Intermittent explosive disorder:* Aggressive impulses resulting in assault or the destruction of property

17. **(B)** Ego-syntonic and ego-dystonic refer to whether thoughts or behaviors are distressing or not distressing to the patient. In this case, the impulses are distressing and would therefore be classified as ego-dystonic. Mood congruency usually refers to delusions or hallucinations in mood disorders and whether they are themes consistent with the mood. Delusions are fixed, false beliefs that are not shared by others.

18. **(B)** Ganser syndrome is a dissociative disorder described by Ganser in three prisoners. It is characterized by approximate answers and talking past the point and is associated with amnesia, disorientation, fugue, and conversion symptoms. Amok and piblokto are dissociative trance disorders that are described as disturbances in consciousness and are indigenous to particular cultures. Malingering is difficult to distinguish in these situations, but in this case a secondary gain is not identifiable. Logorrhea is excessive speech.

19. **(A)** Kayser–Fleischer rings are golden brown or gray-green rings of pigment at the corneal limbus that can be present in a disorder of copper metabolism such as Wilson's disease. Arcus senilis is a light gray ring beginning superiorly and extending to the limbus. It can resemble a corneal arcus, which is associated with hypercholesterolemia, but in an elderly patient it is often a normal finding. Also associated with hypercholesterolemia is xanthelasma, raised yellow areas around the eyelids. Brushfield spots are lighter-colored areas in the outer third of the iris that can be associated with Down syndrome, but can also be a normal variant. Subconjunctival hemorrhage is the finding of blood in the areas of the eye surrounding the iris.

20. **(C)** Hemiballismus is an uncontrolled swinging of an extremity. It is usually sudden, and once initiated it cannot be controlled. Choreiform movements are involuntary, irregular, and jerky but lack the ballistic-like nature of hemiballismus. Athetoid movements, or athetosis, are slow, snakelike movements of the fingers and hands. Myoclonus is a sud-

den muscle spasm, while myotonia is prolonged muscle contraction.

21. **(A)** Magical thinking and ideas of reference are two types of delusions that can be found in psychotic disorders. Magical thinking is the belief that one's thoughts can control outside events. Ideas of reference is the belief that other people or the media are referring to or talking about the person experiencing this delusion. Reaction formation, displacement, and projection are all types of defense mechanisms. Reaction formation is the formation of thoughts that are opposite to anxiety-provoking feelings. Displacement is the transferring of a feeling toward an object that is less threatening, such as the family pet or one's spouse or children. Projection is the false attribution of one's own unacceptable feelings to another.

22. **(A)** Thought broadcasting is the delusion that one's thoughts can be heard by others. It is often seen in schizophrenia. Thought insertion and thought control also can be seen in schizophrenia and are delusions that others can insert thoughts into a patient's mind or that another can control the patient's thoughts or behaviors, respectively. Transference, in strict terms, is the reexperiencing of past experiences with the analyst in the setting of psychoanalytic psychotherapy. In general, this term has come to mean the transferring of emotions and feelings that one has from one's past to the physician or care provider. Echolalia is the repetition of another's words or phrases.

23. **(A)** *Erotomania* is the term used to describe a delusion in which individuals falsely believe that another person is in love with them. Nymphomania is insatiable sexual desire in a woman, and satyriasis is its male counterpart. Thought broadcasting is the delusion that one's thoughts can be heard by others. Alexia is an inability to read.

24. **(D)** This patient demonstrates delusions of grandeur, that is, an elevated sense of one's position or wealth. A delusion of infidelity is

an unfounded belief that one's spouse or significant other is being unfaithful. Micropsia and macropsia are misperceptions of visual stimuli. Objects appear smaller (micropsia) or larger (macropsia) than they are in reality. Palinopsia is the persistence of the visual image after the stimulus has been removed.

25. **(A)** This patient is euphoric and therefore has a heightened sense of emotion and elation. Euthymia is the state of experiencing a normal mood state. Anhedonia is the inability to experience pleasure. Alexithymia is the inability to know or feel one's own emotions. A delusion of infidelity is an unfounded belief that one's spouse or significant other is being unfaithful. Apathy is a disregard for others or the environment.

26. **(A)** Mood is an individual's subjective description of his own internal environment or emotions, whereas affect is the outwardly expressed or observable aspect of an individual's mood. Insight is the ability to understand one's own feelings or behavior. Perception concerns sensory stimuli and is the mental interpretation of these events. Ego-dystonic describes thoughts that are disturbing to a patient.

27. **(B)** A conversion disorder is often a dramatic set of physical symptoms, usually neurologic, that result from unconscious conflicts. Sublimation is a defense mechanism employed to deal with unacceptable feelings or desires that one may possess and to channel these motivations into socially acceptable behaviors. Like sublimation, rationalization is a defense against undesired motivations, but in this case these motivations are concealed by elaborate and reassuring explanations that avoid the actual underlying motives. Dissociation is a defense mechanism that deals with stressors via a breakdown of the usual integration of memory, behavior, and perception.

28. **(D)** La belle indifference is the indifference shown toward a deficit or loss of function classically seen in a conversion disorder. Déjà entendu is the feeling that one is hearing

what one has heard before. It is usually associated with anxiety states or fatigue. Déjà vu is a similar experience but refers to the sensation that something has been seen before. Jamais vu is the opposite of Déjà vu in that it refers to something that should be familiar but seems quite unfamiliar. Folie à deux is a shared delusion aroused in one person by the influence of another.

29. **(A)** Testamentary capacity (the level of competence required to make a valid will) is based on the presence of all of the following: (1) an understanding of the nature of the will; (2) knowledge of one's assets; (3) knowledge of natural heirs; (4) absence of acute psychosis (i.e., delusions), which might compromise rational decision making; and (5) freedom from undue influence or coercion. The validity of the will may be undermined by demonstrating that the individual failed to meet any of the above criteria. The presence of a conservator of person and history of mental illness are important only insofar as they bear upon any of the above-noted factors. A history of mental illness is not sufficient to invalidate one's testamentary capacity. Actus reus refers to the voluntary act of committing a crime and is an element used in determining criminal responsibility. The presence of a judge at the signing of a will is not required.

30. **(B)** Informed consent is crucial in maintaining patient autonomy in decision making. Elements involved in obtaining informed consent include providing the patient with information regarding the risks and benefits of treatment, alternative treatment options (including no treatment), and establishing the competency of the patient to make a voluntary decision. Exceptions to informed consent include: (1) emergency situations in which obtaining informed consent would jeopardize patient safety, (2) patient waiver of informed consent, and (3) situations in which disclosing information would directly harm the patient (also known as *therapeutic privilege* and seldom used). The other choices are not valid exceptions to informed consent.

31. **(C)** Confidentiality is an integral part of the physician–patient relationship and is especially important in establishing the trust of a psychotherapeutic relationship. The physician–patient privilege should be breached only in specific instances such as the patient's waiving of the privilege (i.e., patient initiates litigation, consent to release information is obtained, there is a duty to protect, emergency situation, or in cases in which the court orders release). In this case, the information should not be released unless the patient has waived his physician–patient confidentiality privilege. Lying to or misleading the court is unethical and may subject one to prosecution. The remaining choices fail to maintain confidentiality.

32. **(D)** When a patient has stopped paying his or her bill, the physician should directly address the issue with the patient. Failure to pay one's bills may reflect underlying issues for which the patient has entered into psychotherapy or that are related to psychiatric symptoms. Contacting a collection agency before addressing the issue with the patient is inappropriate. If a patient continues to refuse payment after discussing the issue, the patient should be notified in writing of the outstanding balance, and a referral to a collection agency might be made. To preserve confidentiality, care should be taken to disclose the minimum information needed for collection (i.e., date of service and charge) without referring to diagnosis or treatment rendered. Asking the insurance company to pay you after a check has been disbursed to the patient is futile since the insurance company's obligation toward the insured has been fulfilled. Disclosing the existence of a professional relationship with the patient to his family is a breach of confidentiality. Terminating the therapeutic relationship before exploring the dynamics behind the patient's payment delinquency might harm any future therapeutic alliance.

33. **(C)** The syndrome of approximate answers is known as Ganser syndrome and is characterized by inaccurate but close answers to ques-

tions (e.g., 4 + 4 = 9). It is rare and usually found among prison populations or those attempting to feign mental illnesses. DSM-IV-TR characterizes Ganser syndrome as a dissociative disorder not otherwise specified, but whether it represents a true unconscious process or frank malingering is controversial. "First-break" psychosis is usually associated with symptoms such as gross disorganization of behavior/speech, hallucinations, or delusions. The MSE and history in this case do not confirm the presence of a psychotic process. Amok is a dissociative disorder characterized by a violent outburst or homicidal behavior directed toward another person or object after a perceived insult. The assertion that "an individual is not responsible for a criminal act if he was unable to resist his actions due to a mental illness" is known as the irresistible impulse rule. Koro is a Malaysian term describing a sudden anxiety that the penis will recede into the body and possibly result in the individual's death.

34.   (B) Malingering is the intentional production of symptoms for secondary gain (e.g., to avoid work, to evade criminal prosecution, or to gain financial rewards). A diagnosis of malingering should be suspected in medicolegal cases, in individuals with antisocial personality disorder, when symptoms are out of proportion to objective findings, or when a patient in distress does not cooperate with evaluation/treatment. Factitious disorder can be differentiated from malingering based on the absence of external incentives. In factitious disorder, symptoms are intentionally feigned in order to satisfy an intrapsychic incentive to assume the sick role. Munchausen syndrome is a factitious disorder characterized by repeated acts of feigning illnesses to gain medical attention. Intrapsychic gain obtained by the act of getting medical attention through feigning medical illness in another individual (usually a child or elderly person) is sometimes referred to as Munchausen by proxy. Conversion disorder describes the production of neurologic or other medical symptoms resulting from intrapsychic needs or conflicts. In contrast to factitious disorder

and malingering, symptoms associated with conversion disorder are not consciously produced.

35.   (E) Individuals with malingering tend to be suspicious and uncooperative with diagnostic evaluations. Furthermore, they do not typically follow up with recommended treatment regimens and refuse opportunities to return to social/work activities. Malingerers consciously feign symptoms for financial incentives or to avoid work/social obligations (i.e., secondary gain). In contrast, conversion disorder is the unconscious or involuntary production of symptoms resulting from intrapsychic needs or conflicts. Individuals with conversion disorder are more likely to be friendly, cooperative, interested in evaluations that may "find the answer" and avidly follow up with prescribed treatments. The other choices are not accurate statements distinguishing between malingering and conversion disorder.

36.   (E) Sexual abuse is estimated to occur with an incidence of 0.25% of children per year. Known acquaintances (e.g., fathers, stepfathers, and male relatives) are often the perpetrators. In this vignette, the patient likely has acquired *Neisseria gonorrhoeae* from a male perpetrator. Other physical findings may include injuries to the genitalia (i.e., hymen, vagina) or the perineum. Psychiatric manifestations of sexual abuse may include anxiety, agitation, aggressive/impulsive behavior, and exhibitionism. When sexual abuse of a child is suspected, the first step is to ensure the safety of the child and immediately notify the state's child protective services. Mandatory reporting is required in cases of physical and sexual child abuse. The other choices fail to protect the child and do not satisfy state-mandated reporting statutes.

37.   (A) The insanity defense is used to exculpate individuals from criminal responsibility based on an underlying mental condition. Specific standards for asserting and proving an insanity defense differ among states; however, the American Law Institute Test (can't

appreciate the criminality or wrongfulness of one's actions) is the current standard for insanity defenses in most states. The insanity defense is seldom utilized (less than 1% of felonies), generally unsuccessful (less than 30%), and leads to more time of incarceration compared with individuals found guilty of the original crime. Although in most cases the prosecution and defense are in agreement with regard to the individual's assertion of an insanity plea, it is not required.

38. **(B)** Expert medical witnesses offer opinions regarding a body of knowledge in which they have particularly more familiarity than does the layperson. A fact witness provides only factual information in court. Expert witnesses generally provide a written report to the court and may testify during the trial. Expert witnesses do not work with the jury in establishing a verdict, although the jury typically relies on the testimony given by the expert witness in arriving at their decision. Choice E is a nonsense distracter.

39. **(D)** A physician or therapist is obligated to protect potential victims from imminent harm. This duty may be fulfilled by directly notifying the person at risk, by contacting the police, or by taking other appropriate measures to protect the intended victim. In this case, notifying the police is the most appropriate action to protect the girlfriend. When warning third parties of potential harm, care should be taken to release only that information necessary to protecting them. The remaining choices fail to adequately protect the girlfriend.

40. **(D)** *Tarasoff v. Regents of University of California* is the landmark legal precedent establishing liability to third parties. There have been two rulings regarding the *Tarasoff* case. The original case, *Tarasoff I* (1974), established a "duty to warn" intended victims. The California Supreme Court revised its earlier decision with *Tarasoff II* (1976) which established a "duty to protect." The remaining choices are nonsense distracters.

41. **(A)** Suicide is the second leading cause of death among individuals aged 15 to 24; only accidents account for more deaths in this population. Risk factors for completed suicide include: (1) age > 45, (2) male gender, (3) separated/divorced > married, (4) white race > black race, and (5) Jews/Protestants > Catholics. The lifetime suicide rate in individuals with a diagnosis of a major psychiatric disorder (i.e., schizophrenia, bipolar I disorder, MDD) is estimated at 10 to 15%. Suicide in children younger than age 13 is rare. Women attempt suicide up to four times more frequently than men; however, men are three times more likely to succeed at suicide than are women.

42. **(B)** Physician-assisted suicide involves the doctor's facilitating a person's death by providing the information or equipment necessary to end his or her life. The AMA's Code of Medical Ethics strongly condemns such action as "fundamentally incompatible with the physician's role as healer." Rather, the ethical obligation of the physician is to adequately respond to a patient's end-of-life issues. The AMA's Code of Medical Ethics emphasizes that participation in physician-assisted suicide would have detrimental implications to both society and the practice of medicine. Euthanasia occurs when a physician carries out the killing of a patient in order to relieve intolerable and refractory suffering. Euthanasia is not the mere facilitation of the terminal act, but involves the actual administration of the fatal agent. Like physician-assisted suicide, it is condemned by the AMA's Code of Medical Ethics. Recently, a Michigan physician was found guilty of second-degree murder for giving a lethal injection at the request of a patient suffering from Lou Gehrig's disease.

43. **(B)** Physician–patient confidentiality in the treatment of minors must be maintained unless otherwise mandated by law (e.g., cases of abortion in some states) or when parental involvement is necessary in making complex and life-threatening medical decisions. In this case, the physician must respect the patient's confidentiality but should remain cognizant

of the implications this will have on the family system. Therefore, it is most appropriate to encourage the minor to discuss the issue with her parents. At this point, there is no indication of child harm or neglect that would mandate reporting to child protective services. Testimonial privilege refers to the privilege invoked to protect physician–patient confidentiality when medical information is subpoenaed without patient consent. The remaining two choices fail to maintain physician–patient confidentiality.

44. **(C)** Tangentiality is similar to circumstantiality in its representing speech/thoughts that are logically connected but that drift off the point. Tangentiality differs from circumstantiality in that the speaker never comes back to the point.

45. **(B)** Delusions are disturbances in thought content and are fixed, false beliefs not held by others. They are included in none of the other choices, which are categories of the MSE.

46. **(E)** With this patient's predominantly suspicious, paranoid thought content focused on ideas of reference, he clearly meets criteria for paranoid type.

47. **(A)** The description given clearly describes the criteria of residual type schizophrenia, that is, nonprominent, nonbizarre delusions and/or perceptual disturbances with enough other symptoms of schizophrenia to meet criteria for the disorder.

48. **(A)** Bipolar manic episodes have perhaps the highest rate of response to ECT. The safety of ECT depends on underlying medical conditions, not on the disorder being treated. Its effects are not longer lasting than those of medications.

49. **(C)** This question refers to kindling, the hypothesis that each decompensation in a mental illness leads to increased risk to have another, and likely more severe episode. Conversely, treatment of the decompensa-

tions is theorized to be protective against the above. There is no known effect on the response to ECT or medications in the future.

50. **(B)** Antipsychotic medications are often useful in the treatment of acute mania (especially while waiting for the mood stabilizers to have an effect), and are often also good second-line agents in the long-term treatment of bipolar illness when mood stabilizers have failed. Recent data suggest that olanzapine (Zyprexa), a newer antipsychotic, may have a role in treatment of acute mania. Antidementia medications are not indicated here, nor are antiseizure medications, although many of them have proven to be mood stabilizers. They would, in fact, be contraindicated during ECT. Long-term commitment and psychosurgery such as lobotomy are inappropriately severe approaches.

51. **(B)** Mania has many potential medical causes, including hyperthyroidism, uremia, and CNS infections. The only choice that has two well-established such causes is B.

52. **(A)** PCP, or angel dust, is a powerful hallucinogen that has stimulant effects; it frequently causes a presentation difficult to distinguish from mania and/or psychosis. It is coming back into popular use as a drug of abuse in the form of "illy" or "wet," which is a marijuana joint soaked in formaldehyde and frequently PCP. The other drugs mentioned can cause some manic symptoms in intoxication or perhaps withdrawal, but not with the consistency or acuteness of PCP.

53. **(A)** Age greater than 50 is one of the strongest risk factors for suicide in the setting of depression. Her gender is a protective factor; race has not been shown to be a factor. Lesser risk factors than age, in order of decreasing severity, are means to commit suicide and financial loss.

54. **(E)** Lack of suicide attempt history is her most significant protective factor; a lesser protective factor is social supports. Other factors do not play much of a role.

55. **(E)** Low CSF levels of serotonin are the most consistent and well-documented findings in patients who make suicide attempts. Cortisol is high in depression in general, but not particularly so in patients who attempt suicide. The other choices lack data or have inconclusive data.

56. **(E)** Nonsuppressing dexamethasone suppression tests are one of the most well-documented and common findings in patients with major depression. Other findings have little or no data.

57. **(B)** There are many potential medical causes of depression; the only choice here that lists two well-described such causes is B. Vitamin B_{12} deficiency and adrenal disease, as well as vascular disease, have also been shown to also be potential causes.

58. **(A)** Excessive dental decay is common in patients with anorexia or bulimia who purge by self-induced vomiting. Although the other choices may be present in severe starvation, excessive dental decay is most common and appears earliest.

59. **(B)** Although purging is more common in bulimia, anorexia can be of a purging type. Here, anorexia is suggested by a weight below the 85th percentile. Many patients with anorexia and bulimia also suffer from major depression, but this patient's symptoms are predominantly of an eating disorder. Although the patient may also be suffering from adjustment disorder, given the time frame of her breakup with her boyfriend, again, her symptoms are predominantly those of an eating disorder. There is no evidence of OCD.

60. **(A)** Occupations such as modeling, ballet, and gymnastics, which encourage thinness, have disproportionately high rates of anorexia. Patients with certain personality disorders, including borderline personality disorder, have a higher likelihood of being victims of abuse or trauma. Education and "type A" personalities are not correlated with eating disorders, nor is being a twin.

61. **(C)** This condition has been described only in girls. Diagnostic criteria require symptom onset between ages 5 months and 4 years with apparently normal prior development. Criteria for autism do not require deceleration of head growth. In childhood disintegrative disorder, as in Rett syndrome, development is initially normal. However, in childhood disintegrative disorder, development is normal for at least the first 2 years after birth. In Asperger syndrome, there is no delay in language. Childhood schizophrenia cannot be diagnosed in children meeting criteria for a pervasive developmental disorder who do not have prominent delusions and hallucinations.

62. **(B)** This patient has a clinical course marked by a combination of vocal and motor tics occurring over a time period greater than 1 year. In chronic vocal tic disorder, there are no motor tics. In transient tic disorder, tics last for less than 12 months. The "not otherwise specified" condition is diagnosed when criteria for the specific tic disorders are not met (i.e., onset after 18 years or course less than 4 weeks). Although "repeated sterotyped movements" that are tic-like may occur in pervasive developmental disorders, other realms of dysfunction must be present, such as general impairments in socialization and language capability.

63. **(E)** Childhood schizophrenia is an exceedingly rare condition and there is no mention of psychotic symptoms in this case. Meanwhile, ADHD, conduct disorder, depression, and OCD are not uncommonly found in patients diagnosed with tic disorder.

64. **(A)** Pimozide, a dopamine blocker, has been shown to most clearly suppress tic activity compared to agents affecting other neurotransmitter systems. Although methylphenidate may help this patient's apparent ADHD symptoms, it may also exacerbate his tic disorder. Fluoxetine, topiramate, and clonidine may be effective for comorbid conditions found with Tourette's disorder but have not been found to be specifically helpful for this primary condition.

65. (C) Fire setting in a repeated pattern in children often accompanies other behaviors that are defiant of rules and authority, as in conduct disorder. Although fire setting may occur in children diagnosed with pervasive developmental disorder, mental retardation, or tic disorder, it is much more unusual. Destructive personality disorder of childhood is not a DSM-IV-TR diagnosis, and here serves as a distracter.

66. (D) Secondary enuresis means that the child achieved continence for over a year and then lost it, as the case suggests. Nocturnal means the incontinence happens at night. Primary enuresis means that the patient has never achieved complete continence. Diurnal enuresis is daytime incontinence. Encopresis is the repeated passage of feces into inappropriate places.

67. (E) More than 40 double-blind trials of imipramine have confirmed the drug's efficacy for enuresis. Clonidine is an antihypertensive sometimes used in opiate withdrawal. Haloperidol is a typical antipsychotic. Carbamazepine is an anticonvulsant sometimes used as a mood stabilizer. Diphenhydramine is used for insomnia.

68. (C) Borderline intellectual functioning is defined by IQ in the range of 70 to 85. In mild mental retardation, IQ ranges from 50–55 to approximately 70. In severe mental retardation, IQ ranges from 20–25 to 35–40. Learning disorder not otherwise specified is diagnosed with global learning impairments, but the disability in specific areas of learning is mild and would not result in such low IQ results as in this case.

69. (A) Microcephaly, short palpebral fissures, flat midface, and thin upper lip are all associated with fetal alcohol syndrome (FAS). Cleft palate is not specifically associated with FAS. There are no genetic abnormalities associated with FAS. Congenital blindness is not associated with FAS, although methyl alcohol consumption can cause blindness in adults. Prominent jaw is associated with fragile X syndrome.

70. (D) About 75% of cases of mental retardation are associated with a prenatal cause. Perinatal and postnatal causes account for 10 to 25%.

71. (D) Concerns that fluoxetine could provoke violent behaviors have more recently been attributed to the underlying disorder for which the drug was prescribed. It is the opinion of most psychopharmacologists that fluoxetine and the other SSRIs represent useful medications with relatively few side effect risks. Children tend to have more rapid hepatic metabolism, higher renal clearance, and less body fat, all factors that conspire to increase elimination of these drug classes in children compared to adults. Children tend to be more sensitive to extrapyramidal side effects of neuroleptics than do adults, possibly owing to greater density of dopamine receptors in children's brains compared to adults. Low-potency neuroleptics are associated with sedation that may hinder the academic progress of school-age children. TCAs have not proven themselves to be effective antidepressants in children, possibly owing to immaturity of certain neurotransmitter systems in children compared to adults.

72. (B) Mixed receptive–expressive language disorder does not imply an abnormality in emotional communication such as in displays of aggression toward other children found in reactive attachment disorder. Patients with childhood disintegrative disorder show histories of decline in language and social communication operating that are more profound than in reactive attachment disorder, and there are no criteria noting an association of symptoms of neglect or abuse. ADHD and conduct disorder are most often diagnosed in school-age children who have histories of reactive attachment disorder.

73. (C) The majority of patients diagnosed with borderline personality disorder report histories of sexual abuse. Sexual activity among siblings is the most common form of incest, although parent-to-child incest is the most commonly *reported* form. A history of sexual abuse is in fact a risk factor for being a future victim of sexual abuse. There is no association of childhood sexual abuse and schizophrenia. Abuse of alcohol or other illicit substances at such a young age as this patient is commonly found in victims of childhood sexual abuse.

74. **(D)** Many incestuous fathers act in the face of disappointing and/or conflicted sexual relationships with their spouses. Incestuous fathers and stepfathers all have increased likelihoods of having alcoholism, impulsive or violent behavior, paraphilias such as exhibitionism and pedophilia, and a personal history of being a victim of sexual abuse.

75. **(C)** About one half of all cases of sexual abuse of children represent repeated victimizations.

76. **(D)** This patient has symptoms most consistent with a bipolar mood disorder and therefore would most benefit from lithium or another mood stabilizer such as valproic acid. Lorazepam may be used to treat psychomotor agitation and insomnia of mania but does not generally treat the underlying disorder and has a dependency liability in the long term. Imipramine and fluoxetine, as tricyclic and SSRI antidepressants, respectively, can exacerbate mania. Chlorpromazine, a typical antipsychotic, may help the patient with his mild thought disorder and his psychomotor agitation but may not treat the underlying mood disorder if given alone.

77. **(C)** Atypical depression is characterized by mood reactivity, rejection hypersensitivity, hypersomnolence, increased appetite, and "lead pipe" psychomotor retardation. Severe concentration impairment is a feature of melancholic depression. Patients with either melancholic or atypical symptoms may have either a normal dexamethasone suppression test or psychotic symptoms. A manic response to antidepressant treatment may be indicative of a bipolar syndrome rather than a unipolar depression.

78. **(B)** Although not commonly used because of the risk of side effects, MAOIs are actually the most effective class of drugs for treating atypical depression. SSRIs and TCAs are also effective. Some anticonvulsants are used for the treatment of bipolar disorder, but not unipolar depression. Neuroleptics are used to treat psychotic disorders.

79. **(C)** When changing from an SSRI to an MAOI, one must allow a washout period of about five half-lives for the SSRI to be more than 90% eliminated; in the case of fluoxetine, this is 5 weeks. This precaution avoids serotonin syndrome, which can occur when significant blood levels of both drugs are present. Serotonin syndrome, which can be fatal, is marked by symptoms of tremor, diaphoresis, rigidity, myoclonus, autonomic dysregulation, hyperthermia, rhabdomyolysis, renal failure, and coma.

80. **(D)** MAOIs prevent the peripheral breakdown of tyramine, which may be ingested with certain foods such as beer, red wine, aged cheeses, liver, smoked fish, dry sausage, and fava beans. If too much tyramine builds up in the blood, it may activate peripheral sympathetic nerve receptors and cause a hypertensive crisis. Stiffness and tremor are usually associated with typical neuroleptics and are rare with MAOIs. Bland food is a nonspecific request. Eating food rich in tryptophan, a serotonin precursor, is not a problem. MAOIs are not usually particularly oversedating compared to tricyclic or other "atypical" antidepressants.

81. **(D)** This case deliberately brings together many character traits drawn from "pure" diagnoses of character disorders, including borderline, narcissistic, dependent, obsessive–compulsive, and schizotypal personalities. In clinical practice, a large proportion of patients diagnosable in Axis II do not in fact have any clear-cut character syndrome. Such mixed cases are referred to as personality disorder not otherwise specified. Patients with pure borderline personality disorder are known for their intense personal relation-

ships, self-destructive behaviors, anger management issues, and poor senses of self-image. Narcissistic personality disorder is marked by a grandiose sense of self-worth, entitlement, lack of real empathy, and tendency to use others for one's own ends. Patients with obsessive–compulsive personality disorder are perfectionists, inflexible, and overly demanding of themselves and others. Schizotypal patients are known for their quirkiness and seemingly magical thinking styles.

82. **(D)** Remembering the DSM-IV-TR criteria for schizoaffective disorder can be daunting. Generally speaking, patients who at one time appear to have schizophrenia (i.e., diagnostic criteria for it are met) and at other times appear to have a prominent mood disorder (based on an episode that fulfills either major depression or bipolar disorder with or without psychosis) may be diagnosed with schizoaffective disorder. Technically, the diagnosis requires a period of 2 weeks of psychotic symptoms without affective symptoms. Psychotic disorder not otherwise specified is usually reserved for situations in which the clinician does not have enough historical data to know whether the patient has schizophrenia, a mood disorder with psychotic features, or a medical-related or substance-induced psychosis.

83. **(D)** The elderly are particularly vulnerable to medications known to have psychoactive properties or side effects. This is in part due to the decreased ability of geriatric patients to rapidly metabolize medications, and thus the tendency of the drugs to build up to higher steady-state levels than for younger persons. Additionally, elderly persons are generally more vulnerable to the effects of medications that act on the CNS due to decreased reserve of neurons using particular neurotransmitter systems that may be affected by the drugs. For example, elderly people may be more susceptible to the dopamine-blocking effects of haloperidol that cause parkinsonism because they have a decreased number of dopaminergic neurons that arise from the

substantia nigra. The patient in this case is on a number of medications that may have CNS side effects at high doses, especially in the elderly. However, the highly anticholinergic properties of diphenhydramine (Benadryl) put this patient at particular risk of memory impairment and confusion. Cimetidine and furosemide are conceivable culprits for her confusion due to their minor anticholinergic activity, but are much less likely. Beta blockers like atenolol have been associated with depression presumably associated with blockade of central adrenergic receptors. Additionally, in some vulnerable patients, they may reduce cardiac output enough to cause a functional hypoperfusion of the brain, causing confusion and dizziness. Digoxin may actually decrease sodium ion conduction in CNS neurons enough to produce delirium in some patients.

84. **(A)** Delirium related to blockade of acetylcholinergic receptors is the most common cause of medication-induced delirium in the elderly. Acetylcholine is uniquely involved with memory processes in the brain, and its involvement in the pathophysiology of Alzheimer's disease has been heavily researched. Drugs that alter dopamine neurotransmission are most associated with movement disorder and psychosis-related side effects. Drugs affecting GABA receptors may cause sedation and ataxia, as well as memory disturbances. Fortunately, the diversity of drugs that affect these receptors is much narrower than the broad classes of drugs that block acetylcholine receptors. Drugs affecting serotonin may affect sleep, appetite, and mood, but few nonpsychiatric drugs affect this system. Drugs affecting central norepinephrine transmission may rarely be associated with depression.

85. **(E)** Studies that find no statistical difference between groups when there actually is a difference result in a type II error. In this case, the positive findings at the other universities make the finding at university A less likely to be correct. University A may have needed a larger number of subjects in the study to find

the treatment effect. Type I errors occur more often than type II errors and cause the researcher to conclude that there is a difference between groups when in fact there is none. Standard error is the degree to which the means of several different samples would vary if they were taken repeatedly from the same population. The variance is the sum of the differences of each data point from the mean. Positive predictive value is the proportion of abnormal test results that are true positive, while negative predictive value is the proportion of normal test results that are true negative.

86. **(E)** This patient has signs most consistent with tardive dyskinesia, an extrapyramidal syndrome that usually affects perioral or limb musculature and causes choreiform movements. Its onset is usually several years after being on the medication, and it is more likely to affect older patients. Akathisia is best described as psychomotor restlessness that may have an onset of hours to days after beginning the neuroleptic. Dystonia is an acute reaction to neuroleptics in which particular muscle groups (neck or ocular muscles commonly) contract involuntarily. It can be painful and should be treated immediately with anticholinergics. NMS is a potentially lethal medical emergency in which patients may have global rigidity, mental status changes, fever, cardiovascular instability, elevated creatine phosphokinases, and risk of rhabdomyolysis. Parkinsonism may look identical to Parkinson's disease (tremor, bradykinesia) and may have onset within weeks to months of beginning the medication.

87. **(A)** The basal ganglia, implicated in the yoking of thought to motor action, and in controlling the initiation and quality of motor action, is theorized to be central to the pathophysiology of extrapyramidal syndromes, including dystonia, parkinsonism, akathisia, and tardive dyskinesia. The cerebellum is important in controlling the coordination of motor movements and posture, as well as participating in procedural memory.

The frontal cortex is generally considered to be important for decision making, impulse control, short-term memory, and affect regulation. The midbrain contains nuclei that help ensure CNS homeostasis by regulating neurovegetative, autonomic, and arousal functions. The motor cortex serves as the last stage of cerebral processing of motor information before it descends into the spinal cord. An intact motor cortex is required for initiation of movement.

88. **(B)** The risk of acquiring tardive dyskinesia is apparently cumulative with regard to duration of exposure to a neuroleptic drug. Elderly patients, women, and patients on high doses of medication or combinations of neuroleptics have risks greater than 5% per year.

89. **(A)** Premorbid personality disorders and comorbid Axis I disorders have been shown to increase the risk of acquiring PTSD with exposure to a significant, acute psychological trauma. Exposure to psychological trauma in middle adulthood as opposed to childhood or elderly years is considered the period of least vulnerability to PTSD. Rapid onset of symptoms, short duration of symptoms, and strong social supports are good prognostic indicators for PTSD.

90. **(C)** Erik Erikson is perhaps best known for his description of eight stages of human psychological experience spanning the life span, centered on stage-appropriate developmental conflicts: basic trust versus mistrust (birth to 1 year); autonomy versus shame and doubt (1 to 3 years); initiative versus guilt (3 to 5 years); industry versus inferiority (6 to 11 years); identity versus role diffusion (11 years to end of adolescence); intimacy versus isolation (21 to 40 years); generativity versus stagnation (40 to 65 years); and integrity versus despair (65 and older). Carl Jung developed concepts of the collective unconscious, archetypes, individuation, introversion, and extroversion. Karen Horney's work is notable for an emphasis on the idea that a person's personality traits are the result of an interaction of the person with the environment, and that

"self-realization" is the therapeutic process that removes distorting influences that prevent character growth. Jean Piaget is known for his work using observations of children and adolescents to build a framework describing cognitive stages of development beginning with the sensorimotor stage at birth and ending with the stage of formal operations. Sigmund Freud is the founder of psychoanalysis, notable for such concepts as ego, id, and superego and drive theory.

91. **(D)** About 20% of patients with complex partial epilepsy experience psychotic symptoms at some time.

92. **(B)** Hyperreligious thinking or preoccupation with moral behavior, altered sexual behaviors, hypergraphia or overelaborative communication styles (also referred to as viscosity), and heightened experience of emotions form a classic constellation of personality traits associated with complex partial epilepsy. Urinary incontinence is more often associated with normal pressure hydrocephalus or severe dementia. Sleep disorders, depression, and obsessive–compulsive symptoms may be associated with structural brain injury of frontal and subcortical areas but have not been described as being related particularly to complex partial epilepsy.

93. **(B)** The Glasgow Coma Scale measures level of arousal and ranges from a scale of 3 (deep coma) to 14 (fully alert). The categories assessed are eye opening, best motor response, and best verbal response. Eye opening ranges from a score of 4 (opening spontaneously) to 1 (not opening at all). In this case the eyes open to pain, so a score of 2 is given. Best motor response is as follows: obeys commands, 5; localizes pain, 4; flexion, 3; extension, 2; and no response, 1. In this case, a score of 3 is given for the response. Best verbal response is also based on a scale ranging from 5 to 1. An oriented patient receives a score of 5, and no response receives a score of 1, as in this case. The scores are then added, and in this case are 2 + 3 + 1 = 6.

94. **(D)** At doses of 1,000 mg per day or higher, thioridazine has been associated with pigmentary retinopathy, also known as retinitis pigmentosa. Therefore, doses should not exceed 800 mg per day. Pigmentary retinopathy can cause loss of retinal response to contraction of the visual field. An early sign may be nocturnal confusion. Constipation, dry eyes, and urinary retention are side effects from the anticholinergic properties of thioridazine, but typically are not so severe as to compromise health permanently. Nephrogenic diabetes insipidus is not associated with thioridazine.

95. **(C)** Benztropine 1 to 2 mg IM is useful in the treatment of acute dystonic reactions. Alternatively, diphenhydramine 50 mg IM or IV can be used. If the symptoms do not resolve within 20 minutes, larger doses can be given. Benzodiazepines can also be tried but are not first-line treatment. For acute laryngeal dystonia, 4 mg of benztropine should be given within 10 minutes, then 2 mg of lorazepam IV if needed. None of the other choices are indicated for the treatment of acute dystonia, although switching to a lower-potency neuroleptic might be considered as prophylaxis against further dystonic reactions. Labetalol is an antihypertensive; acetaminophen is an analgesic and antipyretic; and penicillamine is a chelating agent used to treat Wilson's disease.

96. **(A)** The disorder described is diabetes insipidus. Lithium inhibits the effect of antidiuretic hormone (ADH) on the kidney. While haloperidol (an antipsychotic), diazepam (a benzodiazepine), valproic acid (an antiepileptic used as a mood stabilizer), and buspirone (an anxiolytic/antidepressant) may be used to treat various manifestations of bipolar disorder, none of them are associated with diabetes insipidus.

97. **(D)** Clonidine, a central alpha-2 autoreceptor agonist, has been proven useful in the treatment of autonomic hyperactivity associated with opioid withdrawal. Haloperidol, pimozide, and thioridazine are antipsychotics.

Amantadine is used to treat Parkinson's disease and also as an anti-influenza agent.

98. **(C)** Methadone has been proven to greatly reduce the use of heroin when used as a maintenance medication. Patients maintained on doses lower than 40 mg qd of methadone are far more likely to relapse than those on higher doses. Lorazepam and alprazolam are benzodiazepines; sertraline is an SSRI; and lithium is first-line treatment for bipolar disorder.

99. **(B)** TCAs are considered class 1A antiarrhythmics because they possess quinidine-like effects that decrease conduction time through the bundle of His. They have been shown to increase mortality in cardiac patients. TCAs can also increase the heart rate anywhere from 3 to 15 beats per minute, and a patient with compromised cardiac function may suffer from increased oxygen demand. Finally, TCAs are associated with significant orthostatic hypotension, which is further exacerbated in patients with cardiac disease. The SSRIs are safely used in patients with cardiac disease, although attention should be paid to cardiac medicines metabolized through the P450 cytochrome system such as fluoxetine, which could alter medication levels. The butyrophenones and dibenzodiazepines are antipsychotics. Benzodiazepines are not antidepressants.

100. **(D)** Acetylcholine is the neurotransmitter most implicated in cognitive functioning. Anticholinergic effects of medications are frequently implicated in cognitive decline and drug-induced delirium. All of the neurotransmitters listed may be involved in cognition, but acetylcholine is by far the most implicated. Dopamine and histamine are targeted by antipsychotic medications, while serotonin and norepinephrine are thought to be involved in depression.

101. **(B)** Imipramine is a tertiary amine TCA. Tertiary amine tricyclics have high anticholinergic activity. Haloperidol, a butyrophenone antipsychotic, is a high-potency antipsy-

chotic. As a group, high-potency antipsychotics have a lower anticholinergic profile than low-potency antipsychotics. Fluoxetine, an SSRI, can have mild anticholinergic effects. Amantadine, an anti-Parkinson's drug, and clonidine, an antihypertensive, do not possess clinically significant anticholinergic effects.

102. **(B)** Lithium toxicity is characterized early on by dysarthria, ataxia, coarse tremor, and abdominal pain. Later manifestations include seizures, neuromuscular irritability, and impaired consciousness (delirium to coma). Acute dystonias are associated with the use of typical antipsychotics; paranoid delusions are part of the symptom profile of schizophrenia and sometimes of bipolar disorder. Leg pain is not associated with lithium.

103. **(C)** In general, the typical antipsychotics can be continued without significant side effects during ECT, and in fact can lower the seizure threshold, which facilitates ECT. Lithium has been associated with prolonged delirium post-ECT. There are no good data on venlafaxine during ECT. As a benzodiazepine, lorazepam is an antiepileptic and would hinder ECT. Benztropine could cause cognitive difficulties immediately after ECT. Clozapine, an atypical antipsychotic, can cause tardive seizures when administered with ECT.

104. **(A)** A space-occupying lesion is a relative contraindication to ECT. Other relative contraindications include high intracranial pressure, intracerebral bleeding, recent myocardial infarction, retinal detachment, pheochromocytoma, and high anesthesia risk. The other choices are not considered risks.

105. **(E)** There are no absolute contraindications to ECT. The other choices can be considered relative contraindications.

106. **(B)** For extreme agitation, the butyrophenone antipsychotic haloperidol (Haldol) is useful. Benzodiazepines are also useful for this symptom. Phenothiazine antipsychotics can cause autonomic instability when given

to a patient with PCP intoxication. Trihexyphenidyl is used to combat extrapyramidal symptoms associated with antipsychotic use. Trazodone, used commonly for insomnia, and fluoxetine, an SSRI, are antidepressants.

107. **(C)** Supportive care is the best treatment for PCP intoxication that is not complicated by extreme agitation or violence. Haloperidol, a typical antipsychotic, is useful for extreme agitation. Despite urban myths, vitamins and cheese do not have particular therapeutic benefits for PCP intoxication.

108. **(E)** Yohimbine, used to treat impotence, can cause elevated blood pressure and heart rate and should not be used by patients with cardiac or renal disease, glaucoma, or a history of ulcers. In fact, paroxetine and citalopram are antidepressants that can cause impotence. Molindone is an antipsychotic. Diphenhydramine is an antihistamine.

109. **(E)** Clonidine is a centrally acting alpha-2 agonist. In contrast, yohimbine is an alpha-2 antagonist. Clonidine decreases norepinephrine by stimulating the alpha-2 autoreceptor. Yohimbine increases norepinephrine by blocking the alpha-2 autoreceptor.

110. **(C)** This patient is suffering from major depression with psychotic features. Psychosis cannot be treated with antidepressant medication alone, because psychosis should be treated with an antipsychotic such as risperidone. Depression should be treated with an antidepressant such as sertraline. Lithium and synthroid can both effectively augment antidepressants such as paroxetine. Lorazepam, a benzodiazepine, may help with anxiety, but will not be effective against psychosis or depression. Similarly, a combination of lorazepam and clozapine, an atypical antipsychotic, will not treat the depression.

111. **(D)** Benzodiazepines are considered the first-line agents for the treatment of primary insomnia. Short-acting agents such as temazepam are useful in helping patients fall asleep and not remaining drowsy the next day. Diphenhydramine and trazodone are often used for insomnia and are effective medications. However, these can leave patients feeling drowsy the next day. Clozapine and amitriptyline are sedating but have serious side effects and should not be used for primary insomnia.

112. **(A)** Fluvoxamine is an SSRI. As a group, the SSRIs have fewer side effects and are safer than the tricyclics and the MAO "a" inhibitors. Fluvoxamine, imipramine, and phenelzine have all been shown to be effective in the treatment of panic disorder. The first-line agents are the SSRIs because of their better side effect profile. Bupropion, an antidepressant with a dopaminergic mechanism, and deprenyl, an MAO "b" inhibitor, have both been shown to be ineffective in the treatment of panic disorder.

113. **(A)** The tricyclic antidepressants have been shown to increase mortality in cardiac patients because of their quinidine-like effects and tendency to increase heart rate and decrease blood pressure. Sertraline is safe for patients with cardiac disease and affords the fewest drug–drug interactions of the SSRIs. As a class, the amphetamines have been found to be safe in patients with cardiac illness. There may be minor changes in blood pressure and pulse; patients should be monitored closely. Bupropion is safe in cardiac patients. Venlafaxine can increase the blood pressure an average of 8 to 10 mm Hg, but this effect is dose-related. At doses less than 150 mg qd, clinically significant changes are relatively rare. Doses above 300 mg qd are the highest risk, but most patients will tolerate this dose without increases in blood pressure.

114. **(C)** Haloperidol's mechanism of action is dopamine receptor blockade (D_2). Dopamine inhibits prolactin secretion. Because haloperidol prevents dopamine from binding to the dopamine receptor, prolactin secretion is unopposed. The symptoms the patient is experiencing are common effects of elevated prolactin. Haloperidol does not increase ACTH, serotonin, or dopamine levels to clinically

significant levels, and the symptoms described are not associated with ACTH, serotonin, or dopamine.

115. **(I)** Phencyclidine (PCP, angel dust) intoxication produces these symptoms as well as hyperthermia, depersonalization, and hallucinations in auditory, tactile, and visual modalities.

116. **(E)** These symptoms may begin within a day for severe alcoholics in withdrawal, and they can progress to delerium tremens (DTs) by 3 days. DTs are associated with a risk of lethal autonomic collapse.

117. **(C)** These symptoms tend to be mild and last 1 to 2 days post last use in a regular cocaine user. Occasionally, the depression can be great enough to raise the risk of self-injurious behavior or suicide attempts.

118. **(G)** Heroin withdrawal peaks at about 72 hours post last use in dependent users. It is experienced with many flulike symptoms and gastrointestinal complaints, such as cramping, nausea, and constipation. The appearance of piloerection in the syndrome gave rise to the slang term *cold turkey* to describe the action of total cessation of use of the drug.

Cannabis intoxication heightens sensitivity to external stimuli and impairs motor skills. Cocaine intoxication is marked by elated mood, hallucinations, and agitation. Alcohol intoxication involves characteristic behavioral changes, as well as slurred speech, ataxia, and other neurological findings. It can progress to coma if severe. Heroin intoxication is marked by an altered mood, psychomotor retardation, and drowsiness. The syndromes of MDMA and methamphetamine intoxication are similar to those of cocaine intoxication. MDMA users typically report an increased "sense of closeness" with other people. Intoxication by inhalants (volatile substances such as gasoline fumes) is marked by disorientation and fear and is short-lived. Nicotine intoxication is not a category of the DSM-IV-TR. Nitrous oxide intoxication produces euphoria and light-headedness, and usually subsides within hours without treatment. Withdrawal from psilocybin, a hallucinogen derived from mushrooms, is not well-described.

119. **(B)** Clozapine causes agranulocytosis in about 1% of patients. For this reason, weekly blood counts are measured for the first 6 months of treatment, then every 2 weeks thereafter.

120. **(G)** Lithium is associated with clinical hypothyroidism in about 5% of patients, most commonly women. Thyroid supplementation may be added to counter this side effect. Up to 30% of patients may show elevated thyroid-stimulating hormone levels.

REFERENCES

American Medical Association. *Code of Medical Ethics: Current Opinions and Annotations 2000–2001.* Chicago: American Medical Association; 2000

American Psychiatric Association. *DSM-IV-TR Casebook.* Washington, DC: American Psychiatric Press; 2002

American Psychiatric Association. *Diagnostic and Statistical Manual of Mental Disorders,* 4th ed., Text Revision. Washington, DC: American Psychiatric Press; 2000

Benedetti F, Sforzini L, Colombo C, et al. Low dose clozapine in acute and continuation treatment of severe borderline personality disorder. *Journal of Clinical Psychiatry* 1998;59:103–107

Becker AE, Grinspoon SK, Klibanski A, Herzog DB. Current concepts: eating disorders. *New England Journal of Medicine* 1999;340:1092–98

Check JR. Munchausen syndrome by proxy: an atypical form of child abuse. *Journal of Practical Psychiatry and Behavioral Health* 1998;4:340–45

Conley RR. Optimizing treatment with clozapine. *Journal of Clinical Psychiatry* 1998;59:S44–48

Fogel B, Schiffer R, Rao S, eds. *Neuropsychiatry.* Baltimore: Williams & Wilkins; 1996

Friedman M. Current and future drug treatment for post-traumatic stress disorder. *Psychiatric Annals* 1998;28:461

Hyman S, Nestler E. *The Molecular Foundations of Psychiatry.* Washington, DC: American Psychiatric Press; 1993

Arana GW, Rosenbaum JF. *Handbook of Psychiatric Drug Therapy,* 4th ed. Boston: Little, Brown and Company; 2000

Kane JM, Jeste DV, Barnes TRE, et al. *Tardive Dyskinesia: A Task Force Report of the American Psychiatric Association.* Washington, DC: American Psychiatric Association; 1992

Kaplan HI, Sadock BJ (eds.). *Comprehensive Textbook of Psychiatry,* 7th ed. Baltimore: Williams & Wilkins; 2000

Kaplan HI, Sadock BJ. *Kaplan and Sadock's Synopsis of Psychiatry: Behavioral Sciences, Clinical Psychiatry,* 8th ed. Baltimore: Williams & Wilkins; 1998.

Katona CLE, Robertson MM. *Psychiatry at a Glance.* Cambridge, MA: Blackwell Science, Ltd.; 1995

Levenson JL. Neuroleptic malignant syndrome. *American Journal of Psychiatry* 1985;142:1137–45

Lewis M. *Child & Adolescent Psychiatry: A Comprehensive Textbook,* 3rd ed. Baltimore: Williams & Wilkins; 2002

Lezak MD. *Neuropsychological Assessment.* New York: Oxford University Press; 1995

Lishman WA. *Organic Psychiatry: The Psychological Consequences of Cerebral Disorder.* Malden, MA: Blackwell Science, Ltd.; 1998

Lowinson J, Ruiz P, Millman R, Langrod J (eds.). *Substance Abuse.* Baltimore: Williams & Wilkins; 1997

Ollendick TH, Hersen M (eds.). *Handbook of Child Psychopathology,* 3rd ed. New York: Plenum Press; 1998

O'Malley S, Jaffe AJ, Chang G, et al. Six-month follow-up of naltrexone and psychotherapy for alcohol dependence. *Archives of General Psychiatry* 1996;53:217–24

Preskorn SH. Clinically relevant pharmacology of selective serotonin reuptake inhibitors. *Clinical Pharmacokinetics* 1997;32:S1–S21

Price L, Heninger G. Lithium in the treatment of mood disorders. *New England Journal of Medicine* 1994;331:591–98

Schatzberg A, Cole J, DeBattista C (eds.). *Manual of Clinical Psychopharmacology,* 3rd ed. Washington, DC: American Psychiatric Press; 1997

Schatzberg A, Nemeroff C. *Textbook of Psychopharmacology,* 2nd ed. American Psychiatric Press; 1998

Stahl S. *Essential Psychopharmacology,* 2nd ed. Cambridge, England: Cambridge University Press; 2000

Sternbach H. The serotonin syndrome. *American Journal of Psychiatry* 1991;148:705–13

Tasman A, Kay J, Lieberman J (eds.). *Psychiatry.* Philadelphia: W.B. Saunders and Co.; 1997

Yudofsky SC, Hales RD (eds.). *Textbook of Neuropsychiatry and Clinical Neurosciences,* 4th ed. Washington, DC: American Psychiatric Press; 2002